JAPANESE CLASSICAL ACUPUNCTURE

Introduction to

Meridian Therapy

Shudō Denmei
Translated by Stephen Brown, C.A.

EASTLAND PRESS
—— Seattle ——

Originally published as *Keiraku Chiryo no Susume*
Ido No Nippon Company (Tokyo), 1983

English language edition © 1990 by Eastland Press, Incorporated
P.O. Box 12689, Seattle, Washington 98111
All rights reserved.

Library of Congress Catalog Card Number: 90-82526
International Standard Book Number: 0-939616-11-4
Printed in the United States of America

Book design by Gary Niemeier
Photolithoprinted by Thomson-Shore, Inc.
Dexter, Michigan, 1990.

Second printing, 1994

Table of Contents

Foreword to the Japanese Edition

Mr. Shudo has now finished writing the book, *Introduction to Meridian Therapy*. Mr. Shudo has studied and practiced meridian therapy by applying his sharp mind and keen sensitivity. This is an excellent book which explains the fine points of meridian therapy in great detail. I recommend this text because there is so much here that is directly useful in clinical practice.

It is the duty of those who practice medicine to mitigate the ills of society and restore life and enthusiasm in their patients. Meridian therapy must also fulfill this essential role. It is a form of therapy in which disease is understood in terms of changes detected on the meridians and acupuncture points. The objective of meridian therapy is to treat the meridians, and the traditional four examinations of looking, listening, questioning, and palpation are employed to determine which meridians are out of balance. The meridians that are abnormal are identified as being either deficient or excessive, and treatment consists of tonifying deficient meridians and dispersing excessive meridians.

Many acupuncturists today follow the lead of physicians in performing local treatments which focus primarily on the affected area. This is a very limited approach which is not rooted in long years of practice and experience. In contrast to this approach, meridian therapy is a systematic method for identifying the meridians and acupuncture points indicated for treatment, and all disease is treated by tonification and dispersion based on a specific diagnosis. It takes practice to acquire the skills necessary for diagnosis and treatment in meridian therapy but every practitioner can become expert through daily practice. Naturally, innate ability varies from person to person, but the glory of complete mastery is reserved for those with diligence.

Acupuncture and moxibustion are founded on experience. Experience is essential whether in the field of medicine, religion, or athletics. Gushiken, the leading gymnast in Japan today, puts in no less than four hours of practice every day. The experience gained through practice is vital in all sports, be it gymnastics, baseball, or sumo wrestling. There is no way that the necessary skills can be developed without honing one's abilities through regular practice. Many acupuncturists today stop short of becoming expert because they fail to refine their skills through continual practice. To this day I have never failed to practice pulse diagnosis and point palpation. I hope that this book serves to motivate you to practice more, and to continually develop your skills as an acupuncturist.

Okabe Sodo
President, Meridian Therapy Association

Foreword

Acupuncture is one of the modes of treatment within the framework of traditional Oriental medicine which has a continuous history spanning several thousand years. Untold numbers of physicians have practiced acupuncture through its long history, and new and unique approaches have continuously arisen based on the wealth of accumulated experience. Among the ancient civilizations, China developed a system of writing comparatively early, and therefore a rather good record has been left of the various classical approaches to acupuncture. Acupuncture is nevertheless a highly specialized practice, and it is difficult to explain its finer points through the medium of the written word alone. For this reason, the techniques of acupuncture were historically transmitted from master to disciple largely through personal contact.

This need for personal instruction from an experienced practitioner holds true for other traditional skills as well, such as the martial arts. Even if one becomes very knowledgeable about the martial arts, this does not necessarily mean that he is a skilled martial artist. The best way to become proficient at martial arts is to study under a master who is an expert in a particular style. Be that as it may, in this day and age the opportunity to apprentice with a master is rare, and when it comes to gaining practical knowledge and skills in acupuncture, most beginners must content themselves with what can be learned from textbooks and weekend seminars.

This is why the manner in which an approach or technique is presented in a textbook is more critical than ever before. The information must be clear, and the techniques must be readily applicable. To that end, I think that Shudo Denmei has done a remarkable job in this introduction to meridian therapy. In addition to being a very skilled and successful acupuncturist, he is an excellent teacher with a unique ability to share his knowledge and experience. He is both a serious scholar and a dedicated practitioner who has devoted his heart and soul to making his patients well. Although he may yet to have achieved a position of prominence among Japanese acupuncturists, I can recommend him without reservation as one of the best acupuncture teachers today.

Having mastered meridian therapy on his own, Mr. Shudo understands the difficulties faced by the beginner and has a knack for explaining things in a straightforward manner. He is well aware of the problems inherent in learning about something as complicated as acupuncture from a book, and has a good grasp of the obstacles encountered by those unfamiliar with his approach. He has done a wonderful job in presenting his traditional approach to acupuncture in a clear and concise way. I am delighted that Mr. Shudo's book is now being translated into English by Stephen Brown, who himself is knowledgeable about Japanese acupuncture, so that this traditional Japanese approach can be introduced to the West.

This book clearly conveys how acupuncture is practiced in Japan in general, and within the framework of meridian therapy in particular. The fundamental feature of this and many other Japanese approaches to acupuncture is the use of subtle needle stimulation, which is barely (if at all) felt by the patient. This is as an important element of acupuncture which has generally been overlooked by the acupuncture community at large. Many centuries have passed since the technique of acupuncture was imported to Japan from China. During this time, both the instruments and techniques have been refined, and delicate variations have been developed. It is presumptuous to boast that the Japanese variation is better than the original Chinese approach, but there are things about the Japanese approach which are of definite clinical value. It is my hope that more acupuncturists in English speaking countries will be motivated to try this approach for themselves.

In conclusion, I would like to add that I chose to award Shudo Denmei the Manaka Prize in 1987 for this book. This prize is awarded annually by the *Journal of Japanese Acupuncture and Moxibustion* to an acupuncturist in Japan who has made an outstanding contribution to the advancement of acupuncture.

Manaka Yoshio, M.D.
Director, Oriental Medicine Research Center of the Kitazato Institute
Tokyo, 1989

Translator's Preface

Acupuncture in Japan, unlike mainland China, is an alternative form of therapy outside the mainstream of the national healthcare system. In China acupuncture has been closely allied with herbal medicine for at least a thousand years. It has also been standardized during the last half-century as an integral part of the state sponsored medical system. In Japan acupuncture developed separately from herbal medicine and became closely associated with massage, since for centuries acupuncture and massage were the exclusive domain of the blind.

There are marked differences between Japan and China in the way acupuncture is taught, practiced, and received. These differences arose from the widely diverging courses of historical and cultural development in these two countries. The greatest difference between acupuncture in Japan and that in China today may be derived from the economic bases of acupuncture practice. Acupuncture in Japan is a commercial venture as well as a healthcare specialty, and patients are also customers. Japanese acupuncturists compete for business in a free market economy where patients must pay out of their own pockets for acupuncture. This is unlike most other medical expenses, which are covered by national health insurance. The portion of the Japanese population receiving acupuncture is accordingly far smaller than in China. In this intensely competitive environment, the quality of service — or patient satisfaction — has a substantial impact on the way in which acupuncture is practiced.

The age-old fondness of the Japanese for incorporating new and different ideas has given rise to a multitude of approaches to acupuncture. For this reason, it is impossible to identify one system or approach that typifies Japanese acupuncture.

Nevertheless, there are a few common features. The first is a strong emphasis on palpation. Most Japanese acupuncture patients receive a thorough examination by touch as a requisite part of their treatment. Another feature is the use of very thin needles that are inserted with a guiding tube. This method makes it far easier to insert the needles without pain, and provides milder stimulation than do Chinese needles. Japanese patients generally prefer a softer treatment, and have a dislike for strong needle sensation. Finally, one of the most interesting features of Japanese acupuncture is the widespread use of direct moxibustion. Direct application of miniature moxa cones on the skin has been the most popular form of moxibustion for centuries. Direct moxibustion remains the most common adjunct to acupuncture in Japan today. These features of Japanese acupuncture evolved because of the delivery of acupuncture in conjunction with massage and moxibustion in the clinic.

Today the Japanese acupuncture community is dominated by practitioners who place the concepts of modern scientific medicine above the traditional principles of Oriental medicine. For the most part, no systematic method of diagnosis and treatment is taught in the schools, and most acupuncturists rely on their experience to render effective treatment. Therefore, while there is no shortage of gifted practitioners with a lifetime of experience, learning acupuncture in Japan can be difficult and time consuming. Nevertheless, I chose to study acupuncture and Oriental medicine in Japan because I already knew the language, having lived many years in Japan as a child. While inquiring about Oriental medicine in Japan, I learned about meridian therapy, which is today the most prominent school of traditional acupuncture. I was immediately attracted to meridian therapy because I had taken up the study of Oriental medicine primarily because of a fascination with traditional healing arts.

Meridian therapy was developed about fifty years ago by young Japanese acupuncturists who opposed the widespread disregard for traditional principles within their profession. The drive to modernize acupuncture in Japan had caused the profession to lose sight of its valuable traditions, and to forfeit its theoretical foundations for quasi-scientific principles. The originators of meridian therapy spearheaded the movement within the Japanese acupuncture community to reinstate the meridian system as the central concept of acupuncture. They advocated the study the classics of acupuncture, and the application of traditional principles in the clinic. The approach adopted in meridian therapy was all the more compelling because, instead of adding something new or different as is so often done, approaches from the past — such as palpatory diagnosis and subtle needling techniques — were revived to build on the strengths of the Japanese tradition. Thus for the first time traditional Japanese approaches were consolidated to create a systematic and logically consistent approach to acupuncture.

I myself often witnessed the remarkable effects of meridian therapy in the course of my clinical work in Japan. Because it focused on treating the root cause of disease while also effectively treating the immediate symptoms, I became convinced that meridian therapy was superior to the indiscriminate approach of symptomatic treatment that I was being taught in school. However, I was uncomfortable with the narrow-minded attitudes in some circles of meridian therapy that regarded all other approaches to acupuncture as inferior. The original intention of meridian therapy, as set forth by its chief instigator Yanagiya, was not to hold that traditional concepts were infallible, but to strive to understand and apply them in light of our knowledge and experience in the modern age.

This is why I was impressed with Shudo Denmei's articles on meridian therapy featured in the _Journal of Japanese Acupuncture and Moxibustion_. Mr. Shudo's faith in the inherent value of traditional approaches to acupuncture does not compromise his sense of critical judgment. He has the versatility to accommodate both modern and traditional approaches, and to take whatever methods he finds useful and apply them as the situation demands. Not only is his approach highly practical, but he also can communicate his ideas in a clear and simple manner. Mr. Shudo does not pretend to understand the full meaning of the classics. Based on his conviction that only practice and experience lead to insight, he wastes little time in criticizing other approaches, or in arguing about things he does not fully understand. His flexible approach to meridian therapy is far easier to learn and put into practice, and surely holds the key to the future growth of meridian therapy.

Because I was trained in Japan, I developed a deep appreciation for the uniquely Japanese contributions to acupuncture. I find it a shame that the subtle methods of acupuncture developed through the centuries in Japan are practically unknown among acupuncturists elsewhere in the world. If more practitioners worldwide studies the principles of meridian therapy, the invaluable contribution of the Japanese tradition of acupuncture could be preserved and further refined. I am convinced that this would add a new dimension to the ancient practice of acupuncture.

When I was approached by Eastland Press in 1986 to translate a work on Japanese acupuncture, there was no question in my mind that Mr. Shudo's book on meridian therapy was the most suitable for acupuncturists in the West. What I did not know then, not having met Mr. Shudo in person, was how great a teacher of Japanese acupuncture he would be. Once he agreed to have his book translated, he suggested that I modify the text to make it more accessible to Western readers. This revision entailed far more than either of us had imagined. Over the course of the three years that this work has been in progress, Mr. Shudo has generously given of his time and expertise. I have been continually amazed and inspired by his enthusiasm for traditional acupuncture, and his willingness to share everything he has learned during his thirty years of practice. Any other Japanese teacher would have become exasperated by the endless and detailed questions. Mr. Shudo never complained about the burden that this drawn out project placed on his busy schedule. It simply would have been impossible to finish this book without his selfless dedication to the project from beginning to end.

As he advised, I took the liberty of rearranging his book and adding new material and commentary in this English edition. I have attempted to remain as faithful as possible to Mr. Shudo's instructions in conveying his approach to meridian therapy. Nevertheless, the responsibility for any errors or omissions is entirely my own. The main intent of this edition is to familiarize acupuncturists in the West with meridian therapy, and to illustrate how it might be applied in one's practice. Since this material was originally intended for practitioners unfamiliar with traditional concepts, some of it is quite basic in nature. This is, however, consistent with the traditional Japanese approach to learning in which one must constantly return to the beginning. It is hoped that this work will create an impetus for further study and will serve to expand our horizons in the practice of acupuncture. May acupuncturists around the world build on this framework to confirm and expand the application of meridian therapy.

In conclusion, I would like to express my sincere thanks to Dan Bensky of Eastland Press for his continuous support and encouragement in this project. I am also very grateful to the editorial staff at Eastland Press for their valuable input, as well as to Lilian Bensky for her precise and artistic illustrations. I owe thanks to Tobe Yuichiro of the *Journal of Japanese Acupuncture and Moxibustion* for his permission to use all the materials from the Japanese edition. I remain forever indebted to Mr. Shudo for his inspiration, generosity, and patience. Finally, I wish to express my heartfelt gratitude to my father, who by his pioneering spirit laid the foundations for my life's work.

1

Introduction to Meridian Therapy

JAPANESE ACUPUNCTURE AND THE
DEVELOPMENT OF MERIDIAN THERAPY

In contrast to the modern approach in Japanese acupuncture with its disregard for traditional theories, meridian therapy is a system of acupuncture based on the classics developed in the early 1940s in reaction to the "modernizing" trend in acupuncture. Although meridian therapy is grounded in the traditional Japanese approach that developed in the seventeenth century independently of Chinese influence, it is a unique system of classical acupuncture born of the modern era. To appreciate the causes underlying its emergence and evolution, we must first understand the historical forces that shaped the practice of acupuncture in Japan. We will trace the history of acupuncture in Japan from its origins to provide a perspective that places the development of meridian therapy in its broader historical context.

Historical Development of Japanese Acupuncture

Acupuncture arrived in Japan early in the fifth century with the great influx of culture and technology imported from mainland China. Most of the medical knowledge from China first arrived indirectly by way of Korea. During this formative period of the Japanese state waves of Korean immigrants settled in Japan bringing with them various aspects of Chinese and Korean culture. Some of the immigrants had specialized knowledge of acupuncture and herbal medicine. In this manner Japan's first exposure to Oriental medicine came through contact with the Koreans, not the Chinese.

1

In the sixth century Japanese emissaries were sent to Korea to invite learned men in various fields, including medicine, to visit Japan. Korean scholars thus came to educate the Japanese in acupuncture and herbal medicine. Some Korean physicians remained permanently in Japan and began what was to become a lineage of renowned physicians.

In the seventh century the Japanese government established direct contact with China and sent Japanese priests and scholars to the capital of China to study at the very source of culture and learning. During this period many Chinese medical texts were copied and brought back to Japan. These texts were treated with the utmost reverence, and since this medical knowledge was more advanced than any form of medicine then existing in Japan, it was applied as directly as possible.

The Taihō Code, the first written legal system in Japan, was promulgated in 701. It addressed medical practice and education. For example it established an official department of acupuncture and moxibustion, and also designated the three ranks of teacher, practitioner, and student of acupuncture. In the Nara period that followed, all aspects of Oriental medicine including acupuncture were actively promoted and practiced. In the earlier periods when Oriental medicine was first introduced into Japan, it was the Buddhist monks who were most actively involved in the study and practice of acupuncture and herbal medicine. The system of medical education and specialization established in the Nara period led to a reduction in the number of monks serving as physicians. Increasingly, scholars and medical practitioners began to take the initiative in writing texts and advancing medical knowledge. *Ishimpō*, the first Japanese medical text, was compiled in 984 by a prominent physician named Tamba Yasunari. The practice of sending emissaries to China ceased in the mid-ninth century, and Oriental medicine began to follow an independent course of development in Japan.

The stable social order of Japan, based on control by the imperial family, finally collapsed in the twelfth century. The war lords who assumed control promoted trade with China, and medical ideas that had been developed on the continent again reached Japan after three centuries of relative isolation. These ideas exerted a strong influence on the practice of medicine. During the years of political turmoil in medieval Japan the influence of court physicians diminished, and Buddhist monks once more began to play a key role in importing Chinese medical knowledge and adapting new concepts. The monks were also more active in bringing medical care to the general populace. The practice of moxibustion gained popularity during this period because simple treatments were provided at Buddhist temples as part of religious practice.

In the period of political and social chaos preceding the reunification of Japan in the late sixteenth century, medical scholars continued to study texts imported from China and to compile many Japanese texts on acupuncture. Manase Dōsan (1507-1594) was the most renowned physician of this era. Although primarily an herbalist, he contributed greatly to the revival of acupuncture that had lost ground to herbal medicine over the years. Following the reunification of Japan and the restoration of social order, prominent acupuncturists established schools of acupuncture.

Three different approaches to medicine emerged in Japan between the sixteenth and seventeenth centuries, represented by the Gosei school, the Kohō school, and the Rampo school. Each school of thought contended with and influenced the others until the end of the nineteenth century. The Gosei school, started by Dosan Manase, was based on developments in medical thought that were then occurring in China. The Kohō school was inspired by a revival of the medical concepts from the *Discussion of Cold-induced Disorders;* this school rejected many of the newer ideas in Chinese medicine as empty speculation. The Rampō school arose among physicians influenced by Western medicine. Western medicine had begun to make its way into Japan through the Dutch, who had exclusive permission to conduct trade with Japan during its three hundred years of self-imposed isolation in the Edo period (1602-1868).

The development of acupuncture in Japan during the Edo period reflected these three major trends in medicine. Early in this era, a blind acupuncturist named Sugiyama Waichi developed an insertion technique for acupuncture needles using a guide tube. He was awarded the highest official rank as an acupuncturist by the shogun, and his school became the most influential in eastern Japan. Sugiyama's approach soon spread and eventually superseded all others, in part because he established government sponsored schools for the blind. Sugiyama had a profound influence on Japanese acupuncture, and the use of thin needles and guide tubes has since become standard practice among Japanese acupuncturists. Sugiyama built upon the foundations laid down by Manase to popularize acupuncture and moxibustion. Instead of modifying the conceptual basis of Oriental medicine, he introduced new methods and refined existing techniques.

The Mubun school, which was also prominent during the Edo period, had a unique approach. This school used the *dashin* technique, in which a small mallet is used to tap needles into the abdominal area. The Mubun school reached the height of its influence under a monk named Mubunsai. He went against the mainstream of acupuncture by disregarding the traditional system of meridians and acupuncture points and relied instead on the diagnosis and treatment of the abdomen alone. This school was particularly influential in the western part of Japan, because the imperial family (who lived in Kyoto, far to the west of the capitol in Edo) favoured it.

Another group of acupuncturists pioneered an approach that relied on the latest knowledge of anatomy and physiology from the West. As increasing numbers of Japanese physicians began to study Dutch medical texts, many acupuncturists set aside traditional theories and adopted a more pragmatic approach. One of them, Ishizaka Sōtetsu, was a famous acupuncturist trained in the Sugiyama school who had close contact with Dutch physicians. Ishizaka eventually established his own school of acupuncture based on the more accurate knowledge of anatomy taken from Western medicine.

The Meiji Restoration of 1868 marked the end of the feudal era as Japan was opened up to foreign influences. The new government resolved to modernize Japan by modeling itself after the Western powers. This brought sweeping changes to all segments of Japanese society and profoundly affected the practice of medicine. A law was enacted that required all physicians to pass an examination in Western medicine. As a result, practitioners of herbal medicine and acupuncture lost their status as physicians. Although the practice of acupuncture by non-physicians was not actually banned, through the years acupuncture lost ground to Western medicine. Acupuncture had largely become a profession of the blind during the Edo period and the new government allowed this centuries-old institution of social welfare to continue. A new system of occupational training of the visually impaired for acupuncture and massage was established several years after adoption of the new medical system. This placed the largest educational institution of acupuncture under government control, and became the only avenue for formal education in Oriental medicine in Japan.

Thus the Western medical model came to dominate acupuncture. The first law regulating the practice of acupuncture was proposed about a decade after the establishment of the new medical system. But another quarter century passed before an acupuncture licensing law was actually put into effect. In 1911, for the first time in history, the law required acupuncturists to obtain a license from the government to practice acupuncture. This law served to consolidate further the authority of bureaucrats and physicians with Western medical training over the practice of acupuncture.

Political movements arose during the Meiji period among practitioners of herbal medicine to regain the right to practice medicine. These had little influence upon the new government, which was intent on modernization at all costs. Thus experts in traditional medicine were not allowed to participate in setting the standards for education and practice of acupuncture. The government bureaucracy had its own designs for acupuncture, which were to modernize and reduce it to a simpler form, free of cumbersome traditional concepts. In 1918 the government commission on acupuncture education compiled the so-called "revised acupuncture points," which became the standard for licensure. The revised acupuncture points bore no resemblance to the traditional meridians and points, but were arbitrarily arranged according to a grid system superimposed over the surface of the body. With this move to modernize acupuncture, the pendulum of change in Oriental medicine had swung completely to the side of Western medicine.

Despite the political power wielded by administrators who believed in the supremacy of Western medicine, the reality of medical care for the general populace of Japan during the early twentieth century was not so different from what it had been a century earlier. Only the affluent could afford the high cost of Westernized medical care. The great majority of people continued to rely on herbal remedies, acupuncture, and moxibustion as the most accessible and inexpensive forms of treatment. Practitioners of acupuncture and herbal medicine therefore continued to enjoy a broad base of popular support. There was still a handful of practitioners who were serious scholars and adhered strictly to their traditional medical heritage. Even before the government issued its entirely new system of revised acupuncture points, practitioners devoted to the traditional learning began to voice their opposition to the injustice being perpetrated in the name of modernization.

Matsumoto Shirobei was a scholar of Oriental medicine and an advocate of the traditional approach. Matsumoto lost most of his eyesight as a child, and therefore chose to be trained in acupuncture. Despite his visual handicap, Matsumoto immersed himself in the study of the classics and became famous as a talented practitioner at the youthful age of twenty. In 1911 he wrote a very influential book called *The Study of Acupuncture Points*. This was a point location book that drew heavily from the classics, but also described the acupuncture points in terms of Western anatomy. *The Study of Acupuncture Points* was revered among adherents of the traditional approach to acupuncture as a standard of classical knowledge that could withstand criticism from advocates of the Western approach.

Many practitioners of acupuncture and moxibustion resented the government's taking control of the education and practice of acupuncture. Many articles and books were published calling for a revival of the traditional approach, and various societies of traditional medicine were formed in the 1920s. In 1926 Nakayama Tadanao wrote a book entitled, *The New Investigation of Oriental Medicine,* which drew attention to the value of traditional medicine. Although a journalist by trade, Nakayama became a spokesman for Oriental medicine through his association with Sawada Ken. Nakayama's book not only influenced the thinking of practitioners, but also had a significant impact on the general public. In this book he criticized the revised acupuncture points and gave sensationalized accounts of the effectiveness of acupuncture and moxibustion. Sawada, who was already a well-known practitioner of moxibustion, became famous all over Japan because of the book. He was a practitioner of the old school who placed special emphasis on the classics. Many practitioners rallied under Nakayama's banner to make a stand for traditional medicine, which the government had been continually undermining since the Meiji Restoration. It was from this group of acupuncturists who advocated the traditional approach that meridian therapy was eventually born.

The Origin of Meridian Therapy

Among the many advocates of the traditional approach to acupuncture and moxibustion in the 1920s was a young man named Yanagiya Seisuke. Yanagiya was the son of an acupuncturist in northern Japan who moved to Tokyo when he was sixteen to enter the first acupuncture school in Japan established for those with sight. Yanagiya obtained his license at age seventeen. He later changed his name to Sorei, which is the Japanese reading of the first characters in the titles to *Basic Questions* and *Vital Axis* of the *Yellow Emperor's Inner Classic.* Yanagiya took on the work of searching for a new approach to acupuncture based on an understanding of the classics. Perhaps because of his boldness and youth, Yanagiya did not ally himself with other famous practitioners, such as Sawada, who advocated the traditional approach. Instead, he started his own school of acupuncture in 1927 and began to assemble a group of loyal supporters for the cause of classical acupuncture. The core group of his students was later to become the originators of a neoclassical approach to acupuncture called meridian therapy.

After Yanagiya graduated from Nippon University with a degree in Oriental philosophy in 1934, he became even more adamant about the need to change the orientation of the acupuncture profession. He wanted to promote a thorough investigation of the classical literature that would reassess the value of traditional principles and techniques. Yanagiya strongly opposed the total disregard for traditional principles caused by the political dominance of those eager to modernize acupuncture. He was also critical of those who blindly followed traditional approaches taught by older practitioners without critically examining the classical texts on which these practices were supposedly based. Yanagiya contended that the information in the classics was valuable but not infallible. He believed that all classical approaches had to be examined with a critical eye, put into practice, and discussed among practitioners before their worth could be determined.

Okabe Fukuji, one of the earliest students of Yanagiya, left behind a lucrative business in his home town of Toyama to enter Yanagiya's acupuncture school. Okabe displayed exceptional talent from the start. After graduating and obtaining his acupuncture license in 1933, he became an instructor at Yanagiya's request. Okabe was totally committed to the revival of the classical approach to acupuncture. He followed Yanagiya's example by changing his name to Sodo, which means "the way of *Basic Questions*" or ancient texts. Inoue Keiri was another outstanding student who entered Yanagiya's school in 1935. Inoue started his own practice after obtaining a license in 1937. He quickly proved to be a gifted practitioner, and devoted himself to the cause of traditional acupuncture. Okabe and Inoue eventually became the leaders of the group of dedicated, young practitioners who were motivated by Yanagiya's vision of reviving the classical style of acupuncture that had been lost in antiquity.

This youthful group of acupuncturists organized around Yanagiya held bold views of upholding the traditional concepts of acupuncture until they were proven false. They did not become a force in the Japanese acupuncture community until Yanagiya made the vital connection with Takeyama Shinichiro through Komai Kazuo, the most influential acupuncturist in pre-war Japan. Not only was Komai an enormously successful practitioner in Osaka, he was also a distinguished scientist who received his doctorate based on experimental studies in acupuncture. At this time there were only a handful of scientists in Japan who conducted research in acupuncture and moxibustion. Komai selflessly devoted his life to fostering an understanding and acceptance of acupuncture within the Japanese medical community. He founded the Oriental Medicine Research Society, and personally financed the publication of the *Oriental Medical Journal (Tohō Igaku)*. This journal became a forum for the exchange of ideas among practitioners of all types of traditional medicine.

In 1937 Komai invited Takeyama Shinichiro to become the editor-in-chief of the *Oriental Medical Journal*. Takeyama had been a reporter for a large newspaper in Osaka until he became seriously ill. He was unable to get any help from Western medicine, but regained his health through herbal medicine. Being a social activist by nature, Takeyama decided right away that traditional medicine was a cause worth fighting for. Komai's organization was based in Osaka, but Komai wanted to move his headquarters to the capital city of Tokyo. He therefore prevailed upon Takeyama to join forces with Yanagiya, who headed the Tokyo branch of the Oriental Medicine Research Society. Thus Takeyama came under the influence of Yanagiya and took up the cause of classical acupuncture, eventually becoming an acupuncturist himself. Besides being a talented writer, Takeyama was a charismatic organizer. He was largely responsible for setting the stage for the introduction of a classical system of acupuncture. He motivated key members to devote themselves to developing a new treatment system.

In 1939, under the direction of Takeyama, a select group of acupuncturists headed by Okabe and Inoue formed a society for the intensive study of the classics. They wanted to go beyond restoring the status of traditional medicine in Japan. The goal they chose was to establish a new, practical approach to acupuncture firmly grounded in the classical tradition. Okabe and Inoue worked together intently as the dark clouds of World War II began to overshadow every aspect of people's lives in Japan. These acupuncturists rigorously applied the principles of acupuncture set forth in the *Classic of Difficulties* to develop a classical system of treatment that had never before been so clearly defined. This was at a time when most acupuncturists were content to needle a random selection of acupuncture points without any diagnosis. The only method most acupuncturists used was to stimulate tender points, or certain other points thought to be effective for specific symptoms.

Okabe and Inoue and their colleagues formulated a practical and consistent treatment system embodying the spirit of the therapeutic principles outlined in the *Classic of Difficulties*. They called this system meridian therapy because in it the meridians were restored to their rightful place as the central focus of acupuncture. Although the traditional four examinations were still important in meridian therapy, special emphasis was placed on six-position pulse diagnosis in determining the pattern for treatment. The first portion of treatment was called the root treatment. This involved tonifying or dispersing the points associated with the five phases on the limbs to balance the Qi in the meridians. After the meridians were balanced, symptomatic treatment provided additional relief. Meridian therapy thus addressed the underlying cause of a disease, or the excess or deficiency in the meridians, before the symptomatic manifestations.

This new system of acupuncture, distilled from the classics, restored the emphasis on the meridians in Japanese acupuncture and filled a gap for many practitioners who never before had a practical method to guide them in the selection of acupuncture points. Meridian therapy was not an entirely new system, since it was an application of principles outlined in the classics. Furthermore, meridian therapy was not the creation of Okabe and Inoue alone. Yanagiya's vision inspired them, and Takeyama encouraged and promoted their work every step of the way. The work of Okabe and Inoue was also aided by many other like-minded practitioners who tested their conclusions in the clinic. Ironically, just as the foundation of meridian therapy was being laid in the early 1940s, the grand illusion of the Japanese Empire began to crumble, and a nightmare of death and destruction came home to Japan. Yet even as nightly bombing raids leveled Tokyo, a defiant group of traditional acupuncturists continued to meet in that city to develop their system. The inevitable fall of the Japanese Empire came in the summer of 1945, and the founders of meridian therapy, with their fervent desire to revive traditional acupuncture, were among the first to pick themselves up from the devastation and help their compatriots reconstruct their lives.

None of these acupuncturists suspected that the new government, the occupation forces of the United States, would pose the greatest threat in history to the survival of their profession. There were many radical reforms imposed on Japanese society after the war, including demilitarization and land reform. With these changes, the government of occupation headed by General Douglas McArthur attempted to ban acupuncture and moxibustion altogether in the belief that they were unscientific and unsanitary practices. This caused an uproar in the traditional medical community. All differences were set aside for the time being and practitioners of every stripe joined together to defend their right to practice. This movement gained the support of some physicians who had an understanding of, or an interest in, traditional medicine. After a sustained legal battle, a new law was passed in 1948 that guaranteed the right to practice traditional forms of medicine.

Once the crisis had passed the conflict between traditional acupuncturists and those supporting the modern approach resurfaced, and the debate over the future of acupuncture in Japan heated up as never before. The forces of occupation brought a flood of Western influence. Simultaneously the mainstream opinion in the acupuncture community shifted toward the prospect of developing acupuncture as a new therapeutic tool within the context of the Western medical model. Practitioners of meridian therapy tried hard to gain wider acceptance for their approach in the medical community. However, they were unable to overcome the barrier of scientific opinion against the existence of meridians. It may have been too much to expect that physicians trained in Western medicine would accept a system of Qi circulation. However, it was just as unreasonable to ask traditional acupuncturists to ignore thousands of years of precedent and turn their backs on the concepts and principles of the classics. The amount of research on the acupuncture points and their relationship to disease was too small and too distant from the realities of the clinic; scientific research yielded very little data that could be clinically applied. No new treatment system was developed. These practitioners were left with stimulating tenders points along with other point combinations that were thought to effectively treat specific diseases. In addition, because they were neither trained nor authorized to diagnose disease, acupuncturists were totally dependent on the opinions of medical doctors.

Eventually, Takeyama and the practitioners of meridian therapy completely abandoned any hope of gaining influence in the political arena. Instead they devoted their energies to strengthening their organization and training skilled practitioners. Thus acupuncturists who supported the new scientific approach gained the upper hand politically, and it was they who set the new standards for education and licensure. The situation for those entering the acupuncture profession therefore remained largely the same as before the war. Knowledge of Western physiology and pathology was emphasized over traditional concepts, and the average student learned very little about traditional diagnosis and treatment. The training of traditional acupuncturists continued in much the same way as before, with students apprenticing with skilled practitioners after first obtaining their licenses. The number of acupuncturists practicing meridian therapy gradually increased over the years, but not substantially in relation to those practicing the scientific approach.

Today the practitioners of meridian therapy are still a minority within the Japanese acupuncture community, but are still a significant force. Through the activities of the Japan Meridian Therapy Association, Japanese acupuncturists have the option of studying and practicing a traditional approach. In recent years there has been a growing disenchantment with the reductionist approach of Western medicine. There has also been an increase in the influence of traditional Chinese medicine. This has led to more interest in meridian therapy as a classical Japanese approach that has proven its worth in modern times.

How I Came to Practice Meridian Therapy

My teacher, Miura Nagahiko, inspired me to become an acupuncturist. Although Master Miura did not practice meridian therapy, he was an exceptionally gifted practitioner. He was from Ohita in southern Japan and grew up just four miles from where I was born. Master Miura was very bright, and after graduating with honors from the Ohita Teachers' School, he went on to the Advanced Teachers' School in Hiroshima. Master Miura eventually became principal of a local middle school, but he was too much of a free spirit to settle down in a small country school. After a few years he abandoned his career in education and entered the law department of Chuo University in Tokyo. He thus became a lawyer, which was a very special and privileged profession in pre-war Japan.

Master Miura's hard working nature was his undoing. He contracted pulmonary tuberculosis just as he embarked on his new career. Tuberculosis forced him to spend long months in convalescence, and his condition slowly deteriorated. He became interested in acupuncture and moxibustion when the severe coughing and hemoptysis which he had suffered for two months was relieved after just one treatment with moxibustion. As soon as he recovered his health, Master Miura entered the acupuncture school of Yanagiya Sorei. Being close in age and of a similar temperament, he soon became fast friends with Yanagiya. Even though Master Miura became very close to Yanagiya and admired his strong convictions, he never understood the need to develop a system of acupuncture based on the classics.

Master Miura obtained his acupuncture license in 1937 and opened a practice in Tokyo. Since he could not grasp the classical approach espoused by Yanagiya, he practiced the Sawada style, which was very popular at the time. Master Miura was captivated by the acupuncture techniques used in the Sawada school. As I recall, he always seemed to be studying and applying the methods of Shirota Bunshi, Sawada's most eminent student. Master Miura's favorite text was written by Shirota and entitled, *Basic Study of Acupuncture Therapy (Shinkyu Chiryo Kisogaku)*. Practically every page of his copy was filled with red pencil marks highlighting important passages. My teacher's methods were thus based on the approach to acupuncture therapy developed by Sawada.

In 1944 when Japan went on the defensive in the Second World War and bombing raids made it increasingly dangerous to live in Tokyo, Master Miura moved back to Ohita. My father befriended him shortly after his return, and both of my parents received regular acupuncture treatments from him. I was in my early teens during this time and as fortune would have it, an unusual set of circumstances brought me under the influence of Master Miura. In those days there was but one honorable way for a young man to avoid conscription, and that was to excel in school and pass a difficult entrance examination for the teachers' school. Since I was their only son, my parents were eager that I should become a teacher. Master Miura kindly offered his help, and I began going to his place every day for tutoring. I never was very interested in studying before that time, but Master Miura's enthusiasm for scholarship soon led me to study more on my own. He had a way of making various subjects interesting. I began to enjoy reading for the first time in my life, and soon became a voracious reader.

These were trying and desperate times in Japan just before the defeat. Food and basic necessities were in short supply everywhere. Despite these circumstances, or perhaps because of them, I became totally absorbed in reading and studying. This effort, however, proved to be too much of a strain on my frail constitution, and I became very ill. After contracting various diseases, I finally came down with pulmonary tuberculosis, which was rampant in Japan around the end of the war. I was fortunate to be under the care of Master Miura, but due to a lack of nutrition my condition continued to deteriorate. For a while there was some doubt about my survival, but Master Miura never gave up. He continued to treat me, and gradually my condition improved. During this episode I resolved that if I recovered, I would become an acupuncturist just like Master Miura. In time I did recover completely through Master Miura's treatment, and after that I never doubted that I was destined to become an acupuncturist.

After finishing high school I entered a local acupuncture school to become licensed. As an acupuncture student I took an interest in the classical approach to acupuncture, but Master Miura insisted that though the theory was fascinating, meridian therapy was just not a practical approach to acupuncture. In 1949 the first textbook on meridian therapy, entitled *Discourse on Meridian Therapy (Keiraku Chiryo Kowa),* was published. Master Miura suggested that I read the book just for the sake of reference, which I did several times in the years that followed. Although it was not too difficult to follow the general approach outlined in this book, every time I attempted pulse diagnosis, I found it to be impossible. Nevertheless, there seemed to be a simple and beautiful logic to this approach. What could be more convenient than being able to determine everything about the patient from the pulse?

I therefore tried to devise ways of mastering the technique of pulse diagnosis. Master Miura tried to discourage me by saying that pulse diagnosis was an impossible proposition. Furthermore, he said, meridian therapy was simply impractical because needling distal points caused too much pain. Although I understood my teacher's point of view, I still wondered why so many books had been written about pulse diagnosis since ancient times. There also seemed to be many acupuncturists who were practicing meridian therapy with success. If it were all so preposterous, why would any self-respecting acupuncturist write a book on the subject just to disgrace himself before future generations?

After practicing acupuncture for ten years, I had gained enough confidence to take on almost any disease. Still, I felt that something was lacking in my treatments, and that I should give meridian therapy a try. There had to be something to the classical approach, otherwise why would so many intelligent people risk their reputations and livelihoods by devoting themselves to this system? The only way to find out was to try it for myself. The first step in the traditional approach to learning is to follow faithfully a method without passing judgment. Over my teacher's objections, I resolved to study meridian therapy in earnest for ten years to see if it really worked.

In undertaking to learn meridian therapy on my own, I was still faced with one major obstacle: pulse diagnosis, or determining the pattern of Qi imbalance from the pulse. For this reason I started to attend the annual summer seminars on meridian therapy. At the time of my first seminar, I had been suffering from chronic distention of the lower abdomen. Medical tests had shown no abnormality, but when the distention became severe, the discomfort was such that I completely lost my appetite. I was becoming increasingly concerned about this problem, especially when there was no improvement after needling myself in the lower abdomen and back. During the practical portion of the seminar, the instructor briefly examined my pulse and promptly pronounced that I was suffering from Kidney deficiency. All he did was examine my pulse; I had not spoken a word about my condition. Since the instructor was only teaching pulse diagnosis technique, he did not treat me at that time.

I just had to know if this diagnosis was correct and if the prescribed treatment would really work. I therefore needled the main Kidney tonification point, K-7, on both sides just to see what the effect would be. The outcome far surpassed my expectations. In less than a minute the distention that had caused such great discomfort in my lower abdomen began to diminish, as if air were slowly leaking out of a balloon. After a few minutes the distention was gone without a trace, and my lower abdomen felt empty and even slightly depressed. So meridian therapy really did work! I promised myself then and there that I would master pulse diagnosis no matter what it took. Since then, I have continually strived to apply pulse diagnosis in my practice.

Master Miura could not accept my work with meridian therapy for the longest time. About five years before his death, he finally conceded and gave me his blessing saying, "Go ahead and pursue your chosen path and become a master of meridian therapy." My teacher was an unusual character, and he and I were opposites in many ways. He was a yang type who loved wine, women, and study. I am more of a yin type, and although I share my teacher's love for study, I do not have his passion and energy. Nevertheless, it is interesting that, just like my teacher, I have come to practice a completely different style of acupuncture from that first taught to me.

The question of whether meridian therapy really works will be answered more fully throughout this book. It took many years of perseverance before I became totally confident of its efficacy. My sensitivity is far below average, and I tend to be slow at catching onto things. The other acupuncturists who were studying meridian therapy appeared to have very little trouble with pulse diagnosis, but at first, it seemed beyond my grasp. After years of trial and error, I picked up a little hint that made pulse diagnosis accessible to me. There is really nothing to it once you learn how. To see if this hint would work for others, I showed it to some acupuncturists who had never used pulse diagnosis before. They all seemed to pick it up right away. My approach also led to relatively consistent findings. Furthermore, the novice acupuncturists studying under me began to use my approach to pulse diagnosis and meridian therapy in their own practices, with varying degrees of success. These results gave me the courage to present my method to a wider audience.

There are many books about pulse diagnosis and meridian therapy in Japan. Yet in all of these texts the most important details of the method always seem to be missing. Does this mean that the authors are being secretive and are teaching the crucial parts only to their own students? I don't think so. It is more likely that they simply fail to explain those details that are exceedingly obvious. However, there are those who cannot understand anything at all unless all the obvious points are explained. It should therefore be understood that I am writing this book not to discuss the complex theories of classical acupuncture, nor to present greater refinements in technique, but to provide what might be called an idiot's manual to the practice of meridian therapy.

Arguments Against Meridian Therapy

The critics of meridian therapy in the Japanese acupuncture community can be roughly divided into three groups. The first considers meridian therapy to be unscientific and never gives it another thought. The second group includes those individuals who have attempted meridian therapy at some point, but find it difficult to grasp. The third group are practitioners who have a sufficiently thorough understanding of meridian therapy, but who feel that the system is incomplete in some respect and that there are better ways to perform pulse diagnosis and treatment. I believe that this group is in the minority and that most acupuncturists fall into the first and second groups.

> "Meridian therapy is a system of treatment for regulating abnormalities in the physical condition based upon an assessment of the imbalances in the meridians using diagnostic methods unique to acupuncture, and [thereafter] adjusting these imbalances. The traditional four examinations, such as observation, are employed, but pulse diagnosis and palpation receive the greatest emphasis. The imbalances in the meridians are ascertained through [palpation of] the pulse, depressions, indurations, and sensitive points located along the meridians. Once the diagnosis is made, the treatment is indicated. In this way, there is a wonderful unity between diagnosis and treatment. This is the difference between diagnosis of the disease entity in Western medicine and Oriental diagnosis of the pattern [of imbalance]." (Takeyama, 1941)

The validity of meridian therapy may be argued either way, but I feel that no one really has the right to judge this approach until they have tried it themselves. Until then, it seems pointless to answer callous arguments such as how the pulse for the Stomach meridian can still exist after the stomach has been removed. Those who can laugh at this kind of argument already have some knowledge of pulse diagnosis.

The approach to pulse diagnosis and meridian therapy presented in this book should be easy to understand. With practice you should be able to use my method successfully in a few months. Before you examine this method with a critical eye, I would ask that you learn it first and find ways of putting it to work in your practice. I can guarantee that your efforts will not be wasted, and I am confident that learning this approach to acupuncture will benefit you and your patients in many ways.

Some people believe that meridian therapy is a well-defined system of treatment with hard and fast rules. This is not true, however, for it is constantly being refined and developed. Meridian therapy is a system of treatment initially developed by Yanagiya Sorei and his students that is based on the *Classic of Difficulties*. From the beginning different practitioners of meridian therapy have added their own interpretations and refinements. The Japan Meridian Therapy Association was established in 1971 to improve communication and broaden the consensus about the practice of traditional acupuncture among practitioners of meridian therapy. When you begin to study this approach you will realize how practical and yet profound meridian therapy can be.

I am convinced that the path for acupuncturists today lies in absorbing all the useful information medical science has to offer, while continually striving to understand the classics so that the art of acupuncture can be refined by drawing from the best of both traditions. There are those, however, who overemphasize the merits of classical acupuncture and in so doing ignore or make light of modern medicine. This is a very dangerous attitude, and it may well dig the grave for our profession. Modern medicine does have its problems (e.g., the side-effects of drugs), but it is extremely effective in many situations, and it is breaking new ground every day. We must draw from this wellspring of information and use it wherever we can in our practice. We must be ready to refer patients to Western physicians in situations when that type of medical treatment is more effective.

Acupuncture too has its own strengths, and many conditions respond particularly well to it. We must understand both our strengths and our limitations. To that end, we must study Western medicine just as much as the classics of Oriental medicine. Probably none of us is foolish enough to claim that acupuncture is a cure-all. However, from time to time I hear about acupuncturists who say things like, "Don't see a doctor. Take no medicine. My acupuncture works the best." Such a deluded attitude can be found not only among classical acupuncturists, but also in the acupuncture community in general. It is a dangerous attitude that calls for greater prudence.

Finally, there is the issue of sterilization. There are acupuncturists in Japan who ignore common sense and refuse to sterilize their needles. They defend themselves by claiming that acupuncture has been practiced for centuries without sterilization. This is a dangerous rationalization. Standards of sanitation and conditions of medical practice have changed dramatically in modern times. Acupuncture must be practiced in a manner that upholds the highest standards, integrating traditional skills and modern know-how. There is no question that, to ensure the health and safety of the patient as well as the practitioner, acupuncture must be practiced in a way that is consistent with sterile technique as much as possible.

How to Get the Most Out of this Book

Reading this book strictly from the perspective of Western medicine could lead to some confusion. The Stomach in Oriental medicine is different from the gastric organ in Western medicine. It is an entity described in the classics with a much broader range of functions and associations. The Heart, too, is different from the cardiac organ. The Heart is the sovereign organ among the traditional organs that houses the Spirit. Those who are unfamiliar with the fundamental concepts of Oriental medicine should first familiarize themselves with the basic terms before reading this book. Those who wish to learn meridian therapy must have a sound understanding of the special terms used in Oriental medicine. Also, some Oriental medical terms used in the practice of traditional Chinese medicine take on a slightly different meaning when used in the context of meridian therapy. Terms like Liver meridian deficiency, or pattern *(shō/*

zhèng), have a unique connotation in meridian therapy. Every specialty has its own unique terminology, and meridian therapy is no exception. Without a clear understanding of the terminology, it is impossible to discuss, let alone practice, this approach. Although I do not wish to explain the basic concepts of traditional Oriental medicine in depth, in the next chapter I will define or clarify those terms that have a different meaning or are of special importance in meridian therapy.

In the practice of acupuncture, knowledge and technical skill are of equal importance, like the two wheels of a cart. Traditionally, practical ability is more highly regarded in Oriental medicine than theoretical knowledge. Even if a practitioner has a detailed knowledge of the concepts and principles of the classics, it is useless if he lacks the practical ability to apply that knowledge. However, one must still learn the basic principles and study the techniques presented in textbooks. In learning the practical aspects, I advise that you practice each new technique repeatedly until a certain degree of proficiency is attained before proceeding to the next step.

There are many practical textbooks on meridian therapy in Japanese. This book is an amalgamation of these texts to which I have added my own observations and insights. You should be able to use the techniques presented here without undue difficulty by simply reading the text carefully. After practicing these techniques for awhile, you will begin to have more questions; this is the time to consult the classics. The classics of Chinese medicine are worth reading and rereading if one intends to master the classical approach to acupuncture. The *Classic of Difficulties* in particular, as the foundation of meridian therapy, should be studied in depth once you gain some competence in this method.

This book is based only on what I have been able to absorb from the wealth of available knowledge. To avoid confusion, I have attempted to keep the language as simple and direct as possible. I have not written about things I do not understand as if I understood them. This book is not a comprehensive text on meridian therapy, but a beginner's manual. Its purpose will be served if it starts acupuncturists off on the path to acupuncture treatment with a greater awareness of the classics. With this aim in mind, I have used the following format:

- Useful information and explanations from other books have been incorporated in the text, with appropriate references (for full citations, see bibliography).

- When there are significant differences of opinion, all prominent views are presented in no particular order.

- I have sought to clearly point out those methods or techniques that are most effective, based on my own experience.

- Special terms in the text are followed by Japanese and Mandarin transliterations at their first appearance. When both Japanese and Mandarin are given, Japanese is followed by Mandarin. When only one language is given, Japanese and Mandarin can be distinguished by the tone marks over the Mandarin.

- Each chapter ends with an outline of its key points.

2

The Theoretical Foundations
of Meridian Therapy

YIN-YANG AND THE FIVE PHASES

The principles of meridian therapy are drawn from the oldest Chinese medical texts, especially the *Classic of Difficulties*. It is virtually impossible to discuss this traditional approach to acupuncture without touching on the most fundamental concepts of yin-yang and the five phases. These concepts originated in primitive times and were formulated during the growth of Chinese civilization. After becoming established, they were gradually refined by continuous application in all aspects of life.

The yin-yang principle is thought to have its roots in the Chinese calendar. As agriculture grew in importance, the calendar became increasingly necessary to determine the proper time of planting and harvesting. According to Fujiki Toshiro, a Japanese scholar of Chinese history, the principle of the five phases emerged later in history, independent of the yin-yang principle. Over time these two principles were organized into a complementary system which was used both to understand natural phenomena, and to order the conduct of all human affairs including government, economics, medicine, and military strategy. Just as we use the scientific approach to understand the world in our day and age, the principles of yin-yang and the five phases constituted a quasi-science under which Chinese civilization operated.

A basic understanding of yin-yang and the five phases is indispensable to the practice of classical acupuncture. Some people have a hard time accepting the validity of these principles, which appear to be the very symbols of antiquated and unscientific thinking. And yet, although the terms yin and yang may be ancient, the concept which they embody is timeless. The key to their understanding is in finding ways to apply them in organizing one's own experience. This is not as difficult as it may sound. It has been done countless times in the past, and a wealth of literature exists that describes how others have done it. The point is to bring these principles to life in your own experience. Here I will briefly explain these principles for those who are unfamiliar with them.

Yin and Yang

Yin and yang are expressions of two complementary opposites. Yin represents the aspect of quiescence, and yang the aspect of activity. Almost everything can be divided into yin and yang, but the primary dichotomies are day and night, light and dark, hard and soft, male and female, and exterior and interior. It is important to understand that yin and yang, while being opposites, are not two separate entities. Both can be found simultaneously in the same place. It is just like the two sides of a coin: that which is yang viewed from one side is yin viewed from its opposite side. Thus yin and yang are essentially different aspects of the same thing. Whenever a yang quality appears in something, there is always a yin quality to complement it in another part. Yin and yang always coexist within the same sphere.

When I attend acupuncture conferences in Korea many yin-yang symbols are in evidence (Illustration 2-1). This is also known as the Tai Ji symbol, which represents the harmony of yin and yang; it is the central feature of the Korean flag. The lower portion is blue and represents yin; the upper portion is red and represents yang. These colors are very appropriate as the quality of yin is best represented by water, and that

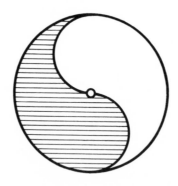

Illustration 2-1
Tai Ji Symbol

of yang by fire. Placing the edge of a ruler on the center point in the figure cuts the Tai Ji symbol in half. Portions of both yin and yang remain in the half circle. Pivoting the ruler on the center point, one can see how the balance of yin and yang changes. Just when yin is at a minimum, yang reaches a maximum. As yang begins to wane, yin begins to wax. Thus the opposing aspects of yin and yang are continuously balancing each other. This also demonstrates that extreme yin eventually transforms into yang and vice versa. In matters of health it is most desirable that the aspects of yin and yang be naturally balanced.

In the human body the lower half is yin and the upper half is yang, the front is yin and the back is yang, the interior is yin and the surface is yang. Among the organs of traditional Chinese medicine, the dense organs are yin and the hollow organs are yang. Yet among the principal five yin organs themselves the Kidney is considered to be the most yin, and the Heart the most yang. From this description it should be apparent that all phenomena can be distinguished as yin or yang, and yet within each such phenomenon there are aspects of yin within yang, and yang within yin. The distinction between yin and yang is essentially one of quiescence and activity.

This brings us to the reason why yin comes first in the term yin-yang. It is yin which first gives rise to yang. Yin and yang originally denoted shade and light respectively. Therefore yin implies something in the dark which lies hidden while yang is something in the light which is apparent. That which is hidden gives rise to that which is visible when light is cast on it. What is visible is always a small portion of everything that lies hidden. For this reason yin can be conceived as enveloping yang instead of simply being in opposition to it. Thus yang is a portion of the whole which is yin. This leads to an extremely important dictum in meridian therapy, i.e., that yin leads and yang follows. This principle has a major influence on the way meridian therapy is performed. Turning one's attention to the yin aspect, or the whole picture, is given precedence over consideration of apparent problems or symptoms, which are yang.

The Five Phases

According to the principles of the five phases, all things are divided into five categories or phases represented by wood, fire, earth, metal, and water respectively. Each of the organs and meridians corresponds to one of the five phases. The wood phase is associated with the Liver and Gallbladder; the fire phase with the Heart and Small Intestine as well as the Pericardium and Triple Burner; the earth phase with the Spleen and Stomach; the metal phase with the Lung and Large Intestine; and the water phase with the Kidney and Bladder. In addition, other aspects and functions of the body are associated with the five phases.

The seasons are representative of the cyclical nature of the five phases. The generating cycle of the five phases follows the sequence of spring, summer, midsummer, autumn, and winter. One wonders how each of the phases came to be associated with particular phenomena, and there are many explanations in the classics. The wood phase is a good example. It is easy to understand how spring and the color green were correlated with wood. Chinese geographical associations account for other correlations: wind that blows from the east in spring, and the fact that lumber is a product of eastern China.

The ancient Chinese classified practically everything in their environment using the five phases. They categorized various body phenomena in accordance with the five phases in order to understand health and sickness. The primary focus was on treating any abnormal occurrence in a way that would bring about harmony among the five phases. Finding an effective treatment was more important than understanding exactly how and why it worked. It seems that these categories and associations were imposed long after useful clinical relationships had been established. This is why it is not very beneficial to seek a scientific or philosophical basis for these categories. All we really need to do is learn the relationships outlined in the classics, and put them to the test in our practice. The five phases are very important in determining the treatment pattern in meridian therapy, and the most useful correspondences from a clinical perspective will be discussed at greater length in connection with the diagnostic procedures in the next chapter.

The most interesting feature of the five phases is the existence of the generating cycle and the controlling cycle. In the generating cycle (Illustration 2-2), wood gives rise to fire, fire to earth, earth to metal, metal to water, and water to wood. Each phase nurtures and promotes the growth of the subsequent phase. (This is similar to the relationship that existed between the United States and Japan in the not so distant past.)

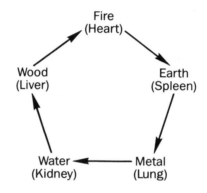

Illustration 2-2
Generating Cycle of the Five Phases

Of the two phases paired together in the generating cycle, the first is called the mother and the second is called the child. A generating relationship between two phases is called a mother-child relationship. Since each of the organs is associated with one of the phases, each organ has two mother-child relationships — as a child in the first, and as a mother in the second. In the figure, the phase from which the arrow originates is the mother, and the phase to which it points is the child. Take the Kidney for example. In the first mother-child relationship, the Lung nurtures the Kidney; the Lung is the mother and the Kidney is the child. In the second mother-child relationship, the Kidney nurtures the Liver; the Kidney is therefore the mother and the Liver is the child. To keep things simple, only the yin organs are listed in the figure.

In the controlling cycle of the five phases (Illustration 2-3), each phase suppresses or keeps another phase in check. In this cycle, wood has control over earth, earth over water, water over fire, fire over metal, and metal over wood. The controlling cycle can be compared to the relationship between the United States and the Soviet Union. It is said that things remain relatively peaceful as long as the balance of power remains even, but as soon as this balance is tipped and one gains the upper hand, there is

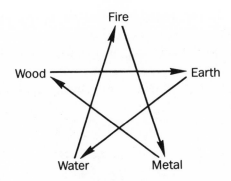

Illustration 2-3
Controlling Cycle of the Five Phases

danger of war. A similar thing happens in the human body when one organ becomes too strong or weak. For example, when the Liver becomes hyperactive, the Spleen is weakened; when the Liver is weak, the Lung and Spleen tend to become hyperactive.

There is no simple explanation for why the generating and controlling cycles work the way they do. But in clinical practice these principles are very useful. For example, suppose a patient complains of a loss of appetite, general lassitude and fatigue, and a craving for sweets. Pulse diagnosis indicates Spleen (earth) deficiency. In this case, quite often the pulse for the Liver (wood), which is in a position of controlling the Spleen, will be excessive. And since the Spleen (earth) cannot perform its normal controlling function over the Kidney (water), the Kidney will also tend to be excessive. When Spleen tonification points are needled, the strength of the pulse should increase at the Spleen position and diminish at the Liver position. If the pulse does not normalize at the Liver position, points to disperse the Liver can be needled. This treatment will serve to improve the patient's appetite. This is not just a theory; it actually works this way in practice.

My feeling about the traditional approach of dividing things into yin and yang and further classifying them in accordance with the five phases is this: in reading the *Classic of Difficulties* I am struck by how the Chinese (especially the author, Bian Que) tried to simplify things as much as possible. In meridian therapy there are only four basic categories of yin meridian deficiency. It might seem simplistic to treat a countless number of patients with just a handful of treatment patterns, yet it works quite well in practice. In this sense, while classification in accordance with the five phases may be slightly arbitrary, it serves our purposes to go ahead and assign four basic categories in the clinic. It is indeed much easier to divide things into endless small categories than to bring things together under a broader category. The difficulty of keeping things simple is quite evident in the clinical setting. Just think how hard it is to give an effective acupuncture treatment by needling only five points. Both yin-yang and the five phases are a means of simplifying things to get closer to the essence of the phenomenon.

The practicality of the yin-yang principle is widely acknowledged among practitioners of Oriental medicine. However, many reject the five phases on the ground that the system is not appropriate in every case, and that some of the associations seem rather far-fetched. It is true that the system of the five phases is far from perfect and we cannot look upon it as the absolute truth. Even so, it has a very practical and time-tested application in selecting acupuncture points, and we would therefore be foolish to discard it. The wiser course would be to first test the usefulness of this system for yourself before discounting its effectiveness on logical grounds.

ETIOLOGY

Etiology in medicine refers to the cause or origin of disease. There are many things which I feel are quite ingenious about Oriental medicine, and etiology is one of them. In Western medicine the cause of disease has been sought in external agents such as germs. It is only recently that much attention has been given to internal causes such as stress. In Oriental medicine, ever since the earliest period when *Basic Questions* was written, the causes of disease have been identified as predisposing factors, internal factors, and external factors. Furthermore, a clear and practical correlation was made between the causative factor and the specific organ or meridian affected. Sometimes one wonders if these correlations are arbitrary, or whether they truly apply in reality. I would like to examine the etiology of traditional Chinese medicine from a practical perspective in order to shed some light on this question.

Predisposing Factors

Predisposing factors pertain to the underlying physical constitution. There are some middle-aged women who come to my clinic and constantly complain about one physical problem or another. On the other hand, I know some spry old men who have never really been sick and just laugh when someone suggests that they see a doctor. Why are there such remarkable differences between people in their physical condition and sense of well-being? Naturally there are some inherent differences in physical strength, since we inherit the genes of our ancestors through our parents. There are people who begin life with a definite physical handicap. The general tendencies toward health or disease are a product of predisposing factors, some of which influence us in our formative stage, and others which affect us after we mature.

"Innate factors are various influences on our lives from the time that we are conceived until we become fully independent adults; this includes our upbringing and spiritual orientation." (Inoue, 1962)

As we live out our adult lives under the influence of various innate, predisposing factors, we are also affected by the climatic and geographical conditions where we live, not to mention our cultural and social environment. These are the acquired factors which become part of our predisposition.

"Acquired factors are the various influences we come under after we begin living life on our own terms. This includes life style or living habits, such as an inclination to study or exercise too much, or to accumulate mental stress, which give rise to certain predispositions." (Inoue, 1962)

Thus predisposition, or the physical tendencies created by predisposing factors, results from a complex blend of influences. This is why the appearance of an internal or external pathogenic influence will cause different reactions in different individuals. Predisposition boils down to individual differences: "Those who become ill have a predisposition which makes them susceptible to illness." (Honma, 1949)

Some practitioners judge predisposition by classifying people into body types based on the correspondences of the five phases. In this approach there are two body types for each of the yin organs (except the Pericardium), one being an excessive type and the other a deficient type. There are thus ten basic body types starting with the Liver (wood) excessive type, and ending with the Kidney (water) deficient type. This method is outlined in *Discourse on Meridian Therapy* by Honma as follows:

Yang constitution: People with a yang constitution have a red complexion regardless of their weight (they can be fat or thin). Their muscles are firm and hard. They have a strong will and a cheerful temperament, and are extroverted. They do not often become ill. When they do, the symptoms are severe, but they recover comparatively quickly.

Yin constitution: People with a yin constitution usually have a weak digestive system and therefore tend to be thin. Even if they are fat, they have a poor complexion and their flesh is soft. Those with thin necks are most susceptible to disease. For those with a yin constitution the course of illness is protracted and often becomes chronic.

Liver excess constitution: People with a Liver excess constitution often have type O blood. Their complexion is dark and bluish, their muscles are firm, and they are endowed with a strong body. They are usually stubborn and unaccommodating towards others. They are hard workers and generally succeed, but, due to a tendency to overwork, their health sometimes fails just before achieving their goal. They tend to eat excessively and this often leads to gastrointestinal disorders. They are also susceptible to strokes and nervous disorders.

Liver deficient constitution: People with a Liver deficient constitution often have type A blood. They are generally congenial and intelligent, but lack mental energy and tend to be nervous and fastidious. Usually their muscles are underdeveloped. Their digestive system is sound despite appearances to the contrary. They are most susceptible to neurasthenia and emotional problems. They generally appear to be weak, but can live a long life if they maintain a healthy life-style.

Heart excess constitution: People with a Heart excess constitution are intelligent and inquisitive as well as very meticulous. They generally have a pear-shaped head and a reddish complexion. They are usually thin but in good health. They appear calm and relaxed on the surface, but when they get excited they can become extremely emotional. They are hard workers and often succeed in intellectual occupations. They are either susceptible to or already have a history of respiratory problems.

Heart deficient constitution: People with Heart deficient constitutions often have reddish complexions, but as the deficiency increases the complexion becomes more pale. They are thin and tend to have a pear-shaped head. They are often quite intelligent, but lack physical stamina. Although they have sharp minds, they may seem somewhat cold. They tend not to socialize and thus often end up alone. They are hard workers but tend to be nervous, single-minded, and stubborn. They must be careful not to work harder than they are physically able. They are susceptible to digestive problems, respiratory problems, and nervous disorders.

Spleen excess constitution: People with a Spleen excess constitution tend to be gourmets and are quite often very overweight. They have a yellowish red complexion and are very talkative and love to eat. They tend to be simple-minded and can seem aloof. They are also weak-willed and have difficulty making decisions. They are susceptible to arthritis and neuralgia. They should be careful about kidney and liver disorders, and should not indulge in excessive sex.

Spleen deficient constitution: People with a Spleen deficient constitution tend to have a yellowish complexion and a weak digestive system. Despite this they always have an appetite. Overeating is particularly detrimental to the health of these individuals and they must learn to control their appetite if they are to live a long life. Usually they have a thin body and are susceptible to lung diseases. Those in this group who have a strong sex drive and overindulge in sex tend to be short-lived. Individuals in this group often develop a Liver excess condition and become nervous and irritable.

Lung excess constitution: People with a Lung excess constitution have a white complexion and tend to be overweight. Their digestive system is relatively strong and they can eat a great deal. They have an unaffected manner and are quite sociable so they get along very well with people and do well in business. Nevertheless, they lack strength of character and are susceptible to heart diseases and neurasthenia.

Lung deficient constitution: People with a Lung deficient constitution have a white complexion and tend to be thin. They usually have a weak digestive system and are particularly susceptible to respiratory problems. They often develop a Liver excess condition which makes them stubborn and short-tempered. They must make an effort to strengthen their digestive system and stimulate their skin (by brushing or rubbing). They should pay attention to the condition of their colon since they are prone to hemorrhoids. They also must be careful about kidney diseases.

Kidney excess constitution: People with a Kidney excess constitution are seldom overweight. They have a blackish complexion and their muscles are very firm and compact. Their appearance or manner may seem harsh or severe but they are actually very warm and sociable. They tend to have a very strong sex drive. Those who have a strong digestive system are fine, but those with a weak digestive system have health problems. They work hard and play hard, but these individuals need to be careful not to end up with a full but short life. They are particularly susceptible to strokes and liver diseases.

Kidney deficient constitution: People with a Kidney deficient constitution generally have a weak sex drive, but their sex drive can become strong when their Liver becomes overactive. They tend to be thin and have a blackish complexion. These individuals are intelligent and prefer intellectual work to physical work. They have a relatively strong digestive system, but their body and limbs tend to be cold. Many of this group have had a severe respiratory illness in their youth and have subsequently regained their health. They can become seriously ill again if they perform physically demanding work for extended periods. Therefore they must know their own limits and do only about eighty percent as much work as others. They must also be careful about urogenital and circulatory disorders.

These are physical and psychological predispositions. A person is judged to have a particular constitution based on information gathered from the four examinations (particularly the looking and palpation examinations). The symptoms or illness of a patient is not a direct indication of the underlying constitution, and one must inquire into the life-style and mental habits of each patient to get a sense of their physical and psychological background, which gives perspective to their current condition. I think these basic body types are a useful tool in determining the treatment pattern when used together with the pulse pattern and symptomology of the meridians. After some years of experience, one should get a sense for the appropriate correlations.

Internal Pathogenic Influences

The basic concept of health and disease in Oriental medicine is that illness cannot occur unless there is an internal imbalance which makes one susceptible to deleterious influences. "Disease comes from over-doing" *(Basic Questions,* chapter 21). This means that excess of any type, be it physical or psychological, disrupts the harmonious functioning of the body and creates susceptibility to disease.

The internal pathogenic influences consist of the so-called seven emotions (joy, anger, grief, sorrow, pensiveness, fear, and fright) and other miscellaneous factors (habitual excesses). Internal pathogenic influences may seem very similar to predisposing factors, but they differ in that they are more the underlying cause of a disease rather than an aspect of one's physical constitution. The seven emotions do not normally cause disease, but a sudden surge of emotion or an otherwise prolonged fixation on any one emotion can be harmful to health. Excesses of emotion, sex, food, drink, and fatigue can all disrupt the balance of yin and yang, impede the circulation of Qi and Blood, and impair the function of the organs. Disease caused by internal pathogenic influences is called 'internal injury.' Each of the seven emotions (and some of the miscellaneous factors) is correlated to one or another of the organs in the system of the five phases, as described below.

Joy: Joy is generally a desirable psychological state, but when it becomes excessive, it can produce psychological stress. When a person becomes overjoyed, there is great excitement. This can lead to insomnia, and in some cases may even cause high blood pressure and angina pectoris. In the Orient a serene state of emotional equilibrium is considered to be the most desirable . Excessive joy is said to injure the Heart. But this is not the only emotion which affects the Heart, as might be expected of the organ that houses the spirit: "Worry and melancholy injure the Heart" *(Classic of Difficulties,* chapter 49), and likewise "Sadness and fear injure the Heart" *(Vital Axis,* chapter 4).

Anger: Excessive anger is said to injure the Liver. This association seems plausible as I often see patients who are irritable, or have loud, angry voices, who present with imbalances of the Liver and Gallbladder. "When anger rises [to the head] and does not descend, the Liver is injured" *(Classic of Difficulties,* chapter 49). Sometimes when I am working in the clinic I become irritated or angry over little things.

Since I cannot vent my anger in that situation, I just have to hold it inside. The expression 'anger rising to the head and not descending' describes this situation perfectly. "The Liver is injured when congestion occurs under the ribs due to bad Blood collecting inside after a fall, or [due to Qi stagnation from] great anger when Qi rises and does not descend" *(Vital Axis,* chapter 4). This passage describes a condition of stagnation or excess in the flanks and upper abdominal regions, either from the accumulation of Blood due to internal hemorrhage after an accident, or from the stifled Qi associated with anger.

Grief and sorrow: Excessive sorrow is said to injure the Lung. There used to be many novels about beautiful women who grieved for years and finally contracted tuberculosis. I find in my practice that patients who are worrisome and always complain about one thing or another, and those who are not satisfied until they have pointed out every little thing that could be wrong with their bodies, often suffer from Lung imbalance. "When there is sadness the Heart is distressed and the lobes of the Lung lift, thus the upper burner becomes blocked" *(Basic Questions,* chapter 39). Both the Heart and the Lung, the most yang of the yin organs, are adversely affected by grief and sorrow.

Pensiveness: Pensiveness is said to injure the Spleen. Pensiveness is included among the emotions here, and implies concern as well as contemplation. Some middle-aged women I know have concerns which cause them to overeat and gain weight. It seems more normal, however, to lose one's appetite when becoming worried about something. Either way, the Spleen is affected. In my experience, pensiveness associated with study seems to affect the Liver more than the Spleen. Whenever I become tired from studying or writing, just touching Liv-8 with the tip of a needle makes me feel much better.

"Overindulgence and fatigue injure the Spleen" *(Classic of Difficulties,* chapter 49). While these factors are not among the seven emotions, they are often related to emotional problems and are exactly the kinds of overdoing which cause disease.

Fear and fright: Fear and fright are said to injure the Kidney. Fear means anything from a timid and fearful disposition to full-blown paranoia. Fright is a nervous state in which one is easily startled or frightened. Together these emotions denote a very weak and vulnerable psychological state.

"When Qi [in the Kidney meridian] is deficient, [a person] is prone to fear" *(Vital Axis,* chapter 10). People with Kidney deficiency often do seem to be more passive and timid than normal individuals. Sometimes they become so timid that they are afraid to leave their homes by themselves. Some patients look as if they would run away during acupuncture treatment unless their spouse stayed close by their side.

"Sitting for a long time in damp places, or getting in water after exertion, injures the Kidney" *(Classic of Difficulties,* chapter 4). It seems that heavy exertion and bathing after perspiring a great deal causes Kidney deficiency. Again, while they are not emotions, fatigue and stress are other internal factors which deplete the Kidney Qi and lead to the corresponding psychological tendency.

We have thus taken a brief look at the internal pathogenic influences with the understanding that, to varying degrees, all of these emotions and activities are a natural part of life. Since we are human, if something makes us mad, we get angry, and if something makes us very sad, we cry. People who never get angry or sad are either very controlled or spiritually enlightened. Individuals who do not express their emotions are not very interesting as people. In any case, when any emotion builds up to an abnormal level, physical functions are affected in accordance with the above mentioned relationships. Although each phase and organ is associated with a specific emotion, there is no need to view these as rigid rules. Every emotion will naturally affect a number of organs. The important thing to understand is that extreme emotions do affect the meridians and can cause functional imbalances in the organs. This is really not so different from the stress theory set forth by Hans Selye. As acupuncturists, we have a way to treat emotional problems and psychosomatic conditions. By tonifying the appropriate points and balancing Qi in the meridians, inappropriate emotions such as irritability and fearfulness can be controlled. This is an approach to psychosomatic medicine which has been practiced successfully for many centuries in East Asia.

External Pathogenic Influences

"These are also known as pernicious influences, and include wind, cold, heat, and dampness, which are environmental factors." (Yanagiya, 1948)

External pathogenic influences are the causes of illness which come from outside the body, and are mainly climatic conditions. Among these influences are the so-called six factors: wind, cold, heat, fire, dampness, and dryness. It may seem strange to view wind or cold as the cause of illness, but there are historical and geographical reasons for this. The continent of China has an entirely different climate from that of Japan, where the weather generally tends to be mild. Although it was May when I visited China, it was so hot the first day that I wanted to take my summer shirt off. The next day I went on a tour of the Great Wall and dressed lightly expecting it to be just as hot. Around noon that day the weather turned windy and cold, and I ended up catching a cold. Therefore in China when the weather is hot, it is boiling hot, and when it is cold, it is freezing cold.

Given this climate, it seems to be a reasonable assumption that such climatic factors can cause illness. It is even more understandable when we realize that in ancient times people had virtually nothing to protect themselves from the elements, unlike the centrally heated and air conditioned structures we have today. The external pathogenic influences are thus a product of a time when geographical and climatic conditions played a major role in the health and well-being of people (Table 2-1).

PATHOGENIC INFLUENCE	Wind	Heat	Dampness	Dryness	Cold
Internal Injury:	Anger	Joy	Pensiveness	Sadness	Fear
Organ Injured:	Liver	Heart	Spleen	Lung	Kidney
Pulse Quality:	Floating & Wiry	Floating & Big	Submerged & Soft		Slow & Tight

Table 2-1 Summary of the Effects of the External Pathogenic Influences

Wind: A light wind is something that can be felt but not seen. Ancient peoples perhaps considered this intangible feature of wind to be capable of causing illness. Among the pathogenic influences, wind seems to have the broadest of meanings, and possesses a decidedly different connotation from the mere meteorological phenomenon of wind.

"When Wind invades the body, it can cause chills and fever, high fever, extreme chilling, one-sided withering, and internal wind" *(Basic Questions,* chapter 42). This passage brings a multitude of conditions to mind. It certainly includes the common cold, which in Japan is called wind *(kaze)*. Many other conditions such as flu, jaundice, cerebral hemorrhage, hemiplegia, facial paralysis, aphasia, and other symptoms of paralysis are likewise attributed to wind. These conditions are often due to internal wind, where heat in a particular organ stirs up wind inside the body to produce a myriad of symptoms. Some people even attribute demonic possession to wind. The concept of wind may sound simple, but it can mean many things and is an elusive pathogenic entity. For clinical purposes, the primary conditions associated with wind are fever with sweating, aversion to wind, and hemiplegia. The last of these is the most serious illness associated with wind.

In the area where I live, the expression "struck by wind" *(kaze ni ataru)* is still used with a spiritualistic connotation. For example, a person might say that he was struck by wind if his knees suddenly became swollen and painful after pulling weeds in a graveyard. Supposedly, a spirit in the grave can attach itself to the person and cause illness or physical problems. In such cases it is said that medicine and acupuncture are not only ineffective, but will aggravate the problem. The person must recite Buddhist sutras or appease the spirit in some way. There are people who actually believe this. Wind in this context means the spirits of dead people, although sometimes it may also include animal spirits or the spirits of the living as well. This belief is very interesting when we consider that people in ancient China must have perceived wind in a similar way. In a sense, wind may have been regarded as the cause of physical disorders which were beyond human comprehension.

According to the classics of Oriental medicine, the external pathogenic influence of wind is most often associated with the Liver and Gallbladder organs and meridians. The pulse quality associated with wind is floating and wiry.

Cold: The invasion of the body by pathogenic cold is said to cause fever and chills, aversion to cold, and headaches. Other, more serious symptoms caused by cold include pain, spasms and contracture of the limbs, and unconsciousness. Cold is generally considered to disrupt the function of the Kidney, which stores the basal Qi that warms the body. In the *Classic of Difficulties,* however, cold is said to disrupt the function of the Lung. Both are true in the sense that the Lung, which is closely associated with protective Qi, is the first to be affected by cold, while persistent cold harms the Kidney, which governs the basal Qi. "Chilling of the body and drinking cold things injures the Lung" *(Classic of Difficulties,* chapter 49). Today we seem to be just as prone to exposure to cold from air conditioning and chilled soft drinks. The pulse quality associated with cold is slow and tight. Manifestations of wind and cold are often found together in the clinic, and descriptions in the classics are not clear in distinguishing these two conditions.

Heat and fire: The external pathogenic influence of heat most often appears during the summer. For the purposes of our discussion it includes the pathogenic influence summerheat. Invasion by heat causes fatigue, headaches, dizziness, and diarrhea, and in extreme cases it can lead to high fever, delirium, and coma. The latter symptoms are typical in cases of heat stroke. Heat is generally considered to disrupt the function of the Heart. The pulse quality associated with heat is floating and big. Heat, like wind and cold, usually appears in combination with other pathogenic influences.

Fire is in many respects similar to heat, but like wind can occur independent of any externally-contracted process as internal fire due to overactivity of an organ. As an external pathogenic influence, fire seems to be more closely associated with direct exposure to the sun or hot flames. In this respect it may be equated with heat exhaustion.

Dampness: When the body is invaded by dampness there is heaviness in the limbs, lassitude, fixed and dull pain, and scanty or difficult urination. In addition, any condition that is aggravated by high humidity is generally associated with dampness. This immediately brings to mind rheumatism, but in the classics a much broader range of conditions is attributed to this influence. Dampness is generally said to disrupt the function of the Spleen, since this organ is responsible for transporting and eventually eliminating dampness. Again, however, there is some inconsistency in the classics inasmuch as the *Classic of Difficulties* states that dampness injures the Kidney. Nevertheless, just as cold can affect both the Lung and Kidney, so too can dampness affect both the Spleen and Kidney. The pulse quality associated with dampness is submerged and soft.

Dryness: The pathogenic influence of dryness depletes the body fluids and causes thirst, dry coughs, and constipation. Dryness is said to disrupt the function of the Lung. Dryness seems to be much less important than the other external pathogenic influences, and the *Classic of Difficulties* does not even list it among the primary pathogenic influences.

PHASES	**Wood**	**Fire**	**Earth**	**Metal**	**Water**
Basic Questions:	Wind	Heat	Dampness	Dryness	Cold
Classic of Difficulties:	Wind	Heat	Overindulgence & Fatigue	Cold	Dampness

Table 2-2   The Five Phases and External Pathogenic Influences: Two Views from the Classics

Differences of opinion have been expressed through the ages concerning the effects and classification of the pathogenic influences (Table 2-2). In some texts, such as the *Classic of Difficulties,* only the four primary external pathogenic influences of wind, cold, heat, and dampness are mentioned, and cold is associated with the Lung. The external pathogenic influences are correlated with the five phases in the earliest texts (see, e.g., *Basic Questions,* chapter 5), but such correlations are not always consistent. In the clinic, however, there is no need to be concerned about which correlation is more correct. In all probability, each of the factors affects several different organ and meridian systems depending on the circumstances and the individual. In Oriental medicine it is far more important to understand the individual differences which make one susceptible to the external pathogenic influences.

The most important point to bear in mind about external pathogenic influences is this: so long as one is not susceptible as a result of predisposing factors or internal pathogenic influences, disease will not occur even if one is exposed to deleterious environmental factors (Illustration 2-4). In other words, illness cannot occur if Qi is circulating through the meridians in a balanced way and all the organs are functioning optimally. This idea seems to have even more validity in this age of technology than it did at the time that the ancient Chinese medical texts were written.

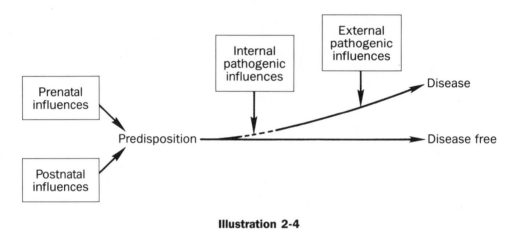

Illustration 2-4
Etiology of Disease

The various etiological factors are summarized as follows in chapter 49 of the *Classic of Difficulties:*

> "Sometimes the meridians [organs] become diseased in and of themselves, and at other times the five pathogenic influences cause injury. How can such cases be distinguished?
>
> It is as follows: Worry and melancholy injure the Heart. Chilling the body and drinking cold [liquids] injure the Lung. When the Qi of anger rises [to the head] and does not descend, the Liver is injured. Overindulgence and fatigue injure the Spleen. Sitting for a long time in damp places, or getting in water after heavy exertion, injures the Kidney. All these are [cases of] meridians [organs] that become diseased in and of themselves.
>
> What are the five pathogenic influences?
>
> They are as follows: Invasion of wind, injury from heat, overindulgence and fatigue, injury from cold, and invasion of dampness. These are known as the five pathogenic influences."

BASIC PRINCIPLES OF MERIDIAN THERAPY

Meridian therapy was developed as part of the revival of the traditional method of acupuncture recorded in the *Classic of Difficulties*. A variety of approaches and techniques of acupuncture, as well as other types of treatment, are detailed in *Basic Questions* and *Vital Axis,* but neither of these texts present such a systematized and self-contained system of acupuncture treatment as that found in the *Classic of Difficulties.* This text is unique in many respects among the oldest of Chinese medical texts, not the least of which is its consistent application of the five phases in almost every aspect of diagnosis and treatment. Accordingly, the object of diagnosis and treatment in meridian therapy is to determine which phase is most out of balance, and to bring it back into balance. An effort is made through all stages of diagnosis to pinpoint the deepest imbalance among the five phases.

Unlike the modern approach to traditional Chinese medicine in which the eight principles comprise the basic diagnostic framework, in meridian therapy the primary emphasis is on the patterns of deficiency and excess in relation to the five phases. The concept of deficiency and excess in meridian therapy is essentially the same as that in other branches of Oriental medicine, since it is derived from the same sources. To practice meridian therapy, however, it is particularly important to have a clear understanding of deficiency and excess because the principal objective of treatment is to correct the Qi imbalance by tonification and dispersion. I will therefore discuss the various approaches to deficiency and excess which are central to meridian therapy, and attempt to clarify the practical implications of these concepts.

Deficiency and Excess

"Deficiency means a loss or lack of normal Qi, [which leads to] a weakening of spirit, a loss of vitality, and a decline of [physiological] function. The Qi of the Triple Burner (source Qi) circulating in certain organs or meridians dwindles, and this causes a decline in resistance to pathogenic influences" (Honma, 1949). "Deficiency is caused by a shortage of normal Qi or source Qi, and disease comes from the inside" (Okabe, 1974).

Deficiency therefore implies a lack of normal Qi in the organs, meridians, or particular areas of the body. There are many levels and manifestations of deficiency, but in meridian therapy a weak or deficient pulse and a lack of spirit are the primary indicators. There are other general indicators of deficiency such as a low energy level, desire for warmth, and pain which responds favorably to pressure, but the presence of these signs merely confirms the overall pattern of imbalance. While it is important to differentiate between deficiency and excess in general, the aim of diagnosis in meridian therapy is to identify specific deficiency and excess within the framework of the five phases. The phase or corresponding organs or meridians with the greatest Qi imbalance must be identified in order to render effective treatment. In the majority of cases, deficiency and excess exist simultaneously, but the signs of deficiency are often masked by manifestations of excess.

"What then is excess? Excess means an abundance of pathogenic Qi. In other words, the pathogenic Qi of a pathogenic influence is active and in excess." (Honma, 1949)

"Excess means a surplus of pathogenic Qi, and it is caused by the effect of external pathogenic influences." (Okabe, 1974)

Excess therefore indicates a state of increased activity in which the normal Qi of the body reacts to a pathogenic influence to produce a hyperactive condition in certain organs or meridians. There are many levels and manifestations of excess, but a strong or excessive pulse and an abundance of spirit are the primary indicators. Other general signs of excess, such as a desire for cold, or pain which is aggravated by pressure, are merely used to confirm the overall pattern of imbalance. Again, excess must be identified in terms of the five phases, and excess tends to occur in combination with deficiency. Determining the pattern of imbalance (deficiency and excess) in the organs or meridians is the first step in meridian therapy.

> "When there is deficiency in one part of the body, another [organ or meridian] will increase its activity to compensate. This is known as reactive excess, or hyperactive yang." (Ikeda, 1977)

Excess can thus occur in an organ or meridian in reaction to external pathogenic influences, as well as in response to deficiency caused by internal pathogenic influences. The former type of excess is called pathogenic Qi excess, and the latter type is called reactive excess. The concept of deficiency and excess in the framework of the five phases is easy to understand using the analogy of a seesaw. When the amount of Qi in two phases is equal, the seesaw is level and there is no deficiency or excess. When the amount of Qi in one phase becomes greater than the other, or if the Qi in one phase is depleted for some reason, the seesaw tips to one side and there is an imbalance. Generally, for every excess in one meridian there is a corresponding deficiency in another.

We must be careful not to confuse deficiency and excess with yin and yang. As explained earlier, yin and yang are like two sides of a coin; yin represents the quiescent aspect, and yang the active aspect. Deficiency and excess are a relative measure of the shortage or surplus of a certain quality or quantity. This is why deficiency and excess can be used to define the state of yin or yang aspects of the body (e.g., heat and cold, Qi and Blood, exterior and interior). It is thus possible to have deficiency or excess of yin or yang. In the body, yin represents the interior, the yin organs, the yin meridians, and the Blood. Deficiency of yin implies deficiency in these aspects of the body. Yang, on the other hand, represents the exterior, the yang organs, the yang meridians, and the Qi. Excess of yang implies excess in these aspects. In meridian therapy, deficiency and excess are primarily used to denote the level of Qi in particular meridians, which in turn relate to certain organs, functions, and aspects of the body. Since treatment directly accesses the meridians, which in turn affects the organs, functions, and other aspects of the body, one need merely diagnose and treat the imbalance of Qi in the meridians.

Tonifying and Dispersing

The easiest way to understand tonification and dispersion as they relate to deficiency and excess is to picture these concepts in terms of a certain optimal quantity:

> "If eight-tenths full is [considered to be] the normal level, when the vessel contains less than this, an appropriate amount is added, and when it contains more than this, an appropriate amount is removed in order to obtain the proper level." (Nagahama, 1978)

Thus, in the simplest sense, tonification and dispersion can be understood as adding or subtracting to achieve the optimum quantity. But tonifying deficiency certainly has a broader meaning than this.

> "Tonification is used to augment the normal Qi, reinforce the life force, and strengthen life functions. In other words, [tonification] means to increase and strengthen the source Qi of the Triple Burner, which plays a central role in effecting recovery from illness." (Honma, 1949)

> "Tonification means to give, increase, or add … What is added, according to classical concepts, is Qi and Blood … This is the wellspring of all nourishment … Normal Qi is that which extends the life force … To tonify is thus to increase the normal Qi." (Yanagiya, 1976)

> "There are three meanings to tonification in practice. The first is the general meaning of drawing and collecting Qi to increase its amount. The second is to gently loosen Qi and Blood which has become stagnant to allow it to flow away so that fresh normal Qi can be drawn in. The circulation of fresh Qi and Blood is thereby encouraged. The third meaning is to add Qi. The first and second [types of tonification] are used when a patient has ample physical strength, but the third [type] is necessary in cases of severe debilitation where Qi must be added from the outside. In this case, warming tonification by moxibustion is the most effective method." (Yamashita, 1971)

Judging from these explanations, tonifying deficiency means to increase the normal Qi (i.e., that which strengthens the life force) which is lacking in certain organs or meridians by drawing the Qi over from another part of the body, or adding it from an outside source. What then does it mean to disperse excess?

> "Dispersing is to take away, control, or kill, [which means to] remove those things which are excessive, harmful, or a hindrance to the body. Pathogenic [Qi] … includes pathogenic influences … as well as unhealthy mental attitudes. Dispersing … means to remove these various pathogenic [factors] and improve the [internal] environment of the body so that the illness goes away … Excess due to internal imbalance must also be dispersed." (Honma, 1949)

> "Dispersion means to take away, reduce, put down, kill, or control. It means to reduce or expel pathogenic Qi, which poses an obstacle to life processes." (Yanagiya, 1976)

Dispersing excess therefore means to expel pathogenic Qi (i.e., anything that hinders the life force) which is in abundance. Dispersing is used both for pathogenic Qi excess and reactive excess.

Basic Approach to Tonifying and Dispersing

The central concept of meridian therapy is set forth in chapter 69 of the *Classic of Difficulties:*

> "It says in the classics to tonify when deficient, disperse when excessive, and use the meridian if neither deficient nor excessive. What does this mean? It means that when deficient, tonify its mother; when excessive, disperse its child. [In treating] first tonify and then disperse afterward. Using the meridian if neither deficient nor excessive means that the disease has originated in a single meridian, and that it has not been attacked by a pathogenic influence [transmitted from] another [meridian]. Thus [points on] that meridian are used. This is known as using the meridian."

This passage can be summarized in four simple rules:

1. When deficient, tonify the mother meridian.
2. When excessive, disperse the child meridian.
3. Tonify first and disperse afterward.
4. Treat only the affected meridian if the imbalance affects only one meridian.

"Tonify the mother when deficient" means, e.g., that when the Lung is deficient, tonify the Spleen, which is the mother of the Lung, or when the Liver is deficient, tonify the Kidney, which is the mother of the Liver. When practicing meridian therapy one must keep in mind the five-phase relationships shown in Illustration 2-2 above.

"Disperse the child when excessive" means, e.g., that when the Liver is excessive, disperse the Heart, which is the child of the Liver, or when the Heart is excessive, disperse the Spleen, which is the child of the Heart.

When there is both a deficient and an excessive meridian, first tonify the deficient meridian. If, after tonifying the deficient meridian the excessive meridian is still found to be excessive, then it should be dispersed. For example, when the Liver is deficient and the Spleen is excessive, first tonify the Liver. After it has been tonified, check the pulses again to see if the two meridians have been corrected. If excess can still be detected in the Spleen, then the Spleen is dispersed. In a case of Lung deficiency and Large Intestine excess, first tonify the Lung, and then disperse the Large Intestine, if necessary. This approach is consistent with the basic tenet of the yin-yang principle: yin leads and yang follows. Deficiency corresponds to yin and excess to yang; treating the yin thus has priority.

Treating only the affected meridian when imbalance exists in only that meridian means that one should do nothing that affects other meridians while treating the affected meridian. This would suggest that one use only the intrinsic point (the five-phase point that corresponds to the phase of the affected meridian), or the source point (for yang meridians), and avoid using points which affect other meridians (i.e., five-phase points that correspond to other phases). For example, if the Lung is deficient and no other meridian is imbalanced, only L-7 (the connecting point of the Lung) and L-8 (the metal point of the Lung) are used to tonify the Lung. Inoue Keiri, a major figure in the development of meridian therapy, maintained that this rule refers to meridians which are neither deficient nor excessive, but are nevertheless symptomatic. This would imply a symptomatic approach to acupuncture, but both interpretations may be correct since the affected meridian is treated in both cases. Moreover, symptomatic treatment is also an important component of meridian therapy, as will be explained later.

KEY POINTS

Yin and Yang

- These represent the active and quiescent natures of things. They are opposite aspects of a whole, such as the interior and exterior. Yin also denotes the hidden portion of the whole and yang the visible portion. It is therefore said that yin leads and yang follows.

Five Phases
- Consist of wood, fire, earth, metal, and water.
- Their relationships to each other are expressed by two cycles, generating and controlling.
- The generating cycle is wood, fire, earth, metal, and water. In this cycle each phase promotes the subsequent phase in a nurturing relationship.
- The controlling cycle is fire, metal, wood, earth, and water. In this cycle each phase controls or inhibits the subsequent phase in an antagonistic relationship.

Causes of Disease
- Predisposing factors are the sum total of factors from one's past which make one resistant or susceptible to disease.
- Immediate causes of disease are classified as internal and external pathogenic influences.
- Disease will not occur from exposure to external pathogenic influences unless one is susceptible due to predisposing factors or internal pathogenic influences.

Internal Pathogenic Influences
- The seven emotions are joy, anger, grief, pensiveness, sadness, fear, and fright.
- The primary miscellaneous factors which lead to internal injury are overindulgence in sex, food, and drink, as well as fatigue.
- Excessive joy, worry, or melancholy injures the Heart.
- Excessive anger injures the Liver.
- Excessive grief or sadness injures the Lung.
- Pensiveness (excessive thinking), overeating, or overworking injures the Spleen.
- Excessive fear or sex injures the Kidney.
- Emotional stability can be regained through appropriate acupuncture treatment.

External Pathogenic Influences
- Wind, cold, heat (summerheat), fire, dampness, and dryness.
- Wind represents those causes of disease which cannot be readily seen. Wind affects the Liver, and its characteristic pulse quality is floating and wiry.
- Cold affects the Kidney and/or Lung, and its characteristic pulse quality is slow and tight.
- Heat affects the Heart, and its characteristic pulse quality is floating and big.
- Dampness affects the Spleen, and its characteristic pulse quality is soft and submerged.
- Dryness affects the Lung.

3

Diagnosis in Meridian Therapy: The Four Examinations

In modern medicine when a patient has a complaint many different types of examinations and tests using modern technology are required to reach a diagnosis. Consider the symptom of coughing. After auscultation, blood tests, culturing sputum, X-rays, and (if necessary) bronchoscopy with a biopsy, one might diagnose the disorder as bronchial asthma, pleuritis, pulmonary tuberculosis, lung cancer, or cardiac insufficiency. Traditional Oriental medicine has its own unique approach to diagnosis known as the four examinations. Even if a practitioner is able to perform pulse diagnosis, he cannot expect to provide appropriate treatment unless he understands all aspects of the four examinations. A medical diagnosis can yield useful information, but it has no direct bearing on identifying the pattern in meridian therapy. In the case of coughing, for example, Lung or Kidney deficiency is the probable diagnosis, but the pattern must be confirmed with information gathered through the four examinations.

> "[In meridian therapy] the condition of the meridians is diagnosed rather than diagnosing to identify the disease [as in Western medicine]." (Honma, 1949)

The four examinations of traditional Oriental medicine are as follows:

1. *Looking:* This means to scrutinize the whole patient from a short distance. Looking is the primary means of gathering information about the patient's prognosis.
2. *Listening and smelling:* Listening to the sounds of breathing and the voice, and smelling the presence of abnormal odors, helps to determine the patient's condition.

3. *Questioning:* This refers to asking the patient about his condition. It includes questions about dietary preferences as well as symptoms associated with the patient's complaint.

4. *Palpation:* This includes palpation of the pulse, abdomen, back, and meridians.

In ancient China palpation was regarded as the crudest and least important of the four examinations. In meridian therapy, however, palpation is considered to be the most important means of diagnosis. Pulse diagnosis in particular is considered to be the primary factor in determining treatment. Nevertheless, all of the four examinations are necessary to obtain a complete diagnostic picture. I will therefore discuss each of the four types of traditional examination in meridian therapy, with special emphasis on pulse diagnosis and palpation.

LOOKING

In the classics, the character used for looking means to look from a distance, rather than close-up. It implies inspecting patients by looking at them from head to toe. To observe the state of the patient's spirit *(shin/shén),* it is best to stand a short distance away.

"Those who gain spirit will thrive, and those who lose spirit will perish" *(Basic Questions,* chapter 13). We must therefore first look for the presence of spirit. Spirit is not nearly as mysterious as it may sound. There are tangible elements that can be observed in a person's appearance and manner which give evidence of spirit. In *Acupuncture by Meridian Therapy,* Okabe Sodo identifies five factors which enable one to judge the presence of spirit in a patient:

1. Whether there is a certain luminescence around the body.
2. Whether there is a sparkle in the eyes.
3. Whether the speech is clear and the behavior is lively.
4. Whether the breathing is deep and even.
5. Whether there is luster in the skin.

Among these factors, the greatest significance is attached to the luster of the skin:

> "[Those whose complexions are] green like the juice from grass will die, [and those] like the wings of a kingfisher will live. [Those with] yellow like a trifoliate orange will die, [and those] like the belly of a crab will live. [Those with] black like soot will die, [and those] like the wings of a crow will live. [Those with] red like stagnant blood will die, [and those] like a cock's comb will live. [Those with] white like a skeleton will die, [and those] like lard will live. *(Basic Questions,* chapter 10)

This means that regardless of the color, those whose complexions are lustrous will recover, and those whose complexions are dull or lusterless are in danger. The truth in this observation is best illustrated by the complexion of cancer patients. When the complexion looks as if a thin mixture of black, dark green, and dark yellow paint were soaked into the skin, it makes you think they do not have long to live. Although it is normal for skin to have a healthy shine, since the amount of luster varies considerably from person to person, it usually serves as only a general indicator of health and vitality.

The patient's skin can be examined for its color and luster anywhere on the body, but there are two places in particular which should be noted. The first is referred to as the cubit skin *(chǐ pí)* in the classics, which means the skin surface on the volar side of the forearm between the acupuncture points L-5 and L-6. This area is very useful for examining the appearance of the skin, especially in those women who wear thick make-up, which makes it hard to judge the complexion by looking at their faces. The second place is in the middle of the forehead, just above the area between the eyebrows. In the classics, this area is called the heavenly garden *(tiān tíng)*. Generally speaking, those whose skin in this area has good color and gives off a light glow, without the excessively polished shine of oily skin, can be regarded as doubly blessed with health and good fortune. Such patients will recover without any difficulty.

"To know [the patient's condition] by looking means to know the disease by observing the five colors [in a person's complexion]" *(Classic of Difficulties,* chapter 61). In the five-phase scheme of color diagnosis, green corresponds to the Liver, red to the Heart, yellow to the Spleen, white to the Lung, and black to the Kidney. This means, for example, that when a person has a blackish complexion without luster, he has a serious Kidney imbalance. Diagnosis of the complexion according to the five colors is useful to keep in mind, but clinically it is not that easy to clearly distinguish colors. Most complexions are a mixture of several colors, and sometimes a person with a blackish complexion shows a Liver imbalance by pulse diagnosis. Some authorities say that those patients whose complexions correlate with other diagnostic findings recover quickly, while those whose complexions do not match other findings are difficult to cure.

There are many other features that should be examined visually besides the presence of spirit and the quality of the complexion, including the eyes, tongue, and posture, as well as the appearance of the affected area. I will not discuss these aspects in detail since they each require considerable study. As with other aspects of diagnosis, for purposes of meridian therapy it is important that the findings of the looking portion of the examination be correlated with imbalances in specific organs or meridians.

LISTENING

The character for listening *(bun/wén)* means both to listen and to smell. Listening is the aspect of examination that applies the auditory and olfactory senses to judge a patient's condition.

"To know [the patient's condition] by listening means to know the disease by listening for the five sounds [in the patient's voice]" *(Classic of Difficulties,* chapter 61). The patient's tone of voice is thus distinguished in accordance with the five phases to determine which organ is affected. The five sounds or notes are impossible to describe in words, and the only way to learn them is to ask someone who is knowledgeable about traditional Chinese music. Aside from the five sounds, which are not commonly known, the five voices and five odors are clinically significant aspects of the listening portion of the examination.

The five voices are commanding, speaking, singing, crying, and groaning. When a patient has a commanding tone in his voice it is a sign of a Liver imbalance. Particularly when a person who is normally mild-mannered becomes imperious and commanding, the Liver meridian has either become excessive or deficient. A commanding voice may be characterized as just a step before anger. Among the five emotions, anger is associated with the Liver; a commanding voice, anger, and the Liver all correspond to the wood phase.

Speaking refers to talking, but in an abnormal way. If a person who is normally quiet suddenly becomes talkative, or a person begins to say strange things, or if the speech is otherwise unclear, these are signs of a Heart imbalance. The Heart is injured when there is excessive joy, and speaking refers to the emotionally-excited state just before extreme joy, when a person is effusive.

Singing refers to a tendency to sing. If a person who rarely sings suddenly starts to sing, or begins to hum tunes incessantly, an imbalance of the Spleen may be indicated. However, a person who normally likes to sing may be considered to have good Spleen and Stomach function.

Crying suggests a whining tone of voice. There are patients who whine about their physical problems throughout the course of treatment. Sometimes this makes you angry because they go on and on and keep repeating themselves, even after you have patiently listened to their complaints. This is typical in cases of Lung imbalances and relates to the Lung being injured by sadness.

Groaning is a voice of distress; patients with a deep, groaning voice are usually seriously ill. Those who make groaning sounds or heave a deep sigh when they have to turn over or move may be suffering from a Kidney imbalance.

The five odors are also used to indicate an imbalance in the organs or meridians in accordance with their five-phase correspondences. The five odors are rancid, burned, fragrant, fleshy, and rotten. Rancid is an oily and fleshy odor that indicates a Liver imbalance. Burned is a charred odor like the smell of burning paper that indicates a Heart imbalance. Fragrant means an unusual sweet odor that indicates an imbalance of the Spleen. A fleshy or fishy smell indicates a Lung imbalance. Rotten is an odor of decay that indicates an imbalance of the Kidney. Sometimes, when simply facing a patient to take their pulse, I am struck by a strong odor which is indistinguishable as either bad breath or body odor. When I examine the tongue of such patients, I invariably find a thick fur of white or yellow color. The pulse often shows a Lung imbalance.

There are many other aspects of listening, including the patient's breathing and bowel sounds. Among the five changes (clenching, melancholy, hiccoughing, coughing and shivering), those things which can be heard are part of the listening aspect of examination. This would include coughing and sneezing, which are associated with imbalances of the Lung, and burping and hiccoughing, which are associated with imbalances of the Spleen. Judging the smell of the feces and vaginal discharge is also traditionally regarded as part of the listening aspect of examination. By thus identifying the sounds and odors issuing from the patient, one can gather some indication of which organ or meridian is affected.

Remember, however, that the sounds and odors that one perceives do not necessarily determine the diagnosis. Even if the patient has a groaning voice and a rotten odor, one should not jump to conclusions. Rather, one should suspect a Kidney imbalance and begin to ask pertinent questions to confirm this finding. Only if other aspects of the examination, particularly the pulse, support the initial findings can one diagnose the pattern with confidence. The listening phase of the examination is therefore a means of getting some sense of the patient's condition, and establishing a direction for other phases of the examination which follow.

QUESTIONING

Questioning is a means by which information about the patient's past and present is obtained, either directly from the patient, or indirectly from a member of the patient's family.

> "To know [the patient's condition] by questioning means to ask which of the five tastes are preferred, and thereby determine where the disease originated and where it lies." *(Classic of Difficulties,* chapter 61)

In the classics the focus of the questioning phase of examination is to find out which of the organs and meridians are affected by asking about the patient's taste preferences and other personal traits. Aside from the five tastes, the five emotions (internal pathogenic influences) and five aversions (external pathogenic influences) also provide clues to the cause of a disease and the organs and meridians involved. The five labors, or physical strains, are likewise useful for judging where a problem originated. Inquiring about the five fluids is useful in cases where they cannot be observed in the course of the looking phase of examination. Here I will briefly explain each of the five-phase correspondences associated with questioning.

THE FIVE TASTES

The five tastes are sour, bitter, sweet, pungent, and salty. The sour taste includes that of citrus fruits as well as vinegar. When a person has a special liking or disliking for sour foods, or if everything seems to taste sour, there is said to be a problem with the Liver, or some imbalance in the Liver and Gallbladder meridians. When a person has a special liking or disliking for bitter foods, or if everything seems to taste bitter, there is a problem with the Heart, or an imbalance in the Heart and Small Intestine meridians. Those who crave sweets or constantly have a sweet taste in their mouths tend to have a Spleen condition, or an imbalance in the Spleen and Stomach meridians. In extreme cases of Spleen deficiency, one will eat raw sugar whenever there are no sweets available.

Pungent refers to a hot or spicy taste, which is typical of peppers. People who love spicy foods tend to have Lung problems, or an imbalance in the Lung and Large Intestine meridians. When I was a child, I remember a neighbor who put an incredible number of red peppers in his miso soup. The soup was literally full of peppers, and when I acted surprised, this man would throw several fried peppers into his mouth just to show off. He happened to be an asthmatic who constantly wheezed, and eventually died of pulmonary tuberculosis. He probably had an extreme case of Lung deficiency.

A preference for salty foods indicates a Kidney condition, or an imbalance in the Kidney and Bladder meridians. Today doctors restrict salt intake for hypertensive patients, but people who have high blood pressure tend to like salty foods. Blood rushing to the head and cold extremities are symptoms associated with Kidney disorders. The former symptom indicates high blood pressure, and the latter denotes low blood pressure. It is unwise for people with Kidney deficiency to totally cut out their intake of salt.

In the classics a shortage of one of the tastes is considered to be as bad as an excess of any one taste. Each of the five tastes nourishes its corresponding organs. Thus, eating foods in a way that balances all of the tastes is the best way to stay healthy. In any case, the five-phase correspondences of the tastes are not only helpful in maintaining health, but are also clinically useful in diagnosis.

THE FIVE EMOTIONS

The five emotions are a very important means of identifying possible internal factors which have caused imbalances to occur. The five emotions are similar to the seven emotions discussed in chapter 2, except that melancholy and fright have been deleted. The five emotions are accordingly anger, joy, pensiveness, sorrow, and fear, each of which is associated with a particular organ or organs.

By the time you start the questioning phase of the examination, you should already have an indication as to whether the emotions are involved by the quality of the patient's voice. The point of questioning is to find out if there is a special problem with any one emotion. I have already discussed the five-phase correspondences of the emotions, but I will briefly touch on this topic once again since it is an important aspect of the questioning phase of the examination.

Anger is associated with the Liver, and excessive anger injures the Liver. It is a sign of Liver or Gallbladder imbalance when a person suddenly becomes hot-tempered or irritated over small things. Hot tempers are especially typical of Liver-excess types. Liver deficiency usually causes a person to become easily frightened. When a person who is normally mild mannered suddenly becomes bossy, this can be interpreted as a sign of reactive Liver excess (i.e., excess resulting from deficiency in another meridian or organ).

Joy is associated with the Heart, and excessive joy injures the Heart. From the standpoint of mental health, joy would seem to be a good thing. I therefore used to think that this particular association was off the mark. But I changed my mind when I read a magazine article which said that the more money people win in horse races or lotteries, the higher their blood pressure becomes. Even joy, when it becomes extreme, can be injurious to one's health.

Thinking is associated with the Spleen, and pensiveness or excessive thinking injures the Spleen. Too much concern or worry impairs the function of the Spleen and Stomach. One often hears of people who worry so much that they stop eating and lose weight.

Sorrow is associated with the Lung, and excessive sorrow injures the Lung. Just before and after the second World War, I often heard of people who grieved a great deal and contracted Lung diseases such as tuberculosis. Excessive sorrow injures the Qi of the thorax. Some patients have a very sad disposition and even start crying as they relate their problems. The majority of such patients have an imbalance in the Lung or Large Intestine meridian.

Fear is associated with the Kidney, and excessive fear injures the Kidney. Patients suffering from Kidney deficiency tend to be fearful and easily frightened. In extreme cases they are afraid to see others and refuse to leave home. This may seem foolish to those of us who are healthy, but it is a serious problem for those who are afflicted with such phobias, some of whom are driven to suicide. Using meridian therapy to alleviate Kidney deficiency can cure such problems. However, the final judgment as to whether or not the problem is one of Kidney deficiency should be based on the pulse. Acupuncture is highly effective for treating phobias associated with Kidney deficiency. I am constantly amazed at how acupuncture serves as powerful psychosomatic medicine when the diagnosis and treatment are appropriate.

THE FIVE AVERSIONS

The five aversions are the five-phase correspondences of the external pathogenic influences based on the discussion in *Basic Questions*. The five aversions are wind, heat, dampness, dryness, and cold. An imbalance in one of the five yin organs is said to cause an aversion to the external pathogenic influence which can injure that organ. When there is a Liver imbalance, one has an aversion to wind. When there is a Heart imbalance, one has an aversion to heat. When there is a Spleen imbalance, one has an aversion to dampness. For example, we often see patients with rheumatism or neuralgia whose condition is aggravated by dampness. They can be said to have an aversion to dampness. When there is a Lung imbalance, one has an aversion to dryness. When there is a Kidney imbalance, one has an aversion to cold. In my experience, those patients who are sensitive to cold usually have either a Lung or a Kidney imbalance. Asking about the patient's preferences for climate or season may provide a useful indication of the imbalances in their meridians.

THE FIVE LABORS

"Walking for a long time injures the sinews, looking for a long time injures the Blood, sitting for a long time injures the flesh, lying for a long time injures the Qi, and standing for a long time injures the bones." *(Basic Questions,* chapter 23)

The five labors are long-term physical strains which injure one or another of the five tissues. In the system of five-phase correspondences, the sinews are related to the Liver, the Blood to the Heart, the flesh to the Spleen, the Qi to the Lung, and the bone or marrow to the Kidney. Thus, walking for a long time causes an imbalance in the Liver, or the Liver and Gallbladder meridians. Looking for a long time tends to cause an imbalance in the Heart, or the Heart and Small Intestine meridians. This particular association seems to apply to those who often overuse their eyes at work, such as computer terminal operators. On the other hand, some practitioners associate overuse of the eyes with Liver imbalances, and walking too long with Heart imbalances. Both associations seem plausible.

With respect to sitting for a long time, an imbalance in the Spleen, or the Spleen and Stomach meridians is indicated. People in occupations involving long hours of sitting, such as tailors, writers, and drivers, tend to suffer from Spleen imbalances. Lying in bed for an extended period of time tends to cause an imbalance in the Lung, or the Lung and Large Intestine meridians. Standing continuously for long hours causes an imbalance in the Kidney, or the Kidney and Bladder meridians. Many people who have jobs that require long hours of standing suffer from Kidney imbalance or Kidney deficiency. For this reason, when a patient finds it difficult to remain standing for long, I suspect Kidney deficiency.

THE FIVE FLUIDS

Asking about abnormalities in the five fluids sometimes provides useful clues as to which of the organs is affected. The five fluids are tears, sweat, drool, snivel, and saliva. Those whose eyes water excessively, or conversely dry out, often have a Liver imbalance. Those who have become sentimental in old age and are brought to tears over things like melodramas on television usually have an imbalance in the Liver meridian. Those who sweat profusely even in cold weather, or those who hardly sweat at all even in the heat of summer, often have an imbalance in the Heart, or the Heart and Small Intestine meridians. Drool is saliva that seeps out of the mouth. Drooling is most often seen in young children and senile people. It is regarded as a sign of an imbalance in the Spleen, or the Spleen and Stomach meridians. Snivel refers to mucous discharge from the nasal cavity. Excessive nasal discharge is a sign of an imbalance in the Lung, or the Lung and Large Intestine meridians. Most patients with allergic rhinitis suffer from Lung deficiency, and this is also true of patients whose nasal passages begin to hurt from lack of mucous secretion. Saliva is related to the Kidney. When there is excessive salivation, or when the mouth becomes dry, it is a sign of an imbalance in the Kidney and Bladder meridians.

The five-phase correspondences of the tastes, emotions, aversions, labors, and fluids are clinically useful clues as to which of the organs and meridians are affected. There is no need, however, to question a patient about each and every one of these. Simply ask about those things which are likely to be relevant in view of other findings. The questioning phase of examination is used primarily to confirm whether the pattern of imbalance found in pulse diagnosis does, in fact, have corresponding symptomatic manifestations. For this reason, there is no need to do an exhaustive and time-consuming interview. If you prefer to have all the information beforehand, give the patient a form to fill out in the waiting room.

PRACTICAL QUESTIONING EXAMINATION

There is a so-called "no-questions diagnostic method" by which a practitioner guesses the patient's problem by looking, listening, and palpating the pulse and abdomen. Yanagiya Sorei, the father of meridian therapy, wrote a book entitled, *Simple Diagnosis Without Questions*. This book details how a practitioner can obtain clues about a patient's condition simply from looking, listening, and palpating. If you focus on a particular method of diagnosis for many years, you will probably become expert at guessing what is wrong with a patient without asking any questions. Patients will be surprised and impressed that you can guess what is wrong with them, and will come to believe that you are equally capable of rendering treatment. This is one way to gain the confidence of your patients. However, it is one thing to guess the patient's symptoms, and another to treat the patient. Needless to say, treatment of the illness is more important. Nevertheless, since diagnosis and treatment go hand in hand, we must utilize all the means at our disposal to acquire information about the patient's condition. Thus, the conscientious practitioner must conduct a thorough inquiry into the patient's illness and history.

Be that as it may, there is rarely enough time for an exhaustive interview at the clinic. We must therefore learn how to ask the best questions for gathering pertinent information in order to administer the appropriate treatment. The skill of a practitioner in questioning directly relates to the accuracy of his diagnosis. The ability to hit the mark is something that comes only through experience. The experienced practitioner is able to quickly narrow the scope of inquiry to focus on the primary imbalance. In many cases, the questioning takes place at the same time as the looking, listening, and palpatory phases of the examination. One example of an efficient questioning examination would be as follows:

An adult male walks into the clinic. After recording the date and personal data, the questioning examination begins.

1. Q: What seems to be the problem?   A: I've got low back pain.
2. Q: Where exactly does it hurt? On the right or the left side, or in the middle?
   A: It hurts on the left side here.
3. Q: When does it hurt the most? Which movements aggravate it?
   A: It hurts the most when I stand up.
4. Q: Does it hurt when you bend backward, bend forward, or twist?
   A: It hurts to bend forward.
5. Q: Is it painful when you wake up in the morning, and then gradually improves through the day?   A: No.
6. Q: Is it painful when you stand up, but improves with movement?
   A: It hurts to bend over, but it's fine when I'm walking.
7. Q: When did this pain start?   A: It started about three days ago.
8. Q: Did it start all of a sudden, or come on gradually?
   A: I felt something funny when I was lifting a load.
9. Q: Is there any numbness in your legs?   A: No.

Physical examination for neurological lesions (such as the Laségue's test and Babinski's reflex) are negative, and the tendon reflexes are normal. Palpation down the lumbar vertebrae reveals a tender point between the spinous processes of the fourth and fifth lumbar vertebrae.

The pulse reveals that the Liver and Kidney positions are deficient, and that the Gallbladder and Bladder positions are excessive. In addition, the Spleen position is slightly excessive. Abdominal palpation shows a lack of muscle tone on the left side, with slight pulsation at S-25 on the left. The questioning thereupon continues:

10. Q: Do you like sour foods?   A: No, not really.
11. Q: Do you sleep well?   A: I often have difficulty falling asleep, and I tend not
    . to sleep well.
12. Q: Has your appetite increased lately?   A: I do have a healthy appetite.

In the above example, question number one concerns the chief complaint. Questions two and nine are for finding points for localized or symptomatic treatment. Questions three through six are for relating the symptoms to specific meridians to determine which meridians should be treated to relieve the pain. Question seven is to find out whether the patient's condition is acute or chronic. In acute cases, symptomatic treatment, treatment of a single meridian, and dispersing techniques are most effective. In chronic cases, however, several meridians must be treated to correct deficiency in the yin meridians, and tonification techniques are most effective. Question number ten concerns the five tastes. Question eleven relates to the symptomology of the Liver meridian, and question twelve to that of the Spleen meridian.

In this manner, the information gathered by questioning is used to determine the pattern of imbalance in the meridians. This is compared with the palpatory findings, especially from pulse and abdominal diagnosis. Questioning often proceeds simultaneously with the physical examination and palpation, and as clues are obtained from these examinations, the questioning is narrowed down to likely problem areas. One need not necessarily ask the questions in the same order, but the relevant questions should be asked in order to gather all the information necessary for arriving at the right diagnosis, which in turn leads to the appropriate treatment. Knowledge of the symptomology of the organs and the twelve meridians from the classics is very useful in framing the questions, as this enables one to ask more relevant questions once the affected meridians are known. There are many texts which list the symptomology of the meridians, and we will discuss this subject in the next chapter. First, however, I would like to turn our consideration to the palpatory examination.

PALPATION

In ancient times when there were no diagnostic instruments as there are today, the physician first employed the looking, listening, and questioning examinations to determine which part of the body was affected, and which of the organs and meridians were involved. Palpation was probably the last step in diagnosis, the stage at which the physician sought to confirm his observations and make the final decisions about rendering treatment. According to a saying attributed to Bian Que, the author of the *Classic of Difficulties,* he who could arrive at the diagnosis without touching the patient was regarded as a superior physician, and he who had to rely on the palpatory examination to determine treatment was regarded as an ordinary physician. Even with all the diagnostic tools at our disposal today, we seem to be less adept at arriving at a diagnosis and formulating an effective treatment than was the ordinary physician in ages past.

Although palpation may be the least sophisticated means of examination according to the classics, it is nevertheless the most crucial stage of diagnosis in meridian therapy. The findings from all the other phases of examination are used primarily to confirm what is felt at our fingertips. Palpation is also crucial as the last step in acupuncture for locating and treating points on the surface of the body.

> "In the palpatory examination we use our hands to palpate the patient's body. Palpation includes three methods: pulse diagnosis, abdominal diagnosis, and meridian palpation." (Honma, 1949)

In the general palpatory examination, in addition to pulse diagnosis (which is most important in meridian therapy), the skin surface of the abdomen, back, and limbs is stroked, pressed, pinched, and tapped to find manifestations of deficiency or excess on the patient's body. Information obtained in this manner is used to confirm the findings from pulse diagnosis, and the abnormal areas on the skin surface themselves become candidates for symptomatic treatment. Unlike medical doctors, we acupuncturists use very few diagnostic instruments. Instead, we have to rely on our sense of touch to arrive at the proper diagnosis and provide effective treatment. For this reason, many palpatory techniques have been devised through the centuries, the mastery of which requires years of practice. It is only right that we dedicate ourselves to honing our palpatory skills if we wish to be regarded as true professionals.

I have heard stories about how traditional physicians in pre-war China were sometimes tested by prospective patients. The patient would deliberately lie about his complaints to mislead the physician, and if he were unable to diagnose correctly, the patient would go elsewhere to see another physician. It is a little frightening, and at the same time amusing, to imagine what it would be like if patients today were so devious. I wonder how many acupuncturists would be able to pass the test and arrive at the right diagnosis!

Meridian therapy is a system of acupuncture based primarily on the *Classic of Difficulties*. This book refers to pulse diagnosis more often than any other type of examination. If we follow the *Classic of Difficulties* to the letter, there would be very little need for any other form of palpatory examination. There is no question that in traditional Oriental medicine pulse diagnosis has always been the most important aspect of the palpatory examination. This tradition is carried a step further in meridian therapy, where the pulse is used as the principal factor in determining the diagnosis and treatment. It is possible to do acupuncture without reference to the pulse, but pulse diagnosis is a preeminently practical way to determine the most appropriate diagnosis and treatment. I will thus begin by explaining in detail how pulse diagnosis is performed in meridian therapy.

Pulse Diagnosis

Pulse diagnosis is the most important aspect of examination in meridian therapy, but what exactly is diagnosed? It is the balance of Qi in the organs and meridians. We palpate the radial artery to see if the organs and meridians are normal or abnormal, and if abnormal, which meridians are deficient or excessive. For example, if the Liver and Kidney meridians are found to be deficient, the Liver and Kidney organs also have the same imbalance. In other words, the functions of the Liver and Kidney are impaired. The nature of the functional impairment is reflected in the energetic state of the meridians, and this can be detected in the pulse. It is unwise, however, to base one's diagnosis solely on the pulse. The final determination of the pattern of imbalance should take into consideration all of the other phases of examination including looking, listening, questioning, abdominal diagnosis, and meridian palpation. Be that as it may, pulse diagnosis is given the greatest weight in determining the pattern of imbalance.

There are two distinct types of pulse palpation used in meridian therapy. The first is the six-position pulse diagnosis outlined in the *Classic of Difficulties,* which compares the strength of the pulse in all six positions on the right and left arms. Six-position pulse diagnosis is used to detect imbalances (deficiency or excess) in the meridians. The other type of pulse palpation is the pulse-quality diagnosis, in which the quality of the pulse (slippery, wiry, thin, etc.) is considered, and the precise position of the pulse is not too important. In six-position pulse diagnosis, the location of the pulse positions must be very exact. Because this type of pulse diagnosis is initially more difficult to learn, I will explain it first.

POSITIONS FOR PULSE DIAGNOSIS

The part of the body used for pulse diagnosis in meridian therapy is the radial artery at the wrist, which is the same location used in Western medicine for taking the pulse. In the classics, this area is called the inch mouth *(cūn kǒu)* or pulse opening *(mài kǒu)*. In its broad sense, the term inch mouth refers to that part of the radial

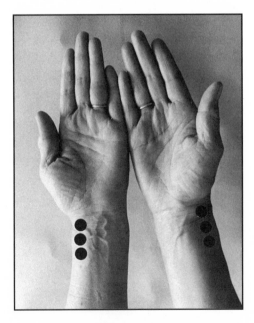

Illustration 3-1
Positions for Pulse Diagnosis

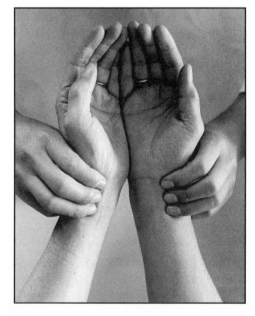

Illustration 3-2
Six-Position Pulse Diagnosis

artery where the pulse is palpated, and in its narrow sense, to the most distal of the three positions of pulse diagnosis. The area over the radial artery just above the wrist is divided into three positions: distal, middle, and proximal. As was just noted, the distal position is traditionally called the inch mouth, or 'inch' for short. The middle position is called the bar top *(guān shàng)*, or 'bar' for short. The proximal position is called the cubit center *(chǐ zhōng)* , or 'cubit' for short. The location of these three positions is actually based on the unit measurement for the entire anterior aspect of the forearm, with the proximal position being two units above the crease of the wrist. The middle position is one unit above the crease, and the distal position is one-tenth of a unit above the crease. This method of locating the pulse, however, is time consuming and complicated. Therefore, the following simplified method is used instead.

First, the middle position is located next to the radial eminence (the distal prominence of the radius) where the radial artery can be felt. The middle position is slightly proximal to the highest point of the radial eminence. Next the distal position is located halfway between the middle position and the palmar crease of the wrist. Finally, the proximal position is located the same distance proximally from the middle position as that between the middle and distal positions (Illustration 3-1).

> "There is a bone [on the lateral side of the wrist] called the high bone [radial eminence]. Do not locate [the middle position] over this bone. After feeling this bone, move the finger toward the proximal position. [Then] press the finger right up against the high bone. Other practitioners say that this [position] is to be found over the high bone, but this is a big mistake." (Manase, 1574)

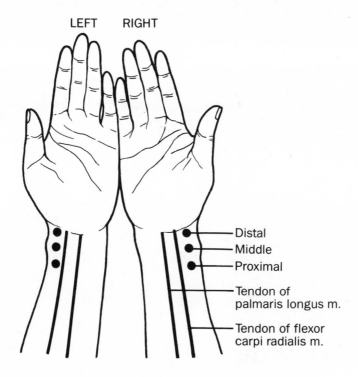

Illustration 3-3
Pulse Positions and Forearm Tendons

The proper method of finger placement for six-position pulse diagnosis is shown in Illustration 3-2. This method is best practiced by bringing the palm of your right hand over the back of your left wrist, and using the index, middle, and ring fingers of your right hand to locate the pulse positions. First locate the radial eminence by placing your middle finger on the radial aspect of the wrist. After locating the highest point of the radial eminence slightly medial to the tendon of the abductor pollicis longus, slide your middle finger just slightly proximal to find a small depression. Then bring the center of the tip of your middle finger over the point on the radial artery adjacent to this depression. This is the middle position. Next put the tip of your index finger on the point between the palmar crease of the wrist and the point under the tip of your middle finger. If a patient's forearm is long and there is some distance between the radial eminence and the palmar crease, the index and middle fingers will be spaced apart. If the forearm is short, you will have to bunch your fingers up against each other. This is especially true when performing pulse diagnosis on children. Finally, locate the proximal position by placing the tip of your ring finger on the point the same distance from the middle position as the distal position. When you do this, your finger-tips should all line up in a straight line, as shown in Illustration 3-2. The fingers will easily align if you practice bringing your fingers up against the tendon of the flexor carpi radialis muscle, which separates the Lung meridian from the Pericardium meridian (Illustration 3-3).

When you face the patient to take the pulses on both wrists at the same time, your right hand holds the patient's left wrist, and your left hand holds the patient's right wrist. Your thumbs should support the back of the patient's wrists around TB-4 (Illustration 3-4). Actually there are many other ways of supporting the patient's wrists during pulse diagnosis, which I shall discuss after explaining the different pulse positions.

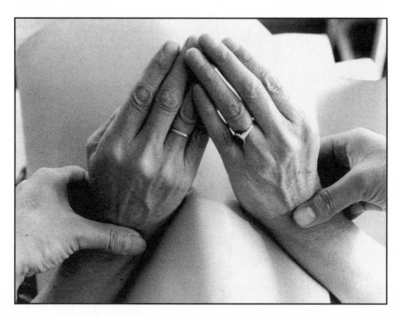

Illustration 3-4
Thumb Position for Pulse Diagnosis

In six-position pulse diagnosis, all of the positions (three on each arm) are palpated at three levels: superficial, middle, and deep. Almost no pressure is applied with the fingers at the superficial level, a moderate amount of pressure is used at the middle level, and a substantial amount of pressure is used to reach the deep level. I will explain how to palpate each of these levels shortly, but first it is important to familiarize yourself with the organ and meridian correspondences for each position and level as shown in Table 3-1. The middle level is not used to diagnose specific meridians, but to check the overall condition of the patient, as explained below.

Left Hand			Right Hand	
Superficial (Yang)	Deep (Yin)		Deep (Yin)	Superficial (Yang)
Small Intestine	Heart	**Distal**	Lung	Large Intestine
Gallbladder	Liver	**Middle**	Spleen	Stomach
Bladder	Kidney	**Proximal**	Pericardium	Triple Burner

Table 3-1 Pulse Positions

HOW TO PALPATE THE PULSES

Palpating the middle level: The first step in pulse diagnosis is to place the index, middle, and ring fingers of both hands on all the pulse positions, right and left, with the thumbs on the back of the wrists. When the fingertips are placed directly over the radial artery and slight pressure is applied, the pulse can usually be felt clearly with all the fingers. The depth or level where the pulse can be felt most clearly in *all* finger positions is called the middle level. The depth of the middle level thus varies from person to person.

> "Because of individual differences one should not assume that the middle level is the same [for everyone]. The middle level is deeper in some people, and shallower in others." (Inoue, 1980)

The strength and quality of the pulse at the middle level reflects the condition of the Stomach Qi, which denotes the overall energy level or function of the middle burner. While the middle level also reflects the functional condition of the individual organs and meridians associated with each position, it is primarily an indicator of the Stomach Qi.

> "In China the central or middle area was designated as the earth position because the center of the four directions is the earth position. Also the central organ of the five organs is the earth organ (which represents the function of the Spleen and Stomach). Accordingly, the middle level of the pulses was described as the earth pulse, or the Spleen and Stomach pulse." (Yamashita, 1982)

The pulse at the middle level is considered to be the same in all six positions. A certain vitality exists in the pulse at the middle level as long as there are no serious disturbances in life processes. Those patients who have very little vitality in their pulse at the middle level, or those whose pulse can only be felt at the superficial or deep levels, are likely to have serious problems. In particular, a patient who has a feeble pulse at the middle level in the middle position on the right (Spleen/Stomach) should be examined carefully; if there is any doubt, he should be referred to a physician for a thorough medical examination.

Palpating the superficial level: After palpating the pulse at the middle level, the pressure on the fingers is relaxed just short of the point at which the pulse can no longer be felt. This is the superficial level. Naturally, the pulse cannot be felt as strongly at this level since the fingers are placed very gently on each position. When strong pulses can be palpated in most positions at this level, it is known as superficial level excess or yang meridian excess. When the pulses are weak in most positions at this level, it is known as superficial level deficiency, or yang meridian deficiency. The strength of the pulses in all positions is compared at the superficial level to determine which of the yang meridians are deficient, and which are excessive.

Palpating the deep level: After palpating the pulse at the superficial level, increase the pressure on the fingers to palpate the deep level. If the pressure is too great, the pulse will weaken or disappear altogether and it will be impossible to compare the strength at different positions. Hold your fingers just above the level at which the pulses begin to fade. This is the deep level where the Qi of the yin organs or meridians is examined. Differentiating whether the deep level is weak or rootless from the end of the deep level can be difficult, especially for beginners. When the pulses are quite strong in most positions at the deep level, it is known as deep level excess, or yin meridian excess. When the pulses are weak in most positions at the deep level, it is known as deep level deficiency, or yin meridian deficiency. The strength of the pulses in all positions is compared at the deep level to determine which of the yin meridians are deficient, and which are excessive (Illustration 3-5).

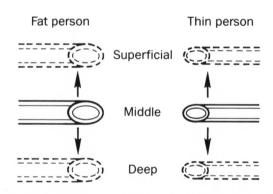

Illustration 3-5
Pulse Levels in Fat and Thin People

"There are people with thick arteries and there are people with thin arteries. Fat people tend to have thick arteries, and yet the distance [from the middle level] to the deep and superficial levels is short. This makes it more difficult to palpate excess and deficiency [in fat people]. Thin people tend to have thin arteries, but the distance [from the middle level] to the deep and superficial levels is often greater. This makes it is easier to palpate [differences in] the pulses." (Honma, 1949)

The role of the thumb in pulse diagnosis: Thus far I have explained the basic finger placement for six-position pulse diagnosis. After learning the proper pulse positions and levels, we must direct our attention to the thumbs. Palpation of the pulse is easier when the focus of attention is shifted away from the fingers on the pulse to the thumb on the back of the wrist. The secret of pulse diagnosis for beginners has been described by experienced practitioners:

"Sit facing the seated patient and palpate the pulses on the right and left side at the same time. When the pulses are palpated with the patient lying supine, the pulses are weaker and more difficult to feel for a beginner. Therefore, palpate the pulses with the patient seated. For patients who cannot sit up, or for those whose pulses are faint even in the seated position, perform some very superficial needling on the upper abdomen. This will make the pulses easier to palpate.

"Position your index, middle, and ring fingers together over the pulse of the radial artery with the radial eminence at the center. Your thumb should go around to hold the opposite side of the wrist in a natural manner. In this way, you palpate the left wrist with your right hand, and the right wrist with your left hand. Do not think of palpating the pulses with the three fingers on the pulse, but rather palpate as if perceiving the pulse with your thumbs. This is the secret to pulse diagnosis.

"Place the three fingers vertically in relation to the artery and put strength in your thumbs. The pulses felt by the three fingers will even out (as if they were one). This is the middle position. This is known as the pulse of the Stomach Qi. We measure the deficiency or excess of the patient's Qi from this pulse. Those whose pulse is weak at this position have a deficient condition, and therefore their illness is difficult to cure." (Araki, 1982)

"Have the patient assume a supine position and place both of their arms on their abdomen in a natural manner. The practitioner must take a wide stance and put strength in his lower abdomen. Strength is not placed in the hands. One must never put strength in the fingers. The thumbs are placed on TB-4, and must be placed accurately. The thumbs are used [to palpate the pulse]. Palpate with the feeling of pushing the thumbs forward." (Inoue, 1962)

These practitioners are talking about the same thing in reference to using the thumb as the focus of strength, and their point is clear. As for positioning the thumbs, however, for people like myself with long fingers, it is sometimes difficult to place them on TB-4. I find it easier to place my thumbs more toward the Small Intestine meridian, and sometimes even on SI-5 (Illustration 3-6). I am of the opinion that everyone should find the place on the back of the wrist which is most comfortable, depending on the length of one's fingers. There is also a method of pulse diagnosis where the thumbs are not used at all. Instead of the thumb, the practitioner's palm holds the back of the wrist so that the thenar eminence is over TB-4, and the hypothenar eminence is over TB-5 (Illustration 3-7). The positioning of the fingers over the artery is

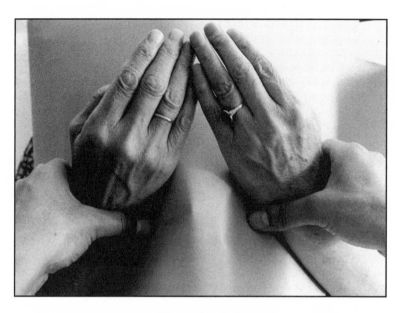

Illustration 3-6
Alternate Thumb Position for Pulse Diagnosis (SI-4)

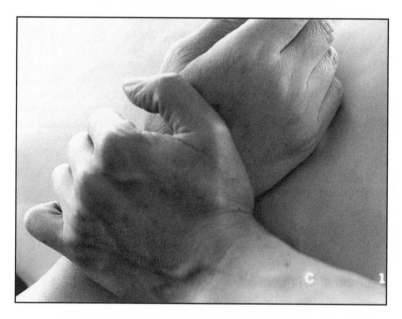

Illustration 3-7
Alternate Palm Position for Pulse Diagnosis

the same, but instead of putting strength in the thumbs, it is exerted from the palms as a whole. This is a useful method for those practitioners with large hands, and is every bit as effective once the practitioner becomes proficient.

When the thumb is pressed into the back of the wrist, leverage causes the greatest pressure to be exerted on the index finger among the three fingers on the

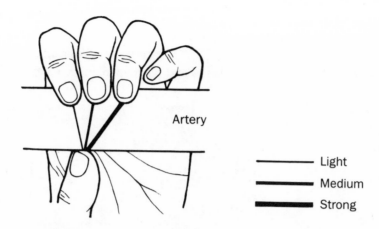

Artery

——————— Light

——————— Medium

——————— Strong

Illustration 3-8
Coordination of Thumb and Fingers in Pulse Diagnosis

artery. One has to press with the thumbs and grasp with the fingers in such a way that slightly more pressure is brought to bear over the proximal positions than over the distal positions (Illustration 3-8). When palpating the distal positions, you must be careful not to allow the patient's wrists to flex too much. The pulses cannot be palpated accurately in this position if the wrist is flexed, because the artery needs to be straight to get an accurate reading. Actually, the wrists should be very slightly extended when palpating this position. When palpating the middle and deep levels, press with your thumbs and pull in a little more on the ring fingers, and avoid the tendency of grasping the wrist mostly with your thumb and forefinger. This can best be accomplished if the practitioner rotates (supinates) his wrists very slightly in addition to grasping with the thumb and fingers. When palpating all the pulse positions at once, it is useful to fix the position of the three fingers in relation to each other, and then to move them up and down simultaneously as if they were glued together. In this way, the pressure exerted by the thumb is brought to bear on all of the fingers as a unit, instead of on individual fingers. To palpate one position in relation to others using this method, e.g., the pulse of the Kidney meridian (left proximal position), simply direct your attention to your right ring finger while holding all the fingers at the deep level with pressure from the thumbs.

This is the standard method for examining the pulses in meridian therapy. If it is still difficult to distinguish which positions are stronger or weaker, try the following things:

1. Examine the pulses with the patient seated.
2. Examine the pulses after superficially needling L-9, the influential point of the pulse.
3. Examine the pulses after superficially needling the abdomen. Needling points such as CV-6 or CV-12 serves to raise the level of Qi, and thus strengthens the pulse.
4. Examine the pulses after superficially needling points on the cranium. Needling points on the cranium such as GV-20, as well as auricular points, serves to raise the level of yang Qi, and thus strengthens the pulse.

In my practice, when the pulses cannot be clearly differentiated, I proceed with the other phases of the examination, and then perform a little needling on the head and auricular points. Then I check the pulses once again. When the pulses are too weak to distinguish their relative strengths and other qualities, I examine the pulses

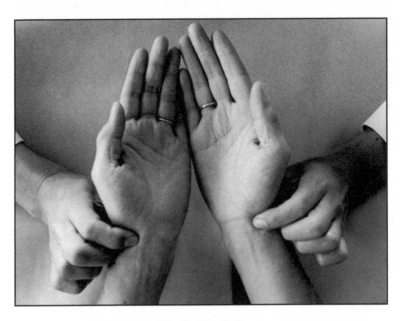

Illustration 3-9
Simultaneous Palpation of Both Distal Positions

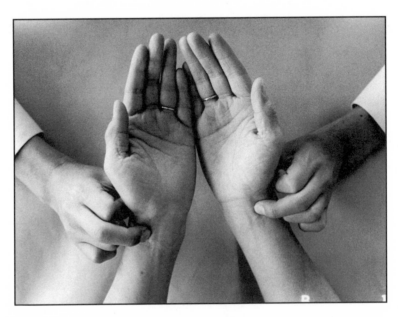

Illustration 3-10
Simultaneous Palpation of Both Middle Positions

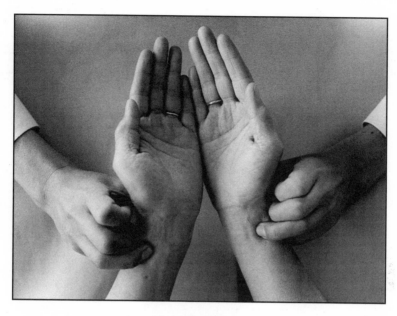

Illustration 3-11
Simultaneous Palpation of Both Proximal Positions

with the patient in a seated position. When the pulses are too strong to differentiate, I have the patient lie down.

It is common for the pulses to be abnormal immediately after a patient gets onto the treatment table. Those patients who are receiving acupuncture for the first time tend to be particularly nervous, and this causes the pulse to be much stronger than normal. In such cases, an accurate reading of the pulse can be ascertained only after treatment has begun and the patient is somewhat more relaxed. The differences in the strength of the pulse at various positions will then be much clearer.

Other methods of six-position pulse diagnosis: Thus far I have explained the standard method of six-position pulse diagnosis, i.e., palpating all six positions at once. However, there are several other ways to perform this technique which I will briefly explain. Some practitioners simultaneously examine the same position on both wrists, successively palpating both distal positions, then both middle positions, and finally both proximal positions (Illustrations 3-9, 3-10, 3-11). This method is similar to the approach that I have developed for beginners. Another widely used method is to examine the pulses on one wrist at a time. Some authorities say that one must first examine the pulses on the left wrist for men, and on the right wrist for women, but I think it matters very little which side is palpated first. To examine the pulse one side at a time from the left, the practitioner takes the patient's left hand in his left hand and uses his right hand to palpate the pulses (Illustration 3-12). It is also possible to palpate one position at a time on one side (Illustration 3-13). When examining the pulses one side at a time with the patient lying supine on the treatment table, in order to take the pulses of the arm on the opposite side, one must either reach over the patient to the other side, or move to the other side of the table. Some practitioners find it easier to palpate the pulses one side at a time or one position at

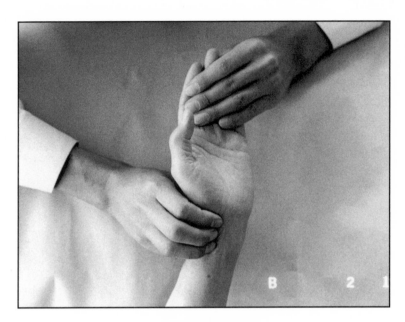

Illustration 3-12
Unilateral Pulse Palpation

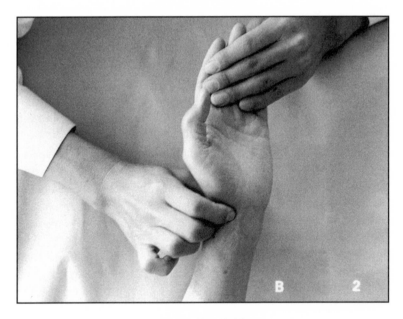

Illustration 3-13
Single-Position Palpation

a time, but this requires an ability to remember the quality of each of the pulses as one moves from one to other.

    There are many other variations of palpating the pulse, but all you have to do is find the easiest method for yourself. Use the method which allows you to palpate the pulse in the most accurate manner. No matter which method you utilize, you must maintain a certain level of consistency so that your fingers palpate the pulse the same way every time. Now I will return to the subject of exactly how and what to feel for in performing six-position pulse diagnosis.

MY APPROACH TO PULSE DIAGNOSIS

Basic policy for pulse diagnosis and treatment: So far I have explored various ways to perform six-position pulse diagnosis, and have suggested that each practitioner choose the method best suited to him or herself. This may sound easy, but in practice pulse diagnosis is quite difficult to master, especially without a teacher. Most beginners have difficulty distinguishing which positions are stronger, and which are weaker. It has been said that when palpating the subtle differences between the positions, if you think it is there, it will appear to be so, and if you think that it is not, it will appear not to be so. Some teachers say that one must palpate the pulses with an empty mind in order to clearly perceive whatever the fingers pick up, but for me emptying the mind only seems to make things more confusing. The beginner is thus faced with a major obstacle at this point. I almost gave up on learning meridian therapy because this obstacle seemed insurmountable. However, since I had promised myself that I would learn meridian therapy, and had practiced acupuncture for many years without pulse diagnosis, I had to find a way. After some trial and error I formulated a plan which allowed me to master pulse diagnosis in stages, and at the same time to immediately apply whatever I learned in my practice. This step-by-step approach to the mastery of six-position pulse diagnosis is as follows:

1. Begin by palpating all positions at the middle level.
2. Palpate the deep level to look for imbalances in the yin meridians.
3. Leave the diagnosis of pulse quality to the very end.

In evaluating the differences in strength of the pulses at the deep level, seek out the deficient positions. In other words, first find the deficient yin meridian. It is said that yin leads and yang follows. Thus, deficiency in one of the yin meridians can be assumed in all pathological conditions. Excess, which most often appears in the yang meridians, is of greatest importance in acute conditions, such as the early stages of a cold. Deficiency in a yin meridian becomes apparent as soon as the illness progresses a bit. After many years of practice, I still feel that this concept of pathology in meridian therapy is quite accurate.

4. Next, tonify the yin meridian which is most deficient. This is the root treatment. For the remainder of the treatment, use the same approach and techniques you ordinarily would. In other words, tonification of the most deficient yin meridian is simply added at the beginning of your treatment.
5. After you become proficient at identifying the deficient yin meridian, start looking for the excessive yin meridians. If there is one, disperse this meridian after tonifying the deficient meridian.
6. Once you have learned to identify the deficient and excessive yin meridians, palpate the superficial level to identify deficient and excessive yang meridians. Tonify

and disperse the yang meridians after treating the yin meridians.

7. After you become proficient at six-position pulse diagnosis, begin paying closer attention to pulse quality. Start by learning to recognize the six basic pulse qualities.

8. After acquiring a good sense of the six basic pulse qualities, learn all of the other pulse qualities.

If pulse diagnosis is learned in steps as outlined above, I have found that given some time, even those like myself without much sensitivity can master it. Those whose tactile sense is not so keen always have to make an extra effort. To the purists, it may seem inappropriate to apply the system of meridian therapy in such a piecemeal fashion, but I feel it is too much to ask of the average person to grasp the entirety of this system at once. Meridian therapy, aside from its remarkable effectiveness for the advanced practitioner, can also be effective at a beginner's level. Patients will benefit from whatever level of meridian therapy you have learned. There is no need to be concerned about doing things perfectly at first.

Looking back, I did not achieve remarkable results after incorporating simple root treatments into my acupuncture practice. Nevertheless, the results improved steadily, and my regular patients also noticed a difference. They began to comment that my treatments seemed to be getting more effective. The benefits of meridian therapy appeared gradually and in a natural way. I feel that my persistence in the step-by-step approach paid off. I recommend it to those practitioners who feel that six-position pulse diagnosis is difficult, or those who think that they have less than average sensitivity. With perseverance you will find that you can master this system one step at a time. It goes without saying that those who feel they are more capable should try to learn the system as fast as they can.

Simplified method for comparing pulse positions: As outlined above, the first step in my approach is to find the most deficient meridian. This may sound simple, but it actually can be quite difficult. Ideally one would palpate all six positions at once, starting with the middle level. Then the fingers would be lifted to palpate the superficial level, and finally the fingers would be pressed into the artery to reach the deep level below the middle level. When I first palpated the pulses in this manner, I could only feel the proximal position pulse at the deep level, and felt nothing at the middle and distal positions. I discovered later that I was pressing too hard at the proximal position. This put too much pressure on the artery, and reduced the amount of blood flow distally. In a similar manner, when a river is dammed upstream it is only natural that the flow is stopped downstream. Even after I realized this, however, I still had a difficult time palpating all six positions at once.

After experimenting with various methods of six-position pulse diagnosis, I arrived at a method of feeling for differences between two positions in a controlling relationship by using the five phases. The controlling relationship is an antagonistic relationship in which one phase inhibits the activity of another phase (Illustration 3-14). If the strength of two positions in a controlling relationship is relatively equal, there is a balance between the two phases represented by these positions. When one phase becomes weaker or deficient, there is an imbalance of Qi, and the controlling phase tends to become stronger or excessive. This can be illustrated as the balance shifting on a seesaw, as explained earlier (Illustration 3-15). Comparing two pulse positions at a time made it possible for me to distinguish the differences between the six pulse positions.

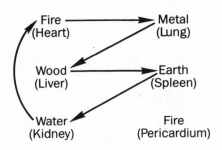

Illustration 3-14
Pulse Positions: Controlling Relationships

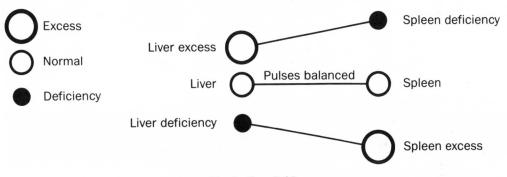

Illustration 3-15
Pulse Positions: Changes in Balance

► Palpating the Middle Level: Even though you are comparing two positions at a time with this method, start by placing your fingers on all six positions at once to palpate the pulses at the middle level. Move all three fingers up and down as a unit on both sides to find the level where the pulses can be most clearly perceived. This is the middle level where the Stomach Qi is felt, and reflects the overall vitality of the patient. The quality of a healthy pulse at the middle level is soft and resilient. This pulse should be felt clearly, and should neither be too hard nor too soft. This is something that takes experience to interpret; even if you don't know exactly what to feel for, just palpate the middle level every time.

► Comparing the Heart and Lung: Start by comparing the positions for the Heart and the Lung. Keep your index fingers on the distal positions of both wrists, and then let go with your middle and ring fingers. Press the index fingers to the point just before the arteries are occluded, and hold them at this level to compare the difference in strength (Illustration 3-16). For the sake of discussion, let us assume that the Heart (left distal) pulse is a little weaker than the Lung (right distal) pulse (Illustration 3-17). If the pulse on either side is difficult to perceive at the deep level, it is possible that the index finger is not directly over the artery. Sometimes the course of the radial

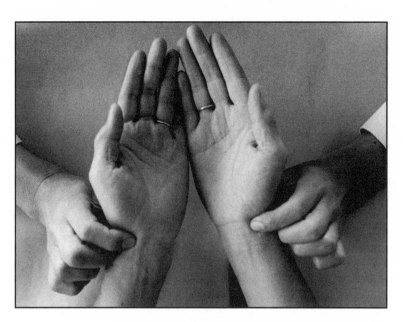

Illustration 3-16
Pulse-Position Palpation: Heart and Lung

artery deviates from the Lung meridian or bifurcates before reaching the wrist (Illustration 3-18). If the pulse is unclear, move your index finger more medially or laterally to see if the pulse can be felt more clearly elsewhere. To detect radially-deviated arteries, it is a good idea to make a practice of first placing the three fingers on the Large Intestine meridian before moving them into position over the Lung meridian (Illustration 3-19). If the pulse in both distal positions is of equal strength, the Qi of the Heart and Lung are balanced.

     ► Comparing the Lung and Liver: Next compare the positions for the Lung and the Liver. Let go of the index finger on the left distal position, and place the middle finger on the left middle position. Compare the strength of the pulses in the right distal and left middle positions (Illustration 3-20). Keep the other fingers off the artery while

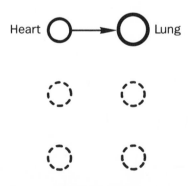

Illustration 3-17
Pulse-Position Comparisons: Step 1 (Heart and Lung)

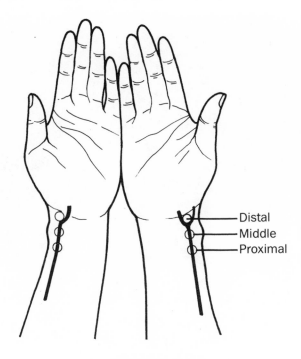

Illustration 3-18
Pulse Positions: Effects of Aberrant Radial Artery

comparing the two positions. Let us assume that the Liver (left middle) pulse is found to be much weaker than the Lung (right distal) pulse (Illustration 3-21).

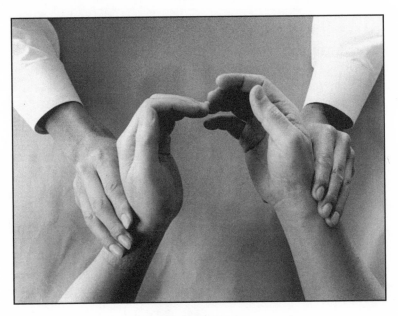

Illustration 3-19
Palpating the Large Intestine Meridian

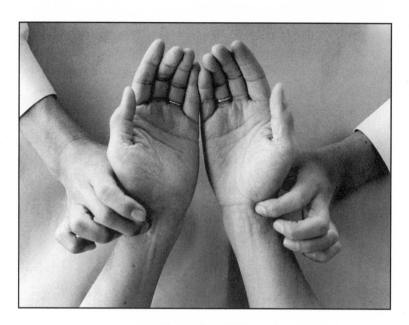

Illustration 3-20
Pulse-Position Palpation: Lung and Liver

► Comparing the Liver and Spleen: Next compare the positions for the Liver and the Spleen. Let go of the index finger on the right distal position, and place the middle finger on the right middle position. Compare the strength of the pulses in the middle positions on the right and left (Illustration 3-22). Comparison of the middle positions has special clinical significance because the difference in these positions determines whether the basic pattern is one of Spleen deficiency, Lung deficiency, or Liver deficiency. Let us assume that the Liver (left middle) pulse is much weaker than the Spleen (right middle) pulse (Illustration 3-23).

► Comparing the Spleen and Kidney: Next compare the positions for the Spleen and the Kidney. The middle finger on the left middle position is released, and the ring finger is placed over the proximal position (Illustration 3-24). The right ring finger

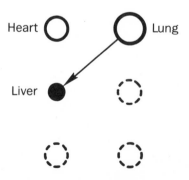

Illustration 3-21
Pulse-Position Comparisons: Step 2 (Lung and Liver)

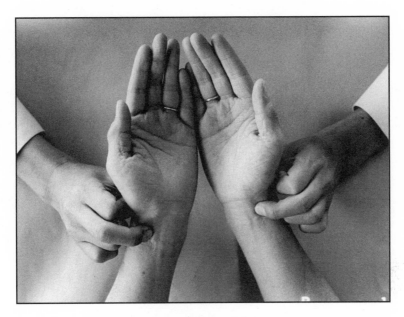

Illustration 3-22
Pulse-Position Palpation: Liver and Spleen

is thus used to palpate the pulse of the Kidney. Perhaps because we tend to use our ring finger less than other fingers, it is hard to get the right amount of pressure with this finger. You should therefore apply a little more pressure over the ring finger. Let us assume for our purposes that the Kidney (left proximal) pulse is much weaker than the Spleen (right middle) pulse (Illustration 3-25). According to the commentary on the fifth chapter of the *Classic of Difficulties* set forth in *The True Meaning of the Classic of Difficulties*, the pressure exerted by the left ring finger is supposed to be the greatest of all six fingers. According to this commentary the weight of pressure brought to bear by the finger on the right distal position should be equal to that of three beans, that on the left distal position to six beans, that on the right middle position to nine beans, that on the left middle position to twelve beans, and that on the right proximal

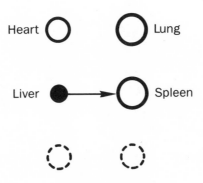

Illustration 3-23
Pulse-Position Comparisons: Step 3 (Liver and Spleen)

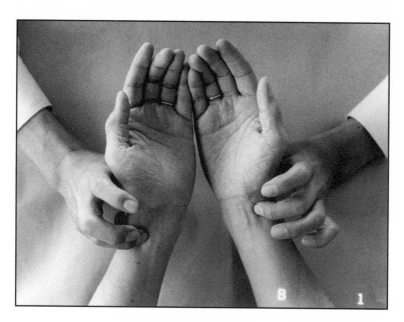

Illustration 3-24
Pulse-Position Palpation: Spleen and Kidney

position to fifteen beans (Illustration 3-26). In other words, the ratio of pressure brought to bear by these five fingers should be one-to-one on the right distal position, two-to-one on the left distal position, three-to-one on the right middle position, four-to-one on the left middle position, and five-to-one on the right proximal position. Although it is not possible to palpate exactly according to these ratios, the point is to increase pressure over the more distal positions.

► Comparing the Kidney and Pericardium: The last positions to compare are those of the Kidney and the Pericardium. A comparison of the water and fire phases could be made between the Kidney and the Heart, but this would mean that the index and ring fingers of the right hand would be used, which would be somewhat different from the bilateral comparisons performed so far. For the sake of consistency, I therefore examine the proximal positions on both sides together. Place both ring fingers

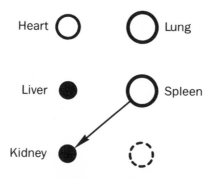

Illustration 3-25
Pulse-Position Comparisons: Step 4 (Spleen and Kidney)

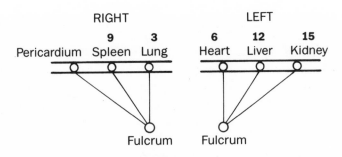

Illustration 3-26
Finger Pressure on Each Position

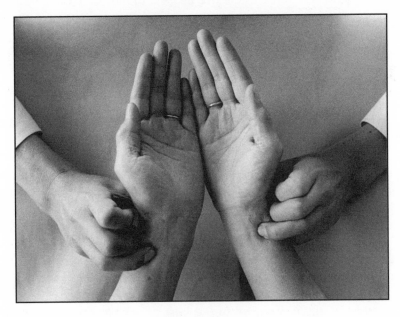

Illustration 3-27
Pulse-Position Palpation: Kidney and Pericardium

on the proximal positions to compare the Kidney and Pericardium (Illustration 3-27). Let us assume that the Kidney (left proximal) pulse is slightly weaker than the Pericardium (right proximal) pulse (Illustration 3-28).

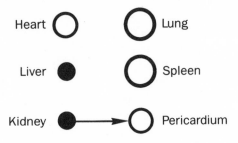

Illustration 3-28
Pulse-Position Comparisons: Step 5 (Kidney and Pericardium)

Reviewing the hypothetical findings from the above examination, the Lung and Spleen are the strongest, the Liver and Kidney are the weakest, and the Heart and Pericardium are normal (Illustration 3-28). This is a perfect example of the balance of pulse strengths that would exist at the middle level of the six positions for a condition of Liver deficiency. Palpating the six positions at the superficial level tends to show an opposite pattern in the balance of pulse strengths. There is a general rule in pulse diagnosis that yin and yang tend to be opposites; thus, here the Large Intestine and Stomach would be weak, and the Gallbladder and Bladder would be strong. I will save the detailed explanation of the basic patterns of yin meridian deficiency for the chapter on treatment, but keep in mind that deficiency and excess tend to double up according to the generating cycle of the five phases. In the above case, earth (Spleen) and metal (Lung) are excessive together, and water (Kidney) and wood (Liver) are deficient together. This classic pattern, in accordance with the generating cycle, does not actually appear very frequently in the clinic. It is nevertheless useful to remember the standard patterns when performing pulse diagnosis. The first step is to learn the five-phase correspondences of the six positions, and to be aware of the generating and controlling relationships among these positions.

Using the step-by-step method I have just described is a good way to learn these relationships, and it also makes six-position pulse diagnosis more accessible. Anyone with an ordinary sense of touch can thereby learn to distinguish subtle differences in pulse strength. As an experiment, I sometimes mark the pulse positions with a pen and have my wife check a patient's pulse to see if we agree. When she palpates the deficient and excessive positions, she is always able to tell which one is deficient. When a patient's condition improves, however, it becomes much harder for her to tell the difference. I suggest the two-position comparison method above for learning six-position pulse diagnosis. Naturally, there will be some stumbling blocks in the learning process since there are a great many idiosyncrasies in pulse patterns, and it can sometimes be difficult to tell in those with very weak or strong pulses. As a beginner it is enough to judge the differences to the best of your ability, and beyond that to trust your instincts.

Further considerations on pulse palpation: When performing six-position pulse diagnosis on both wrists at the same time, the pressure on the right and left sides must be even. Unless the pressure of the fingers in corresponding positions on opposite sides is perfectly even, it cannot be called a true comparison of pulse strength. In practice, however, those who are right-handed tend to place more pressure on the fingers of their right hand, and vice versa. As for myself, I tend to place the greatest pressure on the right middle finger, followed by the right index and ring fingers. One way to become aware of the difference in pressure among the fingers is to inflate the arm band of a sphygmomanometer and press this with each finger to see the actual amount of pressure in mercury. It would be better if there were an even more accurate measuring device available. In any case, it is important to bring, as much as possible, the same amount of pressure to bear on the same fingers on the right and left.

An important factor when trying to keep the pressure even on the fingers of both sides is the positioning of the practitioner's arms and fingers. To exert even pressure, the fingers should ideally be vertical in relation to the artery. The more oblique the angle of the fingers on the artery, the harder it becomes to use the thumb to apply pressure, and the less accurate the palpation. It is difficult to keep the fingers vertical when taking the pulse on both wrists of a supine patient from the side of the treatment table. Unless the practitioner leans over the patient to position the hands

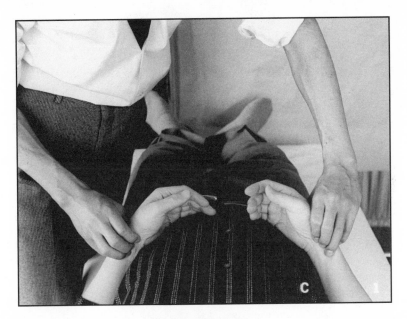

Illustration 3-29
Pulse Palpation from Side of Table

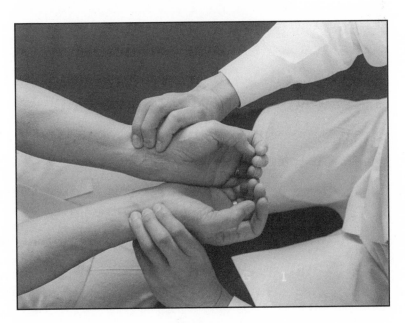

Illustration 3-30
Pulse Palpatioin Facing the Patient

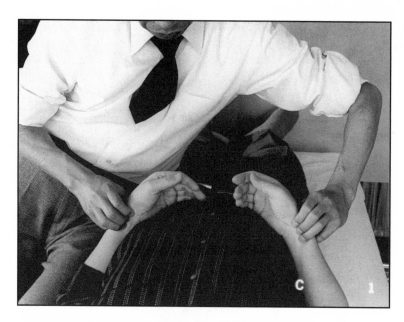

Illustration 3-31
Pulse Palpation from Side of Table

the same way in relation to both wrists, it is very difficult to exert the same amount of pressure (Illustration 3-29).

The most comfortable and accurate way of taking the pulse on both wrists at once is to sit facing the patient (Illustration 3-30). Yagishita, the grand master of acupuncture who inspired the development of meridian therapy, is said to have examined the pulse with the patient seated in a chair with an armrest. To exert equal pressure with both hands on a supine patient, the practitioner must lean over the patient. When on the left side of the patient, he must have the patient close to the left side of the table so that his left hip or thigh is right up against the patient, and his left elbow is extended over the patient (Illustration 3-31). When the differences between the pulses on the right and left are subtle, a change in the position of the practitioner can cause them to be construed in different ways. For this reason, it is important to pay close attention to your body positioning to achieve accuracy and consistency in palpation. It is possible to examine each wrist separately by walking around to the other side of a patient who is lying supine, but this makes my method of comparing positions in a controlling relationship difficult because of the task of comparing pulse strengths from memory.

Thus far I have concentrated on the position of the practitioner in relation to the patient, but some thought should also be given to the positioning of the patient's arms. When examining the pulses bilaterally, with the patient in the supine position, the patient's hands should be brought to the level of the navel, or just below it (Illustrations 3-32 & 3-33). It is not a good idea to raise the patient's hands any higher than the navel, since it is possible that flexion of the elbows could affect blood flow in the radial artery. It is also best for the patient's elbows to remain resting on the table as the pulse is taken. Sometimes a patient will move his right hand toward the practitioner in an effort to be helpful. Although this makes it easier to reach the pulses on the right side, it creates a discrepancy in the positioning of the patient's arms. It goes without saying that for the sake of accurate comparison, the practitioner should not

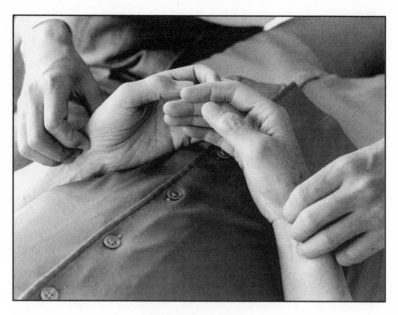

Illustration 3-32
Position of Patient's Arms

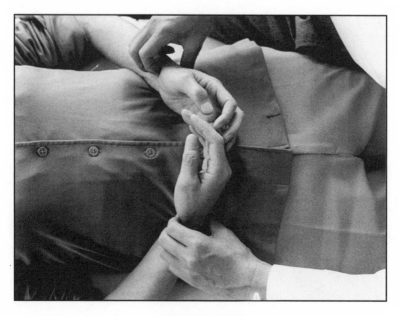

Illustration 3-33
Position of Patient's Arms (from above)

hold the patient's arm in different positions (Illustration 3-34). Positioning the thumb at different places on the back of the wrist should also be avoided, as should the use of the thumb on one side and the palm on the other. When examining the pulses one side at a time, the forearm to be palpated can be raised off the table, but the patient's

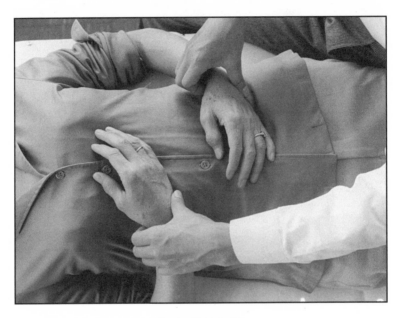

Illustration 3-34
Position of Patient's Arms (incorrect)

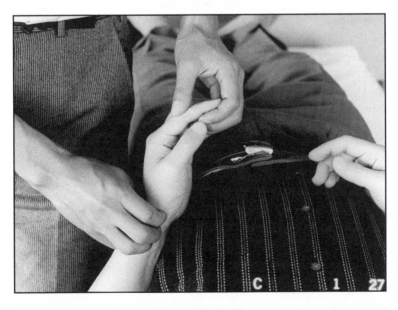

Illustration 3-35
Position of Patient's Arm for Unilateral Palpation (elbow flexed)

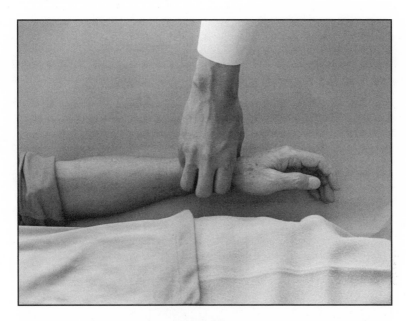

Illustration 3-36
Position of Patient's Arm for Unilateral Palpation (elbow extended)

elbow should not be held in more than ninety degrees flexion (Illustration 3-35). It is also possible to palpate the pulses with the patient's arm lying flat on the table (Illustration 3-36).

These pointers should make six-position pulse diagnosis easier and more accurate. There are times when the difference in pulse strength between positions in a controlling relationship is not very clear at all. This is often an indication that the patient is in fairly good health. In such cases, you may wish to go one step further and use only your most sensitive fingers to compare two positions. For example, if your middle fingers are the most sensitive, you would begin the controlling relationship comparison by placing your middle fingers on the distal positions. Next move your left middle finger to the right middle position, and so on. In this way all of the positions in a controlling relationship would be compared in succession. Since you are using your most sensitive fingers, you should be able to detect subtle differences. I use this method from time to time to distinguish between two key positions which are important in determining the pattern.

> "When placing the fingers [on the pulse] it is easier [to palpate] by using the tips of the fingers more than the pads. There is a difference in the sensitivity of the tips and pads of the fingers, so one should be aware of which parts are most sensitive and use these for palpation." (Okabe, 1966)

> "In pulse diagnosis the sensitivity of the practitioner is most important, so one must test [the sensitivity of] his fingertips. If there is one finger which is not very sensitive, use another, more sensitive finger. We must also take good care of our hands. One must be careful not to injure the hands doing yard work or manual labor.
>
> The main point is to realize that there are differences among practitioners in the sensitivity of their fingers. Some are more sensitive at their fingertips near

their nails, and others are most sensitive at the pads of their fingers. Each person should use the most sensitive part." (Okabe, 1974)

It is true that different parts of the finger are sensitive in different people. As for myself, perhaps because I developed the habit of using my fingertips when

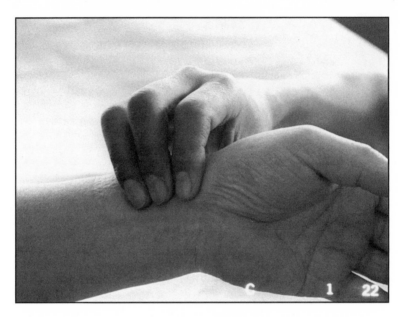

Illustration 3-37
Pulse Palpation Using Tips of Fingers

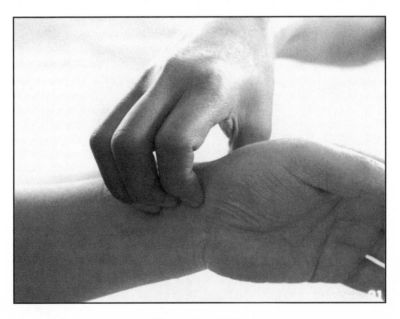

Illustration 3-38
Pulse Palpation Using Pads of Fingers

learning pulse diagnosis, the tips of my fingers are the most sensitive part, and I use them almost exclusively when palpating the pulse (Illustration 3-37). When examining the deep position, however, one must press fairly hard and holding the fingers vertically over the pulse can be very tiring, especially when giving treatments all day long. It may be a good idea to practice palpating the pulse with the pads of the fingers instead (Illustration 3-38). This way the hands will not fatigue as much. It should make little difference whether the tips or pads of the fingers are used since it will eventually become a matter of habit. The important thing is to develop a consistent method utilizing the most sensitive part of your fingers.

Another consideration is the amount of time spent palpating the pulse. One cannot diagnose properly if the pulses are palpated very briefly; on the other hand, it is not good to spend too much time doing pulse diagnosis. Patients may think you are taking a long time examining the pulse because there is something wrong, and their anxiety may even begin to appear in the pulse. Performing six-position diagnosis on both sides at once is the fastest way, and experienced practitioners obtain the information they need in 15-30 seconds. One can check all the levels 2-3 times in about 30 seconds to get a complete picture. Of course, it takes much longer for a beginner, especially those who palpate one arm at a time. The best way to get an idea of how long to palpate the pulse is to observe a practitioner skilled in pulse diagnosis.

> "As a rule, the pulses should be palpated for the duration of 50 [heart] beats for diagnosis. Certainly [one] must not palpate carelessly and miss things. Just focus [your] attention on [your] fingertips. Do not speak, do not look, do not listen, do not smell, and do not think. This is the key principle of pulse palpation." (Yanagiya, 1976)

HOW TO BECOME PROFICIENT AT PULSE DIAGNOSIS

1. Examine your own pulse and that of your family members everyday.

2. Examine the pulse of every patient you see. Pulse diagnosis is like cultivating bonsai plants: even if you don't know what to look for at first, after doing it every day you will eventually learn what there is to know.

3. Examine the pulse before and after every treatment. Treatment brings changes in the quality and strength of the pulse in the six positions. A weak and sunken pulse will gain strength when tonification works, and sometimes a deficient Liver pulse will even become slightly excessive.

4. The best way to learn pulse diagnosis is by hands-on instruction. Attend as many seminars and classes as you can.

5. Keep practicing pulse diagnosis and find ways which work best for you.

So far I have explained in detail how to palpate differences in pulse strength at the deep position in six-position pulse diagnosis. I presented the standard methods as well as my own method for comparing pulse positions that are in a controlling relationship according to the five phases. These methods are quite simple to put into practice, but when put into words they seem more complicated than they really are. I hope that the reader will understand and attempt these methods to find the most workable approach.

But what is a person to do if he still cannot distinguish the pulses in the six positions? If his sensitivity is less than average, he must reconsider his decision to practice acupuncture. As long as one intends to make a profession of acupuncture, one must expect to develop a sensitivity which exceeds that of the average person. One must either try harder and find ways to improve his palpatory skills and increase his tactile sensitivity, or give up the idea of practicing acupuncture altogether. Our sense of touch has to be quite keen not only to palpate the pulses, but to detect differences close to the skin surface, such as indurations and indentations. One's sensitivity can be increased through diligent practice. It is only a matter of persistence and ingenuity. I have presented a simplified version of six-position pulse diagnosis, but it is up to you, the reader, to make it work. Nothing worthwhile can be gained without effort, and I feel that anyone who is unwilling to put forth an earnest effort is unworthy of this profession.

PALPATING THE PULSES AT THE SUPERFICIAL LEVEL

The first and most important thing to palpate in six-position pulse diagnosis is deficient yin meridians, as explained above. The next thing to look for is yin meridian excess in the positions which are in a controlling relationship with the deficient yin meridians. For example, if the Spleen position is found to be the most deficient, one should look for excess in the Liver position. If the Liver pulse is not overly strong, it can be regarded as normal, but if it feels strong and wiry, it is excessive. If an excessive Liver pulse is found together with a deficient Spleen pulse, a pattern of Spleen deficiency and Liver excess is indicated. After learning to identify the deficient and excessive patterns in the yin meridians, one is ready to take on six-position pulse diagnosis for the yang meridians. Since you will have acquired some skill in pulse palpation by this time, the palpation of the yang meridians should be comparatively easy.

As previously noted, the yang meridians are palpated at the superficial level. The key question here is just how much to lift the fingers. Generally speaking, the superficial level is reached by lifting the fingers slowly from the middle position until the pulse can barely be felt. The superficial level is found at that point just before the pulse can no longer be felt.

> "There is a trick to palpating pathogenic Qi excess in the yang meridians. The fingers on the pulse should slowly be raised just to the point where the pulse can no longer be felt. When the fingers are gently vibrated at this point, if there is any pathogenic Qi, it will be felt on the pads of the fingers ... Otherwise [to palpate pathogenic Qi] the fingertips raised to the surface of the skin should be lifted and lowered very slightly in a shaking motion." (Fukushima, 1971)

To palpate the yang meridians, one should hold the fingers gently over the artery. Little if any pressure should be used to palpate the yang meridian pulses; just the weight of the fingers is enough. Instead of placing or holding the fingers over the pulse, a more appropriate description might be to gently touch, as if caressing a baby's cheek. The fingertips held over the pulse in this manner should be moved at a very fine amplitude back and forth at a right angle to the artery. This is the easiest way to perceive the pulse. If you find one position which seems to be a little different, let go of the other positions and repeat the vibration of the fingertip over the position in question. Yang meridian excess is best palpated in this manner.

Excess from pathogenic Qi as well as reactive excess tends to appear most often in the Stomach, Gallbladder, and Bladder meridians. The pulse finding of excess in the yang meridians tends to have a more direct correlation with the patient's symptoms than the same finding in the yin meridians. If the excessive Qi is in the Gallbladder meridian, for example, there are usually corresponding symptoms along the course of the meridian such as headache, neck and shoulder stiffness, lower back pain, or pain in the lower limbs.

Palpating yang meridian deficiency in the pulse is more difficult than finding yang meridian excess. If the pulse at one position cannot be felt at all at the superficial level, it can be regarded as deficient. Comparing the strength of the pulse at the superficial position, however, is not as simple as at the deep position. Pressing deeper to palpate a deficient yang meridian pulse often takes one down to the middle level. The primary focus of six-position pulse diagnosis in meridian therapy is identifying yin meridian deficiency and yang meridian excess; palpating subtle yang meridian deficiencies in the pulse is therefore not so important for the beginner. After many years of practice, you should be able to recognize subtle differences in pulse strengths at the superficial level. The main thing to understand at this stage is that identifying yang meridian excess from the pulse is clinically important because appropriate treatment of such excess is very effective in alleviating associated symptoms such as pain.

COMPARING THE SUPERFICIAL AND DEEP LEVELS

> "Even if [examination of the pulse shows] the Liver is excessive and the Lung is deficient, we cannot assume that the pattern is one of Lung deficiency based only on [a comparison of] the strength [at the deep level]. The difference between the yin and yang [superficial and deep levels] must also be taken into account. If [the pulse in a given position is] weak at both the yin and yang [levels], they are balanced even though weak." (Honma, 1949)

Until this point, I have emphasized the comparison of pulse strength between the positions in a controlling relationship in accordance with the five phases as being the most basic approach in six-position pulse diagnosis. Comparing the strength of the pulses for the yang meridians at the superficial level is not as important, and requires more skill. However, there is one additional aspect of comparing the pulse strength in six-position pulse diagnosis which has yet to be addressed. It is the difference between the superficial and deep levels at each position, i.e., the difference between paired yin and yang meridians, such as the Lung and Large Intestine meridians. When there is an imbalance in a certain phase, the corresponding yin and yang meridians tend toward opposite extremes, i.e., the yin meridian becomes deficient and the yang meridian excessive, or vice versa. Even if the Liver seems to be strong and the Spleen weak, if both the Liver and Gallbladder are strong and both the Spleen and Stomach are weak, these two yin-yang pairs are each balanced between themselves, and thus are not that out of balance. According to Honma, the difference or imbalance between paired yin and yang meridians should be given more weight in determining the pattern, and the excess and deficiency between meridians in a controlling relationship should be taken into account in deciding which points to treat.

If one only pays attention to the differences of strength in the deep position in relation to the five phases, the diagnosis will sometimes be inaccurate. For example, a pulse which seems to show a pattern of Spleen deficiency and Liver excess, when closely examined at the superficial position, often turns out to be Liver deficiency and Gallbladder excess. This usually happens because the pulses are not palpated deeply enough and the middle level reflects the condition of the yang meridians more than the yin meridians. Thus the excess in the Gallbladder meridian is construed to be in the Liver meridian, and the Spleen meridian seems deficient by contrast. Paying attention only to the imbalances among the yin meridians can lead to this kind of mistake. Therefore it is important to palpate the pulses at all three levels and remember the tendency toward opposite extremes of paired yin and yang meridians.

From my own experience with meridian therapy, I think that differences between the yin and yang meridians are not the final word in terms of determining the diagnosis or pattern. Nevertheless, such differences are very important. For the purpose of comparing the difference between the superficial and deep positions, the method of palpating both wrists at once seems easier. Although it is possible to compare one position at a time using one finger, I somehow find this method harder to use. In any case, when there is a marked difference within one yin-yang pair, such as the Liver being very weak and the Gallbladder very strong, the deficient meridian must be tonified. If the Liver is deficient, insert a needle very superficially at Liv-8; while holding the handle of the needle in one hand, examine the pulse with the other. In many cases you can feel the strength increasing in the deep position where the deficiency was palpated. In this manner, a yin meridian deficiency in a yin-yang pair which is extremely out of balance will tend to quickly improve with treatment. Sometimes the excess in the corresponding yang meridian will also improve just by treating the yin meridian deficiency. If the excess yang meridian does not change or becomes stronger, lightly disperse that meridian.

When the difference between the yin meridian and its corresponding yang meridian is very clear, the above approach is most suitable, but quite often a pair of yin and yang meridians will be deficient while the yin-yang pair in a controlling relationship is excessive. In this case, the difference between the meridians in the controlling relationship must be taken into account in formulating the diagnosis. In my experience, it is much easier to rectify an imbalance between one yin-yang pair than it is to strengthen the pulse of a yin meridian which is markedly deficient in relation to another yin meridian in a controlling relationship.

Six-position pulse diagnosis is a way of judging the type of balance or imbalance that exists among the meridians, and there are several angles from which to view this balance. The most fundamental balance is that between the yin meridians, and the comparison of meridians in a controlling relationship is important in determining this pattern. The balance between the yang meridians is more difficult to ascertain, but it has a bearing on the effective treatment of symptoms. The balance between a yin and yang pair of meridians is easier to judge than that between different yang meridians, since the difference in the strength of the pulse is easier to detect at the same position. I suggest starting with the most basic comparisons; thus, begin by examining the balance among the yin meridians at the deep level. Next the beginner may proceed to compare the difference between the yin-yang pairs at those positions that are found to be deficient or excessive. The comparison of yang meridians at the superficial position should be attempted only after the practitioner is able to discern the deficiency or excess of the yin meridians quickly and consistently. The more subtle imbalances can be discerned only after one has become proficient at six-position pulse diagnosis.

PULSE-QUALITY DIAGNOSIS

Pulse diagnosis in meridian therapy is comprised of six-position diagnosis and pulse-quality diagnosis. When only one of these approaches is used to determine the diagnosis and treatment, this cannot be regarded as meridian therapy in the true sense. After acquiring an understanding of six-position pulse diagnosis, one must study the pulse qualities and learn them one by one. This is especially important because the quality of the pulse has a direct bearing on the selection of needling techniques for treatment. If needles are inserted deeply when the pulse is floating, or if needles are retained when the pulse is rapid, the patient will often times feel worse after treatment. This makes patients afraid of acupuncture and they are unlikely to return to the clinic. Providing the appropriate treatment by applying contact needling or superficial needling for those patients who have a floating pulse will bring immediate improvement, and thus strengthen their belief in acupuncture. This is one reason why pulse-quality diagnosis is so important.

To palpate the pulse quality it is best to examine all six positions at once. Pulse-quality diagnosis, in particular, is best performed on both sides at once. If, however, a certain pulse quality is found in just one part or position, one hand or finger may be used. The general pulse quality is usually easier to discern for the beginner than are subtle differences in pulse strength, but actually it is quite difficult to learn to interpret the subtleties of pulse quality. Ultimately, I feel that pulse-quality diagnosis is much more difficult to master than six-position pulse diagnosis. Even so, pulse-quality diagnosis is not beyond the grasp of the average practitioner, especially when learned in stages. Various pulse qualities can be learned over the years through diligent study and practice, by reading texts, asking experts, and examining the pulse before and after every treatment. There is no shortcut to acquiring the power of discrimination which comes from many years of experience. We all have to advance one step at a time.

"Not everyone can distinguish [the basic pulse qualities of] deficient and excessive, floating and submerged, and slippery and choppy from the very beginning ... The starting point of pulse diagnosis is not in thinking, but in palpating the pulses to feel whatever one feels. The basic pulse qualities of deficient and excessive, floating and submerged, and slippery and choppy can be understood after one gets some experience in pulse palpation and reads texts, thinks, and makes comparisons by continuing to apply the same pulse palpation techniques." (Inoue, 1980)

The pulse quality refers to the shape and quality of the pulse, and is also called the pulse condition *(maku shō/mài xiàng)*. The pulse quality is a combination of many factors. The size of the artery (big or small) and its resiliency (hard or soft) are anatomical and physiological characteristics of the artery. The speed of the pulse (slow or rapid) relates to the factor of time, and the level of the pulse (floating or submerged) has to do with its location.

The *Pulse Classic* by Wang Shu-He always serves as the reference point whenever pulse quality is being discussed. This text is a great compendium of pulse diagnosis from the third century upon which all subsequent texts on pulse diagnosis are based. Twenty-four different pulse qualities are listed in the *Pulse Classic*. Unlike the comparison of pulse strength, which is but a single aspect, there are many different aspects of pulse quality. Among the twenty-four classic pulse qualities, six basic qualities are essential. As long as one knows these basic pulse qualities and is able to utilize the information that they provide, meridian therapy can be properly performed without any problem. The beginner must therefore start by studying the basic pulse qualities. Once they are clearly understood, one can proceed to master the other qualities. Just as in learning six-position pulse diagnosis, each person must devise his own way of mastering pulse-quality diagnosis. As for myself, I compiled my own handbook of pulse qualities and also made a simple reference chart. In my pulse-quality handbook, I have listed concise definitions for the different pulse qualities extracted from various texts, and I refer to this handbook whenever I am unsure about a certain quality.

FLOATING	on the very surface and not much deeper
HOLLOW	floating, large, soft and empty in the middle
FLOODING	floating and extremely large
SLIPPERY	smooth and forceful
RAPID	more than five beats per breath
RAPID-IRREGULAR	rapid with occasional skips
WIRY	bowstring
TIGHT	larger and more forceful than wiry
EXCESSIVE	large and long
SUBMERGED	deep beneath the surface close to the bone
HIDDEN	strong when pressed to the bone
LEATHER	submerged, excessive, large and long
THIN	string-like
MINUTE	extremely thin and soft
CHOPPY	thin and slow with occasional skips
SOFT	extremely soft, floating and thin
FRAIL	extremely soft, submerged and thin
DEFICIENT	slow and very soft
SCATTERED	large, floating and irregular
MODERATE	slow, floating and very soft
SLOW	less than four beats per breath
SLOW-IRREGULAR	moderate with occasional skips
CONSISTENTLY-IRREGULAR	regular skips
MOVING	rapid, tight and short

Table 3-2 Pulse Qualities

Since the definitions provided in the classics are not all that clear or easy to memorize, I also made a simple pulse-quality chart with very brief descriptions which I have hung on the wall in my clinic for quick reference (Table 3-2).

The basic pulse qualities:

"There are six basic pulse qualities, which are floating and submerged, rapid and slow, and deficient and excessive. Of course, there are those who include slippery and choppy instead of deficient and excessive. Some authorities also designate floating and submerged, long and short, and slippery and choppy [as the basic pulse qualities]. Whatever the case may be, the pulse of the patient is examined from the perspectives of (1) whether superficial or deep; (2) whether fast or slow; and (3) the force of the pulse, i.e., the amount of tension and its thickness. Thus, a certain pulse can be described as floating but deficient, or as submerged, rapid, and excessive, or otherwise as thin and deficient. When a pulse is described without reference to being floating or submerged, it means that it is neither floating nor submerged, but that it is [strongest] at the middle level. When a pulse is described without reference to being rapid or slow, it means that it is neither rapid nor slow, but that it is around five beats per breath. Also, when a pulse is described without reference to being deficient or excessive, it means that it is not particularly deficient or excessive." (Honma, 1949)

► Floating Pulse:

"The floating pulse can be found when [the fingers are] raised, but it is lacking when pressed. It floats beneath one's hand." *(Pulse Classic)*

"The floating pulse is like a branch floating around on water: when pressed it disappears and cannot be felt by the fingers." (Yama, 1770)

"It is a superficial pulse which can be felt by lightly pressing between the skin and flesh. It is a pulse which can be felt with light pressure, but disappears with heavy pressure." (Honma, 1949)

"The floating pulse is associated with yang and represents [pathogenic influences] invading the exterior. The [choice of] needling techniques for patients with a floating pulse must take the other qualities into account, but [as a rule] the needle should be inserted superficially when there is a floating pulse." (Okabe, 1974)

"A floating pulse can be compared to a ball floating on a pond, with the depth of the pond representing the different levels in pulse diagnosis ... The depth [or vertical range] of the pulse varies according to the individual, but the relative distance from the skin surface to the bone is just about the same [for everyone]. Those whose pulse range is deep have a greater span between the superficial and deep levels, and those whose range is shallow have a smaller span between the superficial and deep levels." (Inoue, 1980)

These descriptions of the floating pulse are more than adequate. The pulse qualities of floating and submerged must be clearly distinguished from the superficial and deep levels of six-position pulse diagnosis. Floating and submerged are pulse qualities which describe different depths at which the middle level can be palpated. The superficial and deep levels of six-position pulse diagnosis refer to the levels of the pulse palpated above and below the middle level and are used to judge the condition of the yin and yang meridians.

A floating pulse is associated with the external pathogenic influence of wind. The basic rule of treatment for a floating pulse is to needle very superficially. Deep insertion is to be avoided, particularly during root treatment, because it can cause an effect which is opposite that which is intended. It is difficult to say just how shallow the needle should be inserted in each case, but it is safe to keep it very shallow, somewhere between just holding the needle tip against the surface of the skin (contact needling) and inserting the needle to a depth of 2-3mm. When performing six-position pulse diagnosis and applying pressure from your thumb to raise and lower the fingers, the floating pulse will seem stronger at the superficial level and very weak or empty at the deep level. When the pulse as a whole seems to be floating close to the surface, one must exercise caution in rendering treatment. The floating pulse is common in patients who are hypersensitive or slightly neurotic. In such cases, it is best to keep the insertion very superficial, and sometimes to avoid inserting the needles altogether. Superficial needling is just as effective as deep needling when applied at the right points.

A patient I once treated really impressed on me the need for shallow needling when there is a floating pulse. The patient was a 35-year-old carpenter. He had been hospitalized 40 days previously with a whiplash injury, but showed little improvement. He was starting to become worried about his job. His chief complaints were neck pain whenever he moved, heaviness of the head, insomnia, loss of balance, and occasional dizziness. His complexion was rather pale and he had a worried expression. His physical build was good, but his appetite was not very good, although he ate the normal amount. His pulse was weak at the Liver and Kidney positions, and the pulse quality was floating and slow. Palpatory examination revealed tenderness under the spinous process of the fifth cervical vertebrae, and at G-20 and G-21 on the left, as well as CV-17 and GV-10.

I knew that the type of insertion for a patient with a floating pulse should be superficial, so I inserted the needles superficially and left them in place. That is, I tapped the needles in with an insertion tube and left them in place without any further manipulation. I needled Liv-8, K-10, B-10, G-20, and G-21. I burned five small cones of moxa on the tender point below the spinous process of the fifth cervical vertebrae. I also needled another tender point nearby on the left inferior border of the spinous process of the fifth cervical vertebrae using a simple insertion technique to a depth of no more than 2cm. I was confident that this would do the trick.

That night I got a call from the patient who reported that the pain had increased and that he was unable to get any sleep. The second time he came in for treatment I examined the pulse quality with special care and found it to be extremely floating. So instead of inserting the needle at Liv-8 as I had before, I just placed the tip of the needle on the point and twisted it very slightly back and forth. When I felt the arrival of Qi, I held the needle on the point and asked the patient how he felt. He replied that his head felt clearer and much better. I therefore repeated this contact needling at the same points I used before, and kept close track of how the patient was feeling. This approach worked beautifully and the patient was able to return to work after the third treatment, just a week after first seeing me. In successive treatments, I started inserting the needles just a little more each time, from about one millimeter to a few millimeters. By this time the patient was beginning to get a sense of how acupuncture worked, and he told me that I could go ahead and insert the needles a little deeper. He did not understand the reason, but he could feel the effect of the needle and could tell the optimum depth. His pulse quality, which had been floating and without strength, became stronger. Ever since this experience, I have paid careful attention to the pulse quality and have adjusted my needling technique accordingly.

When the pulse is floating and strong, especially when it is very tense or wiry, and the patient complains of insomnia, superficial needling at the appropriate points will correct the wiry pulse and alleviate the insomnia. The rule of superficial needling for a floating pulse is a very important one to keep in mind when performing pulse-quality diagnosis.

► Submerged Pulse:

"The submerged pulse is lacking when [the fingers are] raised, but can be found in abundance when pressed. It is said that [this pulse] can be discerned by [applying] heavy pressure." (*Pulse Classic*)

"The submerged pulse is the opposite of the floating pulse in that it beats strongly deep down, but cannot be felt closer to the surface." (Yama, 1770)

"It is a deep pulse which cannot be palpated by lightly touching, but it appears when heavy pressure is applied." (Honma, 1949)

"The basic rule of needling for the submerged pulse is deep insertion. In this case, however, the yang meridians must be examined. If there are deficient yang meridians, these must first be tonified, and after this any excessive yin meridians must be dispersed." (Okabe, 1974)

The submerged pulse is a strong pulse located below what is normally the middle position. It can be found close to the bottom of the pulse range before the bone is reached. When the pulse is even deeper and cannot be felt until pressing almost down to the bone, this is called a hidden pulse.

"The hidden pulse cannot be found in the deep level. Only after reaching the bone can it felt. This pulse is hard to palpate; it appears only by pressing deeply down to the bone." (Yama, 1770)

The hidden pulse thus appears and disappears at the level of the bone, and the submerged pulse is only slightly closer to the surface. The submerged pulse is therefore quite deep. Normally the pulses can be felt by applying slight pressure with the fingers. When the pulse is submerged, however, no pulse can be felt at all, and it makes you think "wait a minute," and press even harder. Only then do you feel it at an even deeper level. Careful palpation of the submerged pulse makes you realize that it is not necessarily such a thin or weak pulse. It is when palpating pulses like these that you will really be amazed how different pulses can be.

A submerged pulse is associated with the external pathogenic influence of dampness. The basic rule for treatment of a submerged pulse is deep insertion, but this does not mean that one may indiscriminately insert the needle deeply. I interpret this rule of deep insertion for the submerged pulse to simply mean inserting deeper than in cases with a floating pulse. The first few needles in particular should not be inserted very deeply. This and other matters related to root treatment and needling technique are discussed in more detail in chapter 5.

► Slow Pulse:

"The slow pulse has three beats per breath. It is extremely slow in coming and going." *(Pulse Classic)*

"The slow pulse is extremely slow and strong. Press down with the fingers, but seek it gently." (Yama, 1770)

"The slow pulse is a pulse which beats only two or three times for each breath of the practitioner." (Honma, 1949)

"[This pulse] denotes coldness. The [needling] technique to be used is to quietly insert and withdraw, as if one were taking leave [of a dear one]. In some cases the needle may be retained." (Fukushima, 1971)

"The slow pulse is yin in nature and appears when yang cannot overcome yin. One approach is therefore to tonify yang. The needling technique for a slow pulse, since it is caused by cold, is to apply the warming needle technique. The warming needle technique means to leave the needle inserted for a long time." (Okabe, 1974)

As described above, the slow pulse is one which beats three times or less per breath. Since the slow pulse is associated with the pathogenic influence of cold, the needle, rather than being removed quickly, is usually left in place. I used to think that three beats per breath meant per each breath of the patient, but in studying various texts to prepare my presentation for a meridian therapy seminar, I found that all of the texts define it as the number of beats of the patient's pulse in relation to the practitioner's breathing. It is written that because the number of beats is based on the practitioner's breath, a practitioner must keep himself in good physical condition so as to be able to breathe evenly and steadily. But what happens if one is slightly ill, or one is an asthmatic? One's breathing would be faster than normal, and therefore many more of one's patients would be diagnosed as having a slow pulse. I feel that it is most accurate to determine whether the pulse is fast or slow based on beats per minute. In practice I go by my instincts when taking the pulse, and when I feel that the pulse is unusually slow or fast, I count the number of beats in relation to one complete breath of the patient to decide whether the pulse is really slow or rapid.

"In a strict sense, if the breathing of the practitioner is used as the standard to determine the number of beats per breath, this means that the determination of slow or rapid varies according to the practitioner. It is more practical to use the breathing of the patient as the standard ... Since the amount of time [different] patients take to breathe one breath will vary, it is not accurate to define a rapid pulse as just being faster than so many beats per minute." (Inoue, 1980)

► Rapid Pulse:

"The rapid pulse is quick in coming and going. It is said that [this pulse] has six or seven beats per breath. It is said that rapid is also described as advancing." *(Pulse Classic)*

"It is a pulse which beats more than five times per breath, and is a yang pulse denoting heat." (Honma, 1949)

"This is a phenomenon which occurs because yin cannot control yang. The needling technique for the rapid pulse, since it indicates heat, is quick insertion and quick withdrawal." (Okabe, 1974)

As described above, the rapid pulse is one which beats more than five times per breath. Since it is an indication of heat, one must employ quick insertion and withdrawal, as if dipping one's fingers into hot water to check the temperature. Like the slow pulse, most texts use the breathing of the practitioner as the standard, but it is really more practical to use the patient's breathing. It does not take very much for the pulse to become rapid in sensitive patients, who tend to go into a state of sympathetic tonus with the slightest bit of anxiety. Such patients occasionally have pulse rates of over one hundred per minute. Once they become accustomed to acupuncture and begin to relax, the pulse slows down considerably. When such patients are first examined, their pulses are extremely rapid if the practitioner's breathing is used as the standard. After the patient lies down for awhile and becomes calm, however, the pulse becomes slow in relation to the practitioner's breathing. Thus, by using the practitioner's breathing as the standard, the indicated needling technique becomes exactly the opposite in a short period of time. If the patient's breathing is used as the standard, however, the breathing will accelerate in tandem with the pulse so that the pulse would not have been judged rapid in the first place.

What happens if the needling techniques of retaining the needle for the slow pulse and quick insertion and withdrawal for the rapid pulse are reversed? I experimented a little by retaining needles in patients with rapid pulses. These patients did not have any fever. The rapid pulse was mostly caused by excitement or apprehension. With respect to the results, there was actually no difference in the majority of cases, but there were a few patients who reported slight nausea or palpitations. In order to get patients with a rapid pulse to relax mentally and physically, it is best to be careful about the depth of needle insertion, and to avoid retaining the needles.

► Deficient Pulse:

"The deficient pulse is slow, large, and soft. When pressed it is lacking. It hides under the fingers, large and empty." *(Pulse Classic)*

"The deficient pulse is without strength and soft, and is also wide, large, and slow." (Yama, 1770)

"It is a pulse which feels weak to the touch. [It indicates] all pulses lacking [in strength]." (Honma, 1949)

"Deficient is a pulse which is palpated as being weak and feeble, and it indicates a deficiency of true Qi. The needling technique used [for a deficient pulse] is tonifition." (Fukushima, 1971)

The definition of a deficient pulse, in addition to lacking strength, includes the qualities of slow, large, and soft. Viewing the deficient pulse just in terms of the basic pulse qualities, however, the single quality of softness seems to be most essential. There is such a thing as a deficient and rapid pulse. Tonification is the needling technique indicated for a deficient pulse.

► Excessive Pulse:

"The excessive pulse is large, long, and slightly strong. When pressed it hides under the fingers, wide and extensive." *(Pulse Classic)*

"It is a pulse which feels strong to the touch, and just like the deficient pulse, it can appear together with floating or submerged and slow or rapid [qualities]. It indicates an excess of pathogenic Qi." (Honma, 1949)

"Among the excesses there is pathogenic Qi excess and reactive excess. This [excessive pulse] is felt as being large and strong and indicates [a condition of] being filled up with pathogenic Qi or imbalances in meridian Qi. The needling technique used [for an excessive pulse] is dispersion." (Fukushima, 1971)

The excessive pulse is therefore a strong pulse which may appear in combination with the other four basic pulse qualities. Dispersion is the technique indicated for an excessive pulse.

Thus far the six basic pulse qualities have been described. It should be clear from this discussion that the pulse quality is examined from three angles to determine its basic quality: its overall level, speed, and strength. An abnormality in the overall level is expressed as floating or submerged, which indicates the depth of the disease (exterior or interior). An abnormality in the speed of the pulse is expressed as either slow or rapid, which indicates whether the body is affected by cold or heat. Finally, an abnormal amount of strength or weakness (softness) in the pulse is expressed as excessive or deficient, which indicates both the force of the disease as well as the physical strength of the patient. In pulse-quality diagnosis, at the very least one must judge the pulse from these three angles.

In six-position pulse diagnosis, on the other hand, one must determine which meridian is most deficient and which is most excessive. Through the two different types of pulse diagnosis used in meridian therapy, the pulses are thus examined from four basic perspectives. In my practice, I first try to grasp the pathological condition of the patient (in terms of the eight principles of yin-yang, interior-exterior, cold-heat, and deficient-excessive) through pulse-quality diagnosis. Then I decide which meridians to treat through six-position pulse diagnosis. Beginners may opt to leave pulse-quality diagnosis to the end, but experienced practitioners should first ascertain the general condition of a patient through the qualities of their pulse.

Pulse diagnosis is always started by palpating the middle level, and this is the best time to judge the qualities of the pulse. After this, the strength of pulse at different positions is compared at the superficial and deep levels to identify imbalances among the meridians. The choice of needling techniques is thus determined first through pulse-quality diagnosis, and then the meridians and points to be treated are selected on the basis of the findings from six-position pulse diagnosis.

Other pulse qualities: If one has a good grasp of the six basic pulse qualities, in addition to six-position pulse diagnosis, this is sufficient for purposes of performing meridian therapy effectively. There is, however, a much greater variety of pulse qualities. The ability to recognize other qualities is useful for reaching a more accurate diagnosis. I will therefore next describe several other pulse qualities, aside from the basic ones, which I frequently encounter in my practice.

► Flooding Pulse:

"[It is] floating and large." *(Pulse Classic)*

"[It is] extremely large and represents heat." (Hongo, 1718)

The flooding pulse is a very wide one which can be felt right at the surface. It is found in patients with fevers, or those with heart conditions. When palpating a flooding pulse, one must be aware of possible cardiac dysfunction. In terms of the seasons, the flooding pulse tends to appear in the summer.

► Wiry Pulse:

"[It feels] as if pressing on the string of a bow, and represents contracture [or a sense of contraction]." (Hongo, 1718)

The wiry pulse feels tight and drawn like a string of an instrument. It is an indication that there is contraction or pain in some part of the body.

► Tight Pulse:

"[It feels] tense like a taut rope, and represents pain." (Hongo, 1718)

The tight pulse is not as thin as the wiry pulse. It can be thought of as a larger version of the wiry pulse.

"[It is] a tense pulse which is not at all vague or diffuse. It is neither choppy nor weak. It can be viewed as a tense pulse with somewhat of a slippery quality." (Inoue, 1980)

The tight pulse is always listed alongside the wiry pulse in the classics, so it is clearly similar to the wiry pulse. It is regarded as a sign of pain.

► Hollow Pulse:

"[It is] hollow in the middle like a green onion, and represents loss of Blood." (Hongo, 1718)

The hollow pulse feels somewhat like pressing a stalk of a green onion in that the inside is hollow while the vascular wall is firm. This pulse can be recognized very easily once you have examined a patient after a massive hemorrhage.

Learning pulse qualities may initially seem easier than six-position pulse diagnosis, but the more you study the pulse qualities, the more complex they become. In some cases the pulse quality is totally different on the right and left wrists, and it is difficult to say which quality should be considered the more significant one for diagnostic purposes. I cannot provide a simple answer, but I will venture to say this much: a position with a pulse quality that significantly differs from other positions requires special attention, and other signs of imbalance in the organs and meridians associated with the abnormal position must be investigated carefully.

Seasonal and pathological pulse qualities: According to the classics, each of the seasons has a corresponding pulse quality. The pulse quality associated with spring is the wiry pulse, which is tense and slightly thin. The pulse quality associated with summer is the flooding pulse, which is large, floating, and slightly soft. The pulse quality associated with autumn is the floating pulse, which floats thin and soft on the surface. The pulse quality associated with winter is the submerged pulse, which is sunken and hard. These qualities are those which are said to normally appear and disappear with the seasons in a healthy individual. Those who are ill have pulse qualities which differ from the norm. When one has a submerged pulse in the summer, for example, it means that the internal condition of the body is close to a state which normally occurs in the winter.

It is also a bad sign if any seasonal pulse quality is extreme during any season. For example, when there is an extremely flooding pulse without any softness during the summer, this indicates a condition of excess. In their extreme forms, all of the seasonal pulses are pathological. In every season the pulse should have a hint of the seasonal pulse quality, but should still retain the softness and buoyancy denoting the presence of Stomach Qi. The pathological pulse qualities associated with the five yin organs are identical to the seasonal pulse qualities associated with the five-phase correspondences. The wiry pulse indicates pathology in the Liver; the flooding pulse in the Heart; the moderate pulse in the Spleen; the floating pulse in the Lung; and the submerged pulse in the Kidney. The moderate pulse is characterized by softness and is regarded as a normal pulse which indicates good health. A moderate pulse quality generally signifies the presence of healthy Stomach Qi, which is palpated in normal pulses, as previously explained.

What then is the ideal pulse quality? In the discussion of pulse diagnosis in the classics, some pulse qualities are said to indicate death in certain situations, and other qualities indicate survival. In ancient times the pulse qualities were used in this fashion to determine the prognosis. The "death pulses" in every case seem to be extreme forms of the various pulse qualities. To put it simply, these pulse qualities all lack Stomach Qi. In contrast to the extreme pulse qualities, the ideal pulse quality is neither too hard nor too soft. The healthy pulse is thus soft but with a certain amount of resiliency, and the beat is steady and rhythmical. It can be said that the pulse quality reflects the condition of the patient's mind and body at that very moment. Although it is possible to explain the various pulse qualities in contemporary medical terms, more significant is that ancient physicians made a very detailed study of the pulses as the primary indicator of health and disease. While it may be true that modern technology can be used to precisely monitor physiological variables including the pulse rate and blood pressure, it is a pity that so many Japanese acupuncturists today make light of the highly refined art of pulse palpation.

Transposed radial artery: A transposed radial artery is a congenital abnormality in the course of the radial artery. Sometimes the radial artery goes around to the dorsal aspect of the arm along the Large Intestine meridian, crossing over to the

Large Intestine meridian just above L-7, instead of staying on the course of the Lung meridian. When no pulse whatsoever can be felt in the normal positions, one can palpate a wider area to find the artery on the other side. The cases which are most misleading are those in which the radial artery branches into two so that a weak pulse can still be palpated in the normal positions. One may therefore conclude that the patient has a deficient condition, or that certain positions are deficient, and treat accordingly; this, however, could be the wrong treatment. For this reason, it is important to make a habit of always checking the dorsal aspect of the wrist before beginning pulse diagnosis. Sometimes the radial artery is transposed on both sides, which makes things a bit difficult.

Once, while examining the pulse of a model patient during a demonstration at a meridian therapy seminar, I found that the patient's pulses were very weak in contrast to his robust appearance. The pulses on both wrists were very weak, and I could not make a good comparison of the pulse positions. I repeatedly examined the pulses between other palpatory examinations, such as abdominal diagnosis and meridian palpation. I could not tell much from the pulses, but I went ahead and treated the patient for Liver deficiency based on the abdominal diagnosis and other palpatory findings. I placed needles at Liv-8 and K-10, as well as some auricular points, and explained what I was doing to the participants. I examined the pulses again, but found that they were still very weak. At that point, my assistant for the day spoke up and said that the model patient had a transposed radial artery. Reexamining the pulses, I felt a large and forceful pulse on the other side. It seems that my assistant had examined the pulses and treated this model before, and had therefore known all about this. I'll never understand why he didn't tell me sooner. I must have been slightly nervous in front of all the participants, because I am usually more careful when I examine the pulse. As a demonstration of diagnosis without questioning, I had gone ahead with the treatment without asking the model about his complaints. After treating him, I found out that he suffered from dizziness and heaviness of the head, so my diagnosis was close to the mark. Nevertheless, it was unnerving to think I that I could have given him the wrong treatment.

How does one go about diagnosing a patient with a transposed radial artery? Even if you are well-aware of the situation, I think it is difficult to base the diagnosis on the pulse. Some practitioners say that when just one side is transposed, those positions which are weak or cannot be felt can be treated as if they are deficient. In other words, they are saying that when the right side is transposed, the patient should be treated for Lung deficiency. This is supposed to increase the strength of the pulse in the weak positions, or to cause the pulse to appear where there was no pulse. In my experience, however, this does not work. Even when an attempt is made to apply the same standards and compare the normal side with the transposed side, the pulse palpated at the normal positions on the transposed side is weak, small, and thin (if it can be palpated at all), and no meaningful comparison is possible. I feel that the best thing to do in such cases is to use other types of examination to ascertain the pattern. The abdominal diagnosis and palpatory examination are very important for this purpose, as is the questioning examination, in order to correlate the signs and symptoms of the patient.

Even if a patient has a transposed radial artery, pulse diagnosis can still be a valuable tool for judging the pulse quality and for finding differences between yin and yang meridians in those positions where the artery is not transposed. If there are any significant differences in the normal positions of a yin-yang pair of meridians, this could be treated as the primary imbalance. Moreover, the pulse quality is always an important indicator of the patient's condition, and the pulses must therefore be examined carefully in every case.

Abdominal Diagnosis

Even though abdominal diagnosis, like pulse diagnosis, is a vital component of the palpatory examination in Japanese acupuncture, outside of meridian therapy it does not seem to get the emphasis it deserves. My own teacher, having been a student of Yanagiya, used to say that "disease resides in the abdomen;" he therefore always examined the abdomen thoroughly and treated abdominal points. While I was studying under him, he would tell me to examine the abdomen and needle those parts which were abnormal, by which he meant those that were tender or indurated. In those days I did not know how to find tender or indurated points, and I had great difficulty in palpating subtle differences on the skin surface. I often felt completely lost with abdominal diagnosis, and to me the abdomen seemed to be too large and unfathomable. If my teacher simply told me to put a needle in the tender point around CV-12, or to carefully inspect the area surrounding CV-9, I could probe around the area to find the most likely point of difference. But searching for tenderness and induration over the entire abdomen seemed like searching for a needle in a haystack. I found it particularly difficult to locate tender points.

There is still much I have to learn about abdominal diagnosis. I decided long ago that every day was a day for learning, and every time I get a chance, I examine an abdomen or flip through various texts on the subject. I am not sure that abdominal diagnosis can be explained in simple terms, but I will do my best to present this complex subject in a clear and simple manner.

HISTORICAL PERSPECTIVE ON ABDOMINAL DIAGNOSIS

Unlike the rest of Oriental medicine, abdominal diagnosis developed very little in China. Instead, it became popular in Japan from the seventeenth century, when it began to develop into a unique diagnostic system in its own right. I never saw the abdomen being examined when I visited China in 1978, or when I attended a seminar in 1980 on Chinese acupuncture presented by a prominent acupuncturist from Wuhan. It seems as if tongue diagnosis takes the place of abdominal diagnosis in China, so carefully do they examine and classify the shape, color, and coating of the tongue. Very few texts of Chinese medicine have anything to say about abdominal diagnosis. Some scholars in Japan have suggested that this is because the Chinese have been more reluctant than the Japanese to expose their abdomens. I am not so sure abdominal diagnosis developed because Japanese were more willing to bare their bellies, but it is true that historically Japanese society has had less inhibition about nudity.

I am of the opinion that the impetus behind the development of abdominal diagnosis in Japan came from the rivaling schools of Sino-Japanese herbal medicine *(kampō)* in the seventeenth century. Although acupuncturists began the practice of abdominal diagnosis, they did not develop a consistent system which survives to this day, as the herbalists did. Abdominal diagnosis was used in both the Gosei school, which was based on then-contemporary Chinese herbal medicine, and the Kohō school, which was a neoclassical movement unique to Japan. In the Gosei school pulse diagnosis was used along with the other traditional aspects of examination to diagnose the condition of the organs and meridians, just as in meridian therapy. In the Kohō school, however, the meridians were disregarded and palpatory findings from the abdomen were considered to be of paramount importance in diagnosis. Purists in the Kohō school did not even examine the pulse. Yoshimasu Todo, the most influential figure in the Kohō school, is famous for his singular reliance on abdominal findings for diagnosis: "The abdomen is the source of life, and therefore the myriad diseases have their root here. The abdomen must always be examined in order to diagnose disease." (Yoshimasu, 1752)

According to Otsuka Keisetsu, the foremost Japanese herbologist in modern times, rather than originating among herbalists, it was acupuncturists who began diagnosing and treating the abdomen exclusively. This reliance on abdominal diagnosis began at about the same time among both the Kohō school herbalists and the Mubun school acupuncturists who practiced a unique form of acupuncture. The originators of abdominal diagnosis could very well have been acupuncturists of the Mubun school in the seventeenth century, who were famous for the Dashin technique in which a small mallet was used to insert needles in the abdomen. Regardless of which group started the practice of abdominal diagnosis in Japan, one thing is clear: abdominal diagnosis as practiced by Japanese herbalists and acupuncturists is a unique system which originated in Japan around the beginning of the seventeenth century. Let us begin our historical examination of abdominal diagnosis with a brief look at the Mubun school.

Abdominal diagnosis in the Mubun School: In 1685 an acupuncturist named Mubunsai published a book entitled, *Compilation of the Secrets of Acupuncture,* which stands apart from other acupuncture texts of its time. In his book Mubunsai maintains that examining the abdomen and treating the abdomen directly is sufficient to cure nine diseases out of ten. Mubunsai divided the abdomen into distinct areas, each of which corresponds to an organ. Pathogenic Qi could be palpated in these areas, and then treated directly on the abdomen where it was located. *Compilation of the Secrets of Acupuncture* explains in detail the relationship between symptomology and abdominal findings in the various diagnostic areas, but does not mention anything about the meridians or acupuncture points. The diagnostic area of the Heart, for example, is explained as follows: "The epigastric region, commonly known as the pit of the stomach, is designated as the domain of the Heart. When pathogenic Qi is in this Heart [area], conditions such as dizziness, restlessness of the tongue, headaches, insomnia, nightmares, palpitations, and chest pain occur."

Each diagnostic area is explained in this manner by directly linking abdominal findings to symptomology. All symptoms can then be treated by needling the corresponding area on the abdomen. There is no mention of other types of diagnosis; in all likelihood, nothing other than abdominal diagnosis was used in the Mubun school. The historical background leading to the development of this method is now obscure, especially since this school of acupuncture, unlike the more popular Sugiyama school, did not survive to modern times. Only the book *Compilation of the Secrets of Acupuncture* remains today as evidence of the existence of this school.

Leaving aside the perplexing questions about the origins and development of the Mubun school, it is interesting to study a diagram from this book which illustrates the diagnostic areas on the abdomen (Illustration 3-39). A close look at the diagram reveals striking similarities to abdominal diagnosis as used in meridian therapy today. The major difference is that abdominal diagnosis in meridian therapy is primarily intended to judge the level of Qi in the yin meridians. Yet despite this basic difference, the scheme is quite similar. It is clear that the abdominal diagnosis used by the Mubun school was loosely based on the *Classic of Difficulties*. Perhaps for this reason the methods of abdominal diagnosis used in meridian therapy today have many things in common with the methods used by that school.

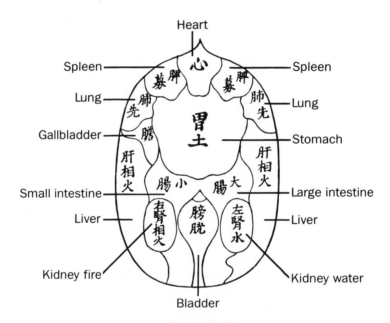

Illustration 3-39
Abdominal Diagnostic Areas: Mubun School

Abdominal diagnosis in the *Precious Record of Acupuncture*: The *Precious Record of Acupuncture* by Hongo Masatoyo was published in 1726, about 50 years after the *Compilation of the Secrets of Acupuncture*. Hongo, unlike Mubunsai, did not recommend diagnosis by palpation of the abdomen alone. Even so, it is clear from his book that palpation of the abdomen had become an important component of diagnosis in other schools of acupuncture. The method of abdominal diagnosis detailed in the *Precious Record of Acupuncture* is similar in many respects to that practiced in meridian therapy today. This is no accident since this text, among the many acupuncture books that were published in the Edo period, is one of the few that is still read by Japanese practitioners today. The reason for its enduring popularity lies in the influence of the great classical acupuncturist Yagishita, who inspired the originators of meridian therapy. Yagishita read and used the *Precious Record of Acupuncture* as his bible of acupuncture, and a day did not go by that he did not refer to it. The method of abdominal diagnosis recorded in the *Precious Record of Acupuncture* is very simple and straightforward:

> "How to Examine the Abdomen and Determine Life or Death — Have the patient lie supine with the legs extended and the hands lying by the thighs. Place your hand under the left breast for men, and under the right breast for women, and have the patient relax. After five or six breaths, slide your hand down to CV-13 and begin to gently press [down the abdomen], examining both sides [of the midline]. Check the left side first for men, and the right side first for women. A feeling of comfort with pressure indicates deficiency, while pain indicates excess. Pain with light pressure means that the pathogenic Qi is in the exterior, while pain with heavy pressure means that the pathogenic Qi is in the interior. When the area between the navel and the ribs is empty [flaccid] and the area below the navel is ample and resilient, this is a good sign of an abundance of Kidney essence. Tightness above the navel and emptiness below the navel indicates Kidney deficiency. Those with abdomens which are even in consistency above and below the navel are healthy. When the abdomen is soft in some places and hard in other places, or when it feels like poking a bag filled with sticks, disease exists even if the patient has no complaint. When the rectus abdominis muscles on both sides are rigid, this indicates a deficiency of normal Qi. To determine life or death, press CV-4 [which is located] three units below the navel. When this area is empty, and palpating with the finger up and down the midline reveals a hollowness which feels like a vertical ditch that the fingers fall into, [the patient] will die."

While there are no references in this passage to the diagnostic areas of the organs (except for the Kidney), the explanation is simple and clear. In view of the fact that this passage is the only discussion of abdominal diagnosis in his book, it is quite obvious that Hongo did not use abdominal diagnosis as the sole means of diagnosis. It is nonetheless quite interesting that Hongo sought vital information about life or death from the abdomen. Traditionally, certain pulse qualities were indicative of death, but basing this determination on the abdomen is consistent with the concept in the *Classic of Difficulties* (chapter 66) that the root of life lies in the lower abdomen:

> "The pulsation [literally, moving Qi] between the Kidneys [located] below the navel is the life of a person. It is the root of the twelve meridians. It is therefore called the source."

Abdominal diagnosis in the *Classic of Difficulties*: The development of abdominal diagnosis in meridian therapy was, without a doubt, based on the *Classic of Difficulties*. This is obviously a far older work than the Japanese texts already discussed, and it is important to understand how abdominal diagnosis is presented in this ancient Chinese classic of acupuncture. In chapter 16, the findings of pulsation, induration, and tenderness on the abdomen are mentioned in reference to diagnosis. For example, the diagnostic findings associated with Liver disease are recorded as follows:

"When the Liver pulse is obtained, as external evidence there is fastidiousness, a greenish complexion, and irascibility. As internal evidence there is a pulsation to the left of the navel, which is either hard or painful when pressed. With this disease there is swelling in the four limbs, dripping urination, difficult bowel movements, and cramping in the [calf] muscles. Those with these [symptoms] have a Liver [condition], and those without do not."

This passage may be paraphrased to make a little better sense as follows:

"When the patient has a wiry pulse, which is the pathological pulse of the Liver, evidence that is apparent from the outside includes fastidiousness, a greenish complexion, and a tendency to become irritable and angry. Evidence within the body is a pulsation to the left of the navel which can be palpated and is hard or painful when pressed. Other symptoms of Liver disease includes edema in the four limbs, dribbling urination, constipation, and cramping in the [gastrocnemius] muscles. When a patient has a wiry pulse together with these signs and symptoms, one can be sure that there is Liver disease. When the pulse is wiry, but none of these signs or symptoms are present, there is no problem with the Liver."

Thus, it is noted that a pathological pulse must be accompanied by corresponding signs and symptoms before a particular diagnosis can be confirmed. The external evidence, internal evidence, and symptoms associated with the pathology of each of the five essential (yin) organs is set forth in this chapter of the *Classic of Difficulties*. However, rather than discuss all of this information at once, I will focus here on just the abdominal signs or "internal evidence" of the five organs. Discussion of the other signs and symptoms of organ imbalances is reserved for chapter 4 below.

As shown in Illustration 3-40, when pulsation, hardness, or tenderness is palpated directly over the navel, there is a Spleen disorder. If it is found in the area around S-25 on the left, there is a Liver disorder, and on the right, a Lung disorder. If it is found around CV-6, there is a Kidney disorder, and around CV-12, a Heart disorder.

As previously noted, however, these findings must be confirmed by a corresponding pathological pulse before a definite diagnosis can be established. In his book, *Acupuncture by Meridian Therapy,* Okabe Sodo discusses the correlation between pulse and abdominal findings in the *Classic of Difficulties:*

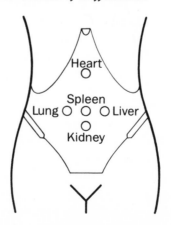

Illustration 3-40
Abdominal Diagnostic Areas: *Classic of Difficulties*

"The pattern can be determined only when the pulse and the external signs reflected in the complexion and pulsation around the navel are consistent. These pulsations are significant only when all the signs correspond. One cannot assume an imbalance in an organ or meridian just by the location of pulsation in the abdomen. If the pulse is wiry, for example, the symptoms of fastidiousness, a greenish complexion, and irascibility must be found in addition to pulsation to the left of the navel. A diagnosis of Liver excess or Liver deficiency can be made only when all of these symptoms are found simultaneously. A finding of pulsation to the left of the navel alone is not enough to diagnose Liver imbalance. It is therefore a mistake to assume that the areas of pulsation [recorded in the *Classic of Difficulties*] are diagnostic areas for the organs or meridians."

Be that as it may, the basic scheme of diagnostic areas used for abdominal diagnosis in meridian therapy is not so far removed from that first outlined in the *Classic of Difficulties*. The difference is in the depth of palpation. In meridian therapy, for the purpose of diagnosis, a palpatory finding of pulsation in the abdomen is not as important as flaccidity or tension on the surface. Even though tenderness and induration are significant, they are considered to be secondary to more superficial abdominal findings in determining the pattern. There is general agreement among practitioners of meridian therapy that pulsation, tenderness, and induration are not very closely related to meridian Qi, which is the main object of diagnostic assessment in determining the pattern of imbalance.

APPROACHES TO ABDOMINAL DIAGNOSIS IN MERIDIAN THERAPY

Since the beginning of meridian therapy about half a century ago, there has been considerable development and refinement in approaches to diagnosis and treatment. Although the fundamental principles of meridian therapy based on the *Classic of Difficulties* have remained unchanged, a number of different approaches have emerged. All practitioners of meridian therapy continue to use six-position pulse diagnosis as the primary means of ascertaining the pattern, but other details of diagnosis and treatment in meridian therapy vary. Abdominal diagnosis is one aspect which has seen a variety of approaches, since slightly different methods were utilized even among the originators of meridian therapy. A real consensus regarding the best approach to abdominal diagnosis has yet to be reached, and we therefore encounter considerable variation when we look at how it is practiced. Be that as it may, since they share a common origin, all of the approaches have many more similarities than differences. Here I shall introduce two of the most widely used approaches to abdominal diagnosis in meridian therapy, beginning with Honma's approach, which is detailed in *Discourse on Meridian Therapy*.

Abdominal diagnosis in *Discourse on Meridian Therapy*: *Discourse on Meridian Therapy* by Honma Shohaku was the first textbook of meridian therapy. This book includes a detailed explanation of Honma's approach to abdominal diagnosis, which is now one of the most widely used approaches among Japanese acupuncturists. My own method of abdominal diagnosis is quite similar to Honma's, since I studied this approach as I came to practice meridian therapy. The chapter on abdominal diagnosis in *Discourse on Meridian Therapy* provides a very detailed explanation of Honma's method, which I shall now summarize (Illustration 3-41).

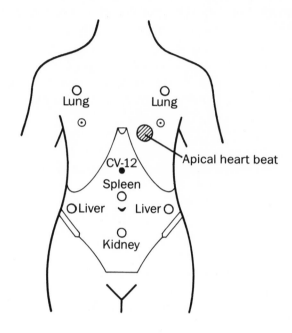

Illustration 3-41
Abdominal Diagnostic Areas: *Discourse on Meridian Therapy*

In order to detect abnormalities in the abdomen, a practitioner must first learn what a normal abdomen is like. When a person is healthy, the skin of the abdomen is smooth and even in consistency from top to bottom, and the abdominal wall is soft and resilient like a rubber ball. The skin of the abdomen should have a proper amount of luster, and should not be excessively dry or moist. The surface of the abdomen should be suitably warm, and no areas of special warmth or coolness should be felt. A healthy abdomen has no points of tenderness, indurations, or strong pulsations.

The standard procedure for abdominal diagnosis is as follows:

1. Before starting abdominal diagnosis the practitioner must be sure that his hands are sufficiently warm.

2. Before starting abdominal diagnosis the patient should be given some time to relax. The practitioner must also be calm and composed.

3. The practitioner should position himself on the left side of the patient.

4. The patient lies in a supine position with the knees straight in a relaxed manner, with the hands next to the thighs. (Patients who are accustomed to having their abdomen examined by medical doctors tend to keep their knees bent, but this is not an examination of the internal organs, so the legs should be fully extended.) The entire torso must be exposed.

5. Once the patient is relaxed, the practitioner observes the respiratory movement over the thorax and abdomen. Any visible movement over the heart, and marked asymmetries of the thorax and abdomen, are noted.

6. The practitioner begins palpating using the palmar aspect of the fingers of the right hand, and the areas around L-1 in the infraclavicular fossae are lightly stroked. Some practitioners use their left hands because they find that it is more sensitive. Usually the pads of the index, middle, and ring fingers are used. The condition of the Lung meridian is palpated in the upper thoracic area around L-1. An abundance of Lung Qi is indicated when the upper thoracic area is large, there is ample flesh, and the area is firm to the touch. A deficiency of Lung Qi is indicated when the skin in this area is dry, the flesh is soft, or the upper ribs can be easily seen or felt.

7.   Next the overall condition of the abdomen is checked by stroking down the midline, passing over the upper abdomen, the navel, and the lower abdomen. (It is a bad sign when a strong pulsation can be felt all the way down the midline from CV-15 to CV-6. Special caution is advised when this is the case, and the patient should be referred to a medical doctor.)

8.   The condition of the Heart meridian is palpated in the epigastric region. The area between CV-15 and CV-12 should be pressed lightly. This area should be soft but resilient, and there should be no pulsation. If there is a strong pulsation or the area is hard, the Heart Qi is deficient.

9.   The condition of the Spleen meridian is palpated in the area between CV-12 and CV-9. The Spleen and Stomach are normal when this area is resilient but not hard. The Spleen Qi is deficient when it feels mushy, or like a plastic bag full of water, or when the patient is extremely ticklish.

10.   The condition of the Kidney meridian is palpated in the hypogastric area around CV-6. There is ample Kidney Qi when this area is resilient and protrudes slightly compared to the upper abdomen. The Kidney Qi is deficient when the area below the navel is depressed or cold, or when a tight band of tension can be felt deep down. A strong pulsation in this area is also a sign of Kidney deficiency. It is normal, however, for a slight pulsation to be felt with the application of light pressure. This is called the "pulsation between the Kidneys" in the *Classic of Difficulties,* and it is considered to be the wellspring of the life force. (When this area is full of strength, one has ample energy, but when the lower abdomen is depressed and without strength, one lacks energy and tires easily. This is the reason why so much emphasis is placed on concentrating one's attention on the lower abdomen in Zen meditation, as well as in most traditional health regimens.)

11.   The condition of the Liver meridian is palpated in the flank regions, the areas on the sides of the abdomen anterior to G-26. When the Liver meridian is normal, the flesh in the flank regions is ample and muscle tone is good. When the flank regions feel empty and lacking in tone, it is a sign of Liver deficiency. It is traditionally said that a lack of muscle tone around Liv-13, which allows the fingers to be easily pressed under the rib cage, is an ominous sign of an impending stroke. This is an accurate observation. It is quite likely that patients with this condition will become paralyzed on the side with abnormal softness within a year. This is the diagnostic area of the Liver meridian, thus flaccidity here indicates Liver deficiency. Treating such patients for Liver deficiency should improve their condition.

The basic procedure for abdominal diagnosis has thus been detailed by Honma. As a very basic standard for a healthy abdomen, it can be said that the epigastric region around CV-14 should be soft, and that the lower abdomen around CV-6 should be firm.

There is a tendency when the epigastric region is tight for the lower abdomen to be soft and depressed. When palpating the lower abdomen of pregnant women, one must exercise some caution. In the early stages of pregnancy, the fetus can be palpated as a soft, movable mass like a water-filled balloon in the lower abdomen. Applying excessive pressure to the lower abdomen of such women can sometimes be injurious. Therefore, when performing abdominal diagnosis, it is best to avoid deep pressure on the lower abdomen of women who are either pregnant or undergoing menstruation.

The skin of the abdomen should have a healthy luster and be appropriately warm. Appearance and superficial texture are very important in abdominal diagnosis. Practitioners who are unpracticed at the gentle abdominal diagnosis of meridian therapy sometimes press too hard. Perhaps they mistake abdominal diagnosis for the palpation of organs in Western medicine and try to feel the organs themselves. If strong pressure is applied right from the start, patients will become defensive, and their abdominal muscles will become tense. This is detrimental to making an accurate diagnosis. To palpate the abdomen in meridian therapy, the hand should be slightly cupped, and the abdomen should be gently stroked with the fingers. Initially, the abdomen should be palpated very gently on the surface to inspect the condition of the skin. This is done for the purpose of detecting deficiency or excess of Qi. After palpating the abdomen over the entire surface, slight pressure is applied with the fingertips to examine the same areas for tenderness, indurations, and pulsations. These more tangible changes are due to prolonged excess or deficiency of Qi. The clinical signs of Western medicine, such as enlargement of certain organs or rebound tenderness, must also be noted. Patients with acute abdominal signs should immediately be referred to a physician.

To summarize, all palpatory findings of the abdomen should be taken into account, but in meridian therapy the color, texture, and resiliency of the skin are the most significant factors for purposes of diagnosis.

Fukushima's approach to abdominal diagnosis: Fukushima Kodo is the leader of one of the largest groups of meridian therapy practitioners, which was originally organized for the visually handicapped. Fukushima himself was the first blind practitioner to master meridian therapy, and is the author of many texts on this subject. Although his approach to abdominal diagnosis is similar to Honma's, there are several differences. In his beginners text published in 1979, *Meridian Therapy Made Simple*, Fukushima provides a very clear presentation of his method of abdominal diagnosis, which I will now summarize.

1. The diagnostic area for the Spleen meridian is around the navel, from CV-7 just below the navel to CV-12 in the upper abdomen.

2. The diagnostic area for the Heart meridian is between CV-13 and CV-15.

3. The diagnostic area for the Lung meridian is the subcostal region just below G-24 and Sp-16 on the right. The corresponding region on the left is also examined for the purpose of comparison.

4. The diagnostic area for the Liver meridian is in the left flank region below the level of the navel, between G-26 and G-29. The right flank region will exhibit the same signs of deficiency as the left flank region when the Liver meridian alone is deficient.

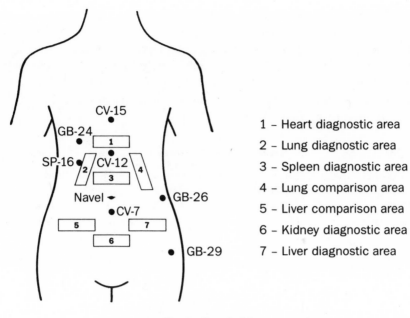

Illustration 3-42
Abdominal Diagnostic Areas: Fukushima Kodo

1 – Heart diagnostic area
2 – Lung diagnostic area
3 – Spleen diagnostic area
4 – Lung comparison area
5 – Liver comparison area
6 – Kidney diagnostic area
7 – Liver diagnostic area

5. The diagnostic area for the Kidney meridian is between CV-7 just below the navel and the superior border of the pubic symphysis. At times, however, Kidney meridian symptoms extend over the entire lower abdomen (Illustration 3-42).

The practitioner must palpate these diagnostic areas to find those which are lacking in luster, tone, and resiliency. Such findings indicate deficiency. The findings on the abdomen must be correlated with six-position pulse diagnosis to determine the pattern. For example, when Lung deficiency is indicated by six-position pulse diagnosis, signs of deficiency should be detected in the diagnostic area for the Lung meridian, and similar signs should be palpated in the diagnostic area for the Spleen meridian. When a pattern of Lung deficiency is diagnosed, the root treatment would be to tonify L-9. Doing this should immediately affect the pulse (i.e., increase the strength at the Lung position) as well as improve the condition of the abdomen in the Lung diagnostic area. Furthermore, tonifying Sp-3 should improve the pulse as well as the condition of the abdomen around the navel. In this way, there is a direct correlation between the pulse and the abdomen.

To begin this type of abdominal diagnosis, the practitioner should place the palm of his right hand over the patient's navel. This means that the index finger is close to the Lung area, and that the little finger is close to the area used for comparison for the Lung. The practitioner's hand should be moved gently over the abdomen to successively palpate the Spleen, Liver, and Kidney areas. What is sought from abdominal diagnosis in meridian therapy are differences in Qi, so the practitioner must not press very hard. The use of excessive pressure makes it difficult to perceive slight differences. The hands should be moved lightly over the abdomen in an effort to detect these subtle differences.

Comparison of approaches to abdominal diagnosis: There is no ironclad rule concerning the location of the diagnostic areas of the abdomen, as is evident from the approaches just described. This is not surprising in view of the fact that it has been less than 50 years since the practice of abdominal diagnosis was resumed by Japanese acupuncturists with the advent of meridian therapy. A comparison of the locations of the diagnostic areas in three approaches to abdominal diagnosis will be useful. The differences are shown in Table 3-3.

DIAGNOSTIC AREA	Liver	Heart	Spleen	Lungs	Kidneys
Classic of Difficulties:	Left of navel	Above navel	Around navel	Right of navel	Below navel
Honma:	Flanks	CV-14	CV-12	L-1	Below navel
Fukushima:	Left lateral abdomen	CV-14	CV-12	Right hypo-chondria	Below navel

Table 3-3 Comparison of Abdominal Diagnostic Areas

As shown in the table, the abdominal diagnostic areas for the Heart, Spleen, and Kidney meridians are just about the same in all three approaches. For the Liver and Lung meridians, however, the diagnostic areas differ. For the Liver meridian, those differences are respectively around S-25 on the left side, the subcostal area anterior to G-26, and the lower flank region on the left side. I use Honma's approach and check the condition of the Liver meridian anterior to G-26 on both sides. I also press S-25 on the left side as well as the right subcostal region for further indications of Liver imbalance. The diagnostic areas for the Lung meridian also vary, and are respectively around L-1, around S-25 on the right side, and the subcostal area on the right side. While any of these areas may be used, I usually find signs of Lung imbalance in the infraclavicular fossae.

As previously noted, there is no definite agreement even among practitioners of meridian therapy regarding the location of the diagnostic areas of the abdomen. Abdominal diagnosis in the modern era was probably not intensively studied by practitioners of meridian therapy until the publication of *Discourse on Meridian Therapy*. The procedure and application of abdominal diagnosis has constantly evolved since that time, and it may be a little premature for us to decide on a particular system at this point. The significance of abdominal findings differs slightly according to the practitioner, but in meridian therapy these findings are mostly used to confirm the diagnosis. There are also other systems of abdominal diagnosis which have a slightly different orientation. I will introduce one such method devised by Maruyama, who is a well-known practitioner of meridian therapy. Approaches like his demonstrate other possibilities in the application of abdominal diagnosis. I look forward to further research and clinical work on abdominal diagnosis by acupuncturists on all fronts so that this invaluable traditional approach can be raised to new heights.

Maruyama's abdominal diagnosis for point selection: A unique method of abdominal diagnosis has been developed by Maruyama Mamoru, a student of Okabe Sodo. Maruyama uses abdominal diagnosis both for point selection and for confirming the diagnosis. His method is a rather complex system of palpating tender points on the abdomen, but this method is of great interest to practitioners of meridian therapy who, because of their reliance on pulse diagnosis, are often unable to objectively demonstrate the effect of their treatment. Maruyama recommends his method as an approach which patients can understand, and in which the effectiveness of specific points can be tested prior to treatment. Below I have excerpted portions of an article which he wrote about his method that was featured in the *Journal of the Japan Meridian Therapy Association*.

The pattern is the criterion for the selection of acupuncture points for root treatment. The pattern is based on findings from the four examinations, but in meridian therapy the findings from pulse diagnosis carry the greatest weight. Once the pattern is determined, I press special diagnostic points on the abdomen to discover points of tenderness. After locating a tender point, I apply finger pressure on the essential points of the corresponding meridian (noted below) on the same side as the tender point. In this manner, I locate an essential point which reduces or alleviates the tenderness at the abdominal points. Its effectiveness in reducing tenderness confirms that this essential point is indicated for treatment. Pressing the effective essential point also reduces tenderness and sensitivity to pinching at sensitive points along related meridians on the arm. Finding three related points on the abdomen, leg, and arm in this way confirms that the diagnosis was indeed correct, and also indicates the most effective points for treatment.

The abdominal diagnostic points I use are as follows (Illustration 3-43):

1. Numbers 1, 2, and 3 are the diagnostic points for the Spleen meridian. Number 2 is located right at CV-8, which is in the navel. Number 1 is located just above the navel, and number 3 is located just below the navel.

2. Numbers 4, 5, 6, and 7 are diagnostic points for the Kidney and Bladder meridians. Number 5 is located at K-16, 0.5 unit lateral to the navel. Numbers 4 and

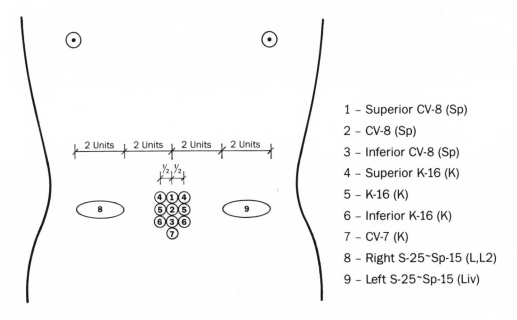

1 – Superior CV-8 (Sp)

2 – CV-8 (Sp)

3 – Inferior CV-8 (Sp)

4 – Superior K-16 (K)

5 – K-16 (K)

6 – Inferior K-16 (K)

7 – CV-7 (K)

8 – Right S-25~Sp-15 (L,L2)

9 – Left S-25~Sp-15 (Liv)

Illustration 3-43
Abdominal Diagnostic Areas: Maruyama Mamoru

6 are points located 1-1.5 units above and below the navel respectively. Occasionally, instead of the above points, tenderness appears at point number 7, which is located at CV-7.

3. Number 8 is the area where the diagnostic point for the Lung and Large Intestine meridians can be located. This area is between S-25 and Sp-15 on the right side.

4. Number 9 is the area where the diagnostic point for the Liver meridian can be located. This area is between S-25 and Sp-15 on the left side. The diagnostic point for the Gallbladder meridian is found at G-26.

After locating a tender point on the abdomen which corresponds with the diagnosis established by six-position pulse diagnosis and other means, a point is sought on the affected meridian which reduces or eliminates the tenderness. Usually an essential point of the affected meridian on the same side is effective in reducing the tenderness, but sometimes an essential point on the other side is more effective. The point most effective in reducing the tenderness at the abdominal diagnostic point is treated with acupuncture as the principal tonification point. Finger pressure on the effective essential point also reduces sensitivity to pinching at certain points on related meridians. The related meridians are those on the arm if the deficient meridian is on the leg, and on the leg if the deficient meridian is on the arm. Therefore, when the Kidney meridian is deficient, aside from tenderness at K-16 being reduced by applying pressure at K-3 or K-7, sensitivity to pinching at L-6 or L-7 is also diminished. This correlation between three points — the abdominal diagnostic point, the essential point on the corresponding meridian, and the point that is sensitive to pinching — confirms the initial diagnosis.

The three related points on the abdomen, leg, and arm are sought on the unbalanced meridian and its related meridian. (Table 3-4).

Unbalanced Meridian	Abdominal Tenderness	Related Meridian
Liver	Liver diagnostic point	Pericardium
Kidney	Kidney diagnostic point	Lung
Bladder	Kidney diagnostic point	Large Intestine
Spleen	Spleen diagnostic point	Heart
Lung	Lung diagnostic point	Spleen
Large Intestine	Lung diagnostic point	Stomach
Gallbladder	Gallbladder diagnostic point	Triple burner

Table 3-4 Maruyama's Abdominal Diagnosis for Point Selection

Thus, when Liver deficiency is indicated by pulse diagnosis and tenderness is detected at S-25 on the left side, finger pressure at Liv-3 or Liv-4 on the left side usually eliminates the tenderness. This also reduces the sensitivity to pinching at P-4, the cleft point of the Pericardium meridian, which is often quite sensitive in cases of Liver deficiency.

This is a very interesting system of abdominal diagnosis characterized by the use of tender points to identify the most effective treatment point on the corresponding meridian. Its difference from the other approaches discussed earlier is that, rather than serving to provide additional information for determining the pattern, Maruyama's method is employed after the pattern has already been ascertained. Palpating tender points on the abdomen, and then locating distal points on the limbs which reduce this tenderness, also serves to confirm the diagnosis. The inventor of the ion-pumping cord, Dr. Manaka Yoshio, has developed a system of abdominal diagnosis for treating the extraordinary vessels which is likewise based on the palpation of tender points. There are thus practitioners outside of meridian therapy who use methods of abdominal diagnosis similar to Maruyama's. I do not use Maruyama's method much in my own practice, but examining his method does lead to an important point about abdominal findings and treatment: when the appropriate treatment is rendered, there will be improvement in the condition of the abdomen. It is important that you obtain, during the initial stage of treatment, immediate and reproducible results in the abdomen and pulse. In other words, signs of imbalance detected in the pulse and abdomen should be corrected to some extent before the root treatment, which is directed at balancing the Qi in meridians, can be considered complete.

Alarm points in abdominal diagnosis: We cannot end this chapter on abdominal diagnosis without touching on the subject of alarm *(bo/mù)* points, which are the oldest diagnostic points on the abdomen. With the exception of L-1, all of the alarm points are located on the abdomen. Findings at the alarm points, including tenderness, induration, depression, lack of resiliency, and sensitivity to pinching, can provide useful information for judging the condition of the corresponding meridians. The problem with using alarm points for diagnosis lies in the complexity of their distribution, and the close proximity of some of the points to each other. For example, CV-3, CV-4, and CV-5, the alarm points of the Bladder, Small Intestine, and Triple Burner meridians respectively, are all located next to each other on the conception vessel. Traditionally, these points were not used in formulating a diagnosis, as is done today with abdominal diagnosis in meridian therapy. The significance of the alarm points and the associated *(yu/shù)* points on the back is explained in the following manner in the *Classic of Difficulties* (chapter 67):

> "Yin diseases go to the yang [aspect] and yang diseases go to the yin [aspect].
> The alarm points are therefore located on the yin [aspect] and the associated
> points on the yang [aspect]."

There is thus a cross connection between the yin and yang aspects of the body. Yang diseases or symptoms appear on the front of the body or the abdomen. According to the above passage, the alarm points, located on the abdomen, are connected with yang diseases. Yang diseases usually manifest as imbalances in the yang meridians. If the alarm points are in fact related more to the yang meridians, they are not especially useful for judging yin meridian deficiency, which is the main thrust of meridian therapy. While findings of tenderness or induration at specific alarm points are very useful for symptomatic treatment after the diagnosis is established, they do not lead to a diagnosis in and of themselves. Findings at alarm points are generally useful for reference in the selection of points, or as indicators of correct treatment. In this sense, the use of alarm points can be considered similar to that of the diagnostic points used by Maruyama.

MERIDIAN PALPATION

Meridian palpation is important as the final step of the palpatory examination. Meridian palpation must be distinguished from palpation done for the purpose of point location. Although there is a close relationship between them, they are two different steps. Careful palpation of the affected meridian for the purpose of point location is very important, but the meridians are first palpated prior to locating the points as a means of confirming the initial diagnosis. The significance of meridian palpation is that it is the final step of the palpatory examination and is used to confirm the effect of Qi imbalances on the distal portions of the affected meridian. Meridian palpation often reveals differences which have a direct bearing on the selection of acupuncture points. The more exacting palpation to locate the points is done just prior to needle insertion; this step is based in part on the information gathered from meridian palpation. I usually perform meridian palpation after determining the pattern of imbalance based on the four examinations, particularly pulse and abdominal diagnosis.

Let us say, for example, that I find the Lung and Spleen positions are weak (a sign of Lung deficiency) according to six-position pulse diagnosis, and that the abdominal findings confirm this impression. I then begin meridian palpation by stroking along the course of the Lung meridian on the arm. I examine the Lung meridian on both sides for unusual depressions, protrusions, warmth, or coolness. Then I press key points such as the cleft point (L-6), the connecting point (L-7), and the source point (L-9) to check for tenderness or induration. After examining the Lung meridian on both arms, I examine the course of the Spleen meridian on the legs in the same manner. While performing meridian palpation, I also take a close look at the surrounding skin surface to see if there are visible differences which might indicate if the meridian in question is in a more deficient or excessive state compared with adjacent meridians. Through meridian palpation I generally detect some difference or indication of imbalance in the affected or related meridian which confirms my diagnosis. In practice, however, one rarely finds a clear sign of imbalance, such as a marked depression or protrusion, along the entire length of a meridian. What one usually finds are only small areas, or a few points with a slight difference. Meridian palpation is actually much more difficult than it sounds because it requires a great deal of experience and refined palpation skills to locate subtle differences over a large area.

There is another technique of meridian palpation known as pinching diagnosis in which the skin is lightly pinched up along the course of a meridian or over specific points. This technique was mentioned earlier in connection with Maruyama's approach to abdominal diagnosis. In Maruyama's method, a pressure point is sought on the affected meridian which alleviates tenderness at related abdominal points, and simultaneously reduces sensitivity to pinching at sensitive distal points on a related meridian. When there is an imbalance in a meridian, there is often increased sensitivity to pinching along related meridians. One point is often surprisingly sensitive to pinching compared to adjacent points. Aside from a lowered pain threshold in small areas of the skin, by pinching, localized differences can sometimes be detected in the texture of the skin. Practitioners skilled at pinching diagnosis are able to detect abnormalities on the meridians very quickly and accurately. I often use this palpation technique, but sometimes sensitivity to pinching appears over a wide area overlying the path of several meridians, which makes it difficult to judge which meridian imbalance is responsible for the reaction. Sometimes meridian palpation yields findings which are either inconsistent or in conflict with the perceived pattern. In such cases, the findings from pulse and abdominal diagnosis are always given precedence. With some experience, the practitioner will be able to zero in on relevant information without becoming unduly concerned about every little finding.

KEY POINTS

Looking Examination: Imbalances in the meridians are diagnosed based on the patient's complexion.

* Those with luster in their skin are easy to treat, and those without are difficult to treat.
* The best place to examine the skin is on the forehead and the anterior aspect of the forearms.

Listening and Smelling Examination: Imbalances in the meridians are diagnosed based on the sounds and odors emanating from the patient.
* A commanding manner or tone of voice is a sign of Liver meridian imbalance.
* Effusiveness is a sign of Heart meridian imbalance.
* Suddenly starting to hum or sing a song is a sign of Spleen meridian imbalance.
* A whining voice or constant complaining is a sign of Lung meridian imbalance.
* A groaning voice is a sign of Kidney meridian imbalance.

Questioning: Imbalances in the meridians are diagnosed by asking the patient questions about their preferences and symptoms.
* Those who prefer a sour taste tend to have Liver meridian imbalance.
* Those who prefer a bitter taste tend to have Heart meridian imbalance.
* Those who prefer a sweet taste tend to have Spleen meridian imbalance.
* Those who prefer a pungent taste tend to have Lung meridian imbalance.
* Those who prefer a salty taste tend to have Kidney meridian imbalance.

Palpatory Examination: pulse diagnosis, abdominal diagnosis, and meridian palpation.
PULSE DIAGNOSIS
    ► Generalities
* Assesses the patient's overall condition as well as the pattern of meridian Qi imbalance.
* There are six positions which are the distal, middle, and proximal positions on each arm.
* There are three levels: superficial, middle, and deep.
* The first step is to assess the Stomach Qi at the middle level, which is where the pulse can be palpated at its strongest in all positions.
* The balance between the yang meridians is examined at the superficial level, reached by raising the fingers to the point just before the pulse can no longer be felt.

- The balance between the yin meridians is examined at the deep level, reached by pressing with the fingers to the point just before the pulse weakens and disappears.
- The tips of the three fingers must contact the artery at a right angle.
- When pressing down on the artery with the three fingers, the thumbs (or thenar eminences) are used to exert pressure. The thumbs are usually placed on TB-4, but can be more radial if that is more comfortable.
- When the pulse is hard to discern, examine the pulse with the patient seated, or otherwise insert needles superficially in the abdomen, cranium, or at L-9.
- Do not spend too much time examining the pulses.

► Six-position pulse diagnosis

- There are several ways to perform six-position pulse diagnosis. The most direct method is to palpate all six positions at once. Another common method is to palpate one wrist at a time. A simpler method is to compare the same positions bilaterally using one finger on each side.
- One method of mastering six-position pulse diagnosis is to start by concentrating solely on determining which yin meridians are deficient. When this can be done, then one can feel for excessive yin meridians, and after that one can proceed to feel for yang meridian excess and deficiency.
- A simplified method of finding deficient yin meridians is to compare positions in the controlling relationships of the five phases as follows: **1.** Compare the Heart (left distal) and Lung (right distal) positions. **2.** Compare the Lung (right distal) and Liver (left middle) positions. **3.** Compare the Liver (left middle) and Spleen (right middle) positions. **4.** Compare the Spleen (right middle) and Kidney (left proximal) positions. **5.** Compare the Kidney (left proximal) and Pericardium (right proximal) positions.
- To master six-position pulse diagnosis at the superficial level, first learn to palpate yang meridian excess. Yang meridian imbalances have a direct relationship to the patient's symptoms.
- When there is a marked difference in the force of a pulse between the superficial and deep levels for paired yin and yang meridians, that phase can be considered to have the greatest imbalance. Yin meridian deficiency together with excess in its paired yang meridian is relatively easy to correct.

► Mechanics

- When examining the pulses on both wrists with the patient supine, the patient's upper arms should remain on the table and the wrists should be placed on the abdomen next to the navel. The practitioner must lean over the patient and extend his left elbow over to the other side.
- The practitioner should be aware of which fingers are most sensitive, and must find a way to consistently apply even pressure on both sides.

- When palpating subtle differences crucial to the diagnosis, use the two most sensitive fingers.
- In order to master pulse diagnosis, examine pulses every day, examine the pulses of every patient before and after treatment, and study with experts.

▶ Pulse Qualities. There are twenty-four pulse qualities:

- Six of these are known as the basic pulse qualities: floating and submerged, slow and rapid, and deficient and excessive. Concentrate only on these in the beginning, and then learn additional pulse qualities one by one.
- The floating pulse can be felt at the very surface of the skin by just lightly placing the fingers over the artery. It indicates a wind condition, and the appropriate needling technique is superficial insertion.
- The submerged pulse can only be felt at the deep level, and it indicates a damp condition. The appropriate needling technique is deep insertion.
- The slow pulse beats less than four beats per minute. It indicates a cold condition, and the needles should be retained.
- The rapid pulse beats more than five beats per minute. It indicates a condition of heat, and the needles should be inserted and withdrawn quickly.
- The deficient pulse is soft and without strength. Tonification techniques should be utilized.
- The excessive pulse is large and strong. Dispersion techniques should be utilized.
- The seasonal pulse qualities are wiry in spring, flooding in summer, floating in fall, and submerged in winter. The healthy pulse should bear a hint of the appropriate seasonal quality.

ABDOMINAL DIAGNOSIS

- First learn what the abdomen of a healthy person is like: soft but resilient without any points of tenderness, hard areas, or pulsations.
- For abdominal diagnosis the patient must lie supine with both legs extended.
- The practitioner stands on the left side of the patient and allows time for the patient to relax before beginning to palpate the abdomen. The practitioner's hands must be suitably warm.
- First observe the breathing movements in the chest and abdomen.
- The condition of the Lung is examined around L-1 in the infraclavicular fossa.
- The condition of the Heart is examined around CV-14 in the epigastric region.
- The condition of the Spleen is examined between CV-12 and the navel.
- The condition of the Kidney is examined around CV-6 in the hypogastric region.
- The condition of the Liver is examined in the area between Sp-15 and G-26 in the flank region.

MERIDIAN PALPATION

• Examines the condition of the meridians by stroking, pressing, and lightly pinching along the course of the meridians.

4

Determining the
Pattern of Imbalance

Many factors must be taken into account when determining the pattern of imbalance, since the pattern has a direct bearing on how the treatment is performed. Although in meridian therapy the findings from palpation of the pulse and abdomen are of primary importance, all of the findings from the four examinations must still be considered. The information obtained through questioning which pertains to the signs and symptoms is particularly useful because of the specific pathological manifestations traditionally associated with each organ and meridian. A familiarity with the symptomology of the organs and meridians thus makes it easier to distinguish the pattern of imbalance. If the pattern can be discerned from the pulse and abdomen alone, it may be unnecessary to listen to the complaints of the patient, but the palpatory examination does not always provide sufficient information. For the best results, the pattern of imbalance should be established and confirmed from as many angles as possible.

I sometimes encounter cases where the pulse is so weak that it is difficult to tell which position is deficient and which is excessive. It seems as if all the positions are deficient. If the chief complaint happens to be loss of appetite and an inability to keep food down, I would treat the patient for Spleen deficiency. In most cases this brings rapid improvement. The symptoms of loss of appetite and an inability to keep food down suggest that there is a weakness or deficiency of Qi in the Spleen and its associated meridian. This is a very direct application of the symptomology of the organs and meridians to determine the pattern of imbalance and the method of treatment. Needless to say, it is much better to use the symptomology to confirm the findings from the pulse or abdomen, but even when the results of the palpatory examination are unclear, a knowledge of symptomology alone can often be applied to render an effective treatment.

SYMPTOMOLOGY OF THE ORGANS AND MERIDIANS

The symptomology of the organs and meridians recorded in the classics of acupuncture was derived from experience with pathological manifestations and Qi imbalance in localized areas of the body, as well as the body as a whole. Classical symptomology consists of groupings of symptoms associated with imbalances in particular organs or meridians, each of which is related to specific parts of the body. Although there is no definitive list of symptoms, those recorded in the classics do give us a general idea of the groupings of symptoms most commonly associated with particular organs and meridians. Let us take a look at the groupings in the earliest classics starting with the symptomology of the five yin organs.

Symptomology of the Five Yin Organs

The groupings of symptoms associated with the five yin organs are the simplest categorization of pathological manifestations. They are particularly useful in meridian therapy because in this school of acupuncture the basic pattern of imbalance is always defined in terms of a deficiency of a yin organ or meridian. This is a very helpful rule, especially as the classics often fail to specify whether symptoms associated with an organ are those of excess or deficiency.

The symptomology of the yin organs automatically implies pathology of the yin aspect. The Li-Zhu school of Chinese medicine holds that the yin always tends toward deficiency, and the yang toward excess. This school is based on the teachings of Li Dong-Yuan (1180-1228) and his student's student, Zhu Zhen-Xiang (1281-1358). It took a critical view of the dominant school in China at that time, which emphasized the therapeutic strategy of cooling fire. The Li-Zhu school regarded the Spleen and Stomach as the most important organs, and emphasized warming of the middle burner in treatment. This school gained prominence during the Yuan dynasty and has had a major influence on medicine in both China and Japan ever since.

In meridian therapy the notion that the yin always tends toward deficiency and the yang toward excess is taken to mean that the yin organs and meridians have a tendency to become deficient, and the yang organs and meridians to develop excessive conditions. Since the symptomology of the five yin organs is very important in confirming a diagnosis of pathology in the yin meridians, I have listed below the symptoms found in chapter 22 of *Basic Questions,* followed by those found in chapter 16 of the *Classic of Difficulties.*

SYMPTOMOLOGY OF THE LIVER

"With Liver disease there is pain in the flank regions which extends to the lower
abdomen, and the person is easily angered. When [the Liver is] deficient, the

eyes become blurred and cannot see, and the ears cannot hear. One is very fearful as if about to be captured. When the Qi [of the Liver] rushes upward, there is headache, loss of hearing, and swelling in the cheeks." *(Basic Questions)*

"When a Liver [wiry] pulse is felt, as external signs there is fastidiousness, a greenish complexion, and a tendency to become angry. As internal signs there is a pulsation to the left of the navel, and [this area] is either hard or painful when pressed. With this disease there is swelling of the four limbs, oliguria, constipation, and cramping in the calf muscles. Those with these [signs] have Liver [disease] and those without [these signs] do not." *(Classic of Difficulties)*

SYMPTOMOLOGY OF THE HEART

"With Heart disease there is pain in the middle of the chest, fullness in the hypochondria, and pain in the flank region. The chest, [upper] back, and intrascapular regions are painful, as is the medial aspect of the arms. When [the Heart is] deficient, the chest and abdomen feel bloated, and there is pain in the flanks which extends to the lower back." *(Basic Questions)*

"When a Heart [flooding] pulse is felt, as external signs there is a red complexion, dry mouth, and a tendency to laugh. As internal signs there is a pulsation above the navel, and [this area] is either hard or painful when pressed. With this disease there is restlessness of the heart, heart pain, heat in the palms, and dry heaves. Those with these [signs] have Heart [disease] and those without [these signs] do not." *(Classic of Difficulties)*

SYMPTOMOLOGY OF THE SPLEEN

"With Spleen disease there is a feeling of heaviness in the body, a tendency to be hungry, atrophy of the muscles, and loss of strength in the legs. When walking there is difficulty in raising the feet, cramping and spasms, and pain in the soles. When [the Spleen is] deficient, there is fullness of the abdomen and borborygmus and loose stools with undigested food." *(Basic Questions)*

"When a Spleen [moderate] pulse is felt, as external signs there is a yellowish complexion, belching, a tendency to think too much, and a fondness for eating. As internal signs there is a pulsation over the navel, and [this area] is either hard or painful when pressed. With this disease there is distention and fullness of the abdomen, food is not digested, a feeling of heaviness in the body, aching in the joints, fatigue and lethargy, a desire to lie down, and an inability to pull the limbs in toward the body. Those with these [signs] have Spleen [disease] and those without [these signs] do not." *(Classic of Difficulties)*

SYMPTOMOLOGY OF THE LUNG

"With Lung disease there is coughing and wheezing, Qi rushing upward [to the head], and pain in the shoulders and upper back. There is sweating, and pain in all the areas from the genital region and buttocks down to the feet. When [the Lung is] deficient, there is shallow breathing and shortness of breath, loss of hearing, and a dry throat." *(Basic Questions)*

"When a Lung [floating] pulse is felt, as external signs there is a white complexion, a tendency to sneeze, melancholy and lack of joy, and a desire to cry. As internal signs there is a pulsation to the right of the navel, and [this area] is either hard or painful when pressed. With this disease there is shortness of breath, coughing, wheezing, and shivering from fever and chills. Those with these [signs] have Lung [disease] and those without [these signs] do not." *(Classic of Difficulties)*

SYMPTOMOLOGY OF THE KIDNEY

"With Kidney disease there is bloating of the abdomen and swelling in the calves. There is coughing and wheezing and a feeling of heaviness in the body, as well as night sweats and aversion to wind. When [the Kidney is] deficient, there is pain in the chest and in the upper and lower abdomen. The limbs are chilled and one is unable to feel joy." *(Basic Questions)*

"When a Kidney [submerged] pulse is felt, as external signs there is a blackish complexion, a tendency to be fearful and frequent yawning. As internal signs there is a pulsation below the navel, and [this area] is either hard or painful when pressed. With this disease there is Qi rushing upward [to the head], tension and pain in the lower abdomen, diarrhea with a feeling of heaviness in the bowels, and a feeling of cold and rebellion in the lower extremities. Those with these [signs] have Kidney [disease] and those without [these signs] do not." *(Classic of Difficulties)*

Symptomology of the Six Yang Organs

There is less written in the classics about the symptomology of the six yang organs than there is about the five yin organs or the twelve meridians. Perhaps the lack of information about imbalances in the yang organs is due to the tendency of yang organ symptoms to manifest in the meridians. Thus, it can be said that the symptomology of the yang organs is basically that of the yang meridians. The symptoms of the six yang organs set forth in chapter 4 of the *Vital Axis* are listed below. Looking over this list, it is apparent that the symptoms of the meridians have been mixed in with those of the organs. It should also be noted that most of the symptoms associated with the yang organs resemble those for diseases of the same organs in modern medicine.

SYMPTOMOLOGY OF THE LARGE INTESTINE

"With disease of the Large Intestine the bowels hurt as if they were cut, and there is the sound of water. When one is also exposed to cold in the winter, there is diarrhea and pain around the navel, and it is difficult to stand for very long. The symptoms [associated with disease of the Large Intestine] resemble those of the Stomach."

SYMPTOMOLOGY OF THE STOMACH

"With disease of the Stomach the abdomen becomes distended and there is pain between the stomach and heart which may spread to the hypochondria. There is a loss of communication between the throat and diaphragm so that food and drink do not go down."

SYMPTOMOLOGY OF THE SMALL INTESTINE

"With disease of the Small Intestine there is pain in the lower abdomen and pain which extends from the lumbar spine to the scrotum, and there is colicky pain with elimination [of stool or urine]. There may be a sensation of heat anterior to the ear, or that area may be very cold, or the superior aspect of the shoulders may feel very hot accompanied by a feeling of heat between the little and ring fingers. A depression along the course of the meridian is also a sign [of disease of the Small Intestine.]"

SYMPTOMOLOGY OF THE TRIPLE BURNER

"With disease of the Triple Burner the abdomen becomes distended with gas and the lower abdomen is extremely hard. There is an inability to urinate with intense pain, and there is retention [of fluids], resulting in edema."

SYMPTOMOLOGY OF THE BLADDER

"With disease of the Bladder the lower abdomen primarily becomes swollen and painful, and [although] pressing this area with the hand produces a desire to urinate, one is unable to urinate. The shoulders become hot or there is a depression along the course of the meridian. There is also either heat or a depression along the posterior border of the fibula and the lateral margin of the little toe."

SYMPTOMOLOGY OF THE GALLBLADDER

"With disease of the Gallbladder there is sighing, a bitter taste in the mouth, and regurgitation of bile. Pounding is felt in the epigastric region, and the person is fearful as if someone were trying to capture him. There is a sensation of something being caught in the throat and one must expectorate from time to time."

Symptomology of the Twelve Meridians

Comparing the symptomology of the organs and their associated meridians, it is doubtful that a clear distinction was made in the classics between symptoms of the organs and those of the meridians. Since an organ and meridian of the same name are so closely linked, it may be natural that there is some overlap in their symptomology. The symptomology of the meridians is often expressed in terms of whether the condition is one of deficiency or excess. For example, modern Japanese texts list the following symptomology for Lung meridian deficiency: weakness or difficulty in breathing, dryness of the throat, chilling or numbness of the hands and feet, pain or loss of sensation in the skin (Honma, 1949); chills, cold and/or numb hands and feet, dyspnea, dryness of the throat, pain in the skin. (Araki, 1982)

One might ask why these particular symptoms are associated with deficiency of the Lung meridian. Are they exclusive and unalterable, or might not other symptoms be added to the list? Many practitioners of meridian therapy use such groupings of symptoms as a matter of course in determining the pattern of imbalance, but how do we know that they are correct? To answer these questions, it is worthwhile to go back to the very origins of classifying symptoms according to meridians in order to obtain a clearer picture of how acupuncturists in ancient times understood the symptomology of the meridians. In chapter 10 of *Vital Axis* there is a complete list of the symptomology of the twelve meridians. This list is particularly well-known since it was reintroduced more than a thousand years later in *Elaboration of the Fourteen Meridians*. All subsequent classifications of meridian symptomology are probably based on this one, and it therefore deserves careful examination.

An exciting discovery was made in China a few years back which sheds some light on the origin of the symptomology of the meridians. In 1973, medical manuscripts predating the *Yellow Emperor's Inner Classic* were excavated from the tomb of a former Han-dynasty prince at Ma Wang Tui in Hunan province. The manuscripts, which are inscribed on strips of silk buried in 168 B.C., are thought to reflect medical concepts which were prevalent at least a century before that time. Until the discovery of these manuscripts, the *Yellow Emperor's Inner Classic* was thought to be the oldest text of Chinese medicine extant, but now the manuscripts from Ma Wang Tui give us a glimpse of the formative period of Chinese medicine a few centuries before that work appeared. They thus allow us to trace the process of development of Chinese medical concepts.

The ideas presented in the medical manuscripts from Ma Wang Tui bear a close resemblance to those in later texts, but there are some distinct differences. Only eleven meridians are described in these manuscripts, the Pericardium meridian being absent. Furthermore, the meridians all originate independently from the Heart, instead of being an interconnected system for the circulation of Qi.

The medical manuscripts from Ma Wang Tui are also of monumental significance in reconstructing the history of Chinese medicine because they clarify terms used in later texts which were previously obscure. For example in the passages from chapter 10 of *Vital Axis* quoted below, the phrases "when disturbed, disease occurs" *(shì dòng zé bìng)* and "when giving rise to disease" *(sǔo shēng bìng)* appear repeatedly in reference to the symptomology of the meridians. These phrases were poorly understood until the discovery of the Ma Wang Tui manuscripts shed some light on their meaning:

> " 'When disturbed, disease occurs' refers to abnormal conditions arising when the meridian [Qi] is disrupted, and the progress of this disturbance can be checked by treating the meridian involved ... 'When giving rise to disease' refers to conditions in which the disruption [of Qi] in the meridian progresses beyond a certain point [and involves the organs]." (Kuwahara, 1976)

Whether the meridian pathology results from an external disturbance or from a disease which arises from within, symptoms always appear in relation to the affected meridian. Although the symptoms are listed as those of the meridians, since the meridian is internally connected with a pair of organs, symptoms associated with the organs are also included. We can get a better understanding of how the symptomology of the organs and meridians evolved by comparing the symptomology of the meridians recorded in *Vital Axis* with that in the manuscripts from Ma Wang Tui. For this purpose, I will present the symptomology from both sources for each meridian, followed by my own commentary.

Among the medical manuscripts from Ma Wang Tui, there are three sections which detail the course of the meridians and their symptomology. These sections have been named the *Moxibustion Classic of the Eleven Meridians on the Arms and Legs, Moxibustion Classic of the Eleven Yin and Yang Meridians,* and *Treatment of Fifty-two Diseases.* Among these texts, the symptomology of the meridians recorded in *Moxibustion Classic of the Eleven Yin and Yang Meridians* (hereafter referred to as the *Moxibustion Classic)* will be presented together with that found in chapter 10 of *Vital Axis.* Those portions of the symptomology recorded in *Vital Axis* which are not found in the *Moxibustion Classic* are italicized for the sake of comparison. Also, because some passages from the *Moxibustion Classic* are illegible due to the extreme age of the silk manuscripts, they are denoted by ellipsis marks (...).

SYMPTOMOLOGY OF THE LUNG MERIDIAN

Moxibustion Classic: Arm Greater Yin Meridian

> "When disturbed, disease occurs and there is palpitations, cardiac pain, and pain in the supraclavicular fossa. In extreme cases one crosses his arms over the chest and shivers violently. This is known as depletion [or collapse — *jüe*] of the arms. These are diseases that can be treated on the hand greater yin meridian. When giving rise to disease, there are the five diseases of chest pain, gastric pain, heart pain, pain in the four limbs, and Qi stagnation."

Vital Axis: Arm Greater Yin Lung Meridian

> "When disturbed, disease occurs and there is *distention and fullness of the lungs, wheezing and coughing, and* pain in the supraclavicular fossa. In extreme cases one crosses his arms over the chest and the vision is blurred. This is known as depletion of the arms. When that which controls the Lung gives rise to disease, there is *heat in the face, wheezing and coughing, dryness in the throat, irritability and fullness in the chest, pain along the lateral aspect of the arm,* depletion, *and heat in the palms.* When the Qi is excessive, there is *pain in the shoulders and intrascapular region, wind-cold causes sweating, and when attacked by wind there is frequent urination and yawning.* When the Qi is deficient, there is *pain and coldness in the shoulders and intrascapular region, shortness of breath and inability to breathe deeply, and a change in the color of the urine."*

Author's Commentary:

It is difficult to learn all the symptoms of each meridian just by reading a list of words. When I was first learning the symptomology of the meridians, I drew in the location of all the symptoms on a figure of the body, and marked them with a simple notation for easy reference. A picture appeals to one's visual sense and makes it easier to remember the various symptoms associated with each meridian. Another way is to use tables, which helps organize the material in your mind, and thereby aids in memorization. Throughout this section the symptoms associated with each meridian are organized in tabular form by location in order to make them easier to memorize.

Pain, numbness, and coldness in the arm are symptoms along the course of the Lung meridian. Heat in the palms not only occurs in connection with Lung meridian disorders, but also the Heart and Pericardium meridians. When there is internal heat together with colds or lung disorders (such as pulmonary tuberculosis), the palms and soles of the feet often do feel uncomfortably warm. Lung meridian deficiency is common in these patients. Pain in the supraclavicular fossa is a symptom related to problems of the cervical spine, cervicobrachialgia, and thoracic outlet syndrome. Tenderness and induration in the supraclavicular fossa is often associated with Lung meridian imbalances.

Symptoms associated with the Lung as an organ include wheezing, coughing, and distention and discomfort in the chest. Shortness of breath and an inability to breathe deeply is a common complaint, and patients with Lung disorders often complain that they have to stop and catch their breath from time to time. The *Moxibustion Classic* also lists the organ symptoms of chest, heart, and stomach pain, which are not found

Area	Symptom
General	Yawning
Head	Flushing
Throat	Dryness
Upper Back	Sweating from exposure to wind-cold
	Pain and a sensation of cold
Upper Body	Heat in the palms
	Pain along the anterolateral aspect of the arms
	Pain in shoulders and supraclavicular fossa
	Tendency to hug oneself due to feeling cold
Lungs	Shortness of breath, inability to breathe deeply
	Wheezing and coughing
Chest	Distention and fullness of the chest
	Irritability
Genitourinary	Frequent urination
	Change in the color of urine

Table 4-1
Symptomology of the Lung Meridian

in *Vital Axis,* but would seem to be valid.

Pain and cold in the shoulder and intrascapular region are common symptoms of Lung imbalances. When the pulse reflects Lung deficiency and there is strong tension in the shoulders or on the medial border of the scapula, one can almost be certain of Lung deficiency. I often treat sudden changes in the frequency of urination as a Lung imbalance. Sweating secondary to exposure to wind or cold is a common symptom when one contracts a cold or influenza. Heat in the head is also a common symptom associated with Lung imbalance. Other symptoms I have observed in patients with Lung imbalance include sore throat, hemorrhoids, pain in the lower abdomen, pain in the ileocecal region, and skin disorders.

SYMPTOMOLOGY OF THE LARGE INTESTINE MERIDIAN

Moxibustion Classic: Tooth Meridian

> "When disturbed, disease occurs and there is toothache and swelling of the cheeks. These are diseases that can be treated on the tooth meridian. When giving rise to disease, there are the five diseases of toothache, swelling of the cheeks, yellowish eyes, dryness of the mouth, and pain in the upper arm."

Vital Axis: Arm Yang Brightness Large Intestine Meridian

> "When disturbed, disease occurs and there is toothache and swelling in the cheeks. When that *which controls the thin fluids* gives rise to disease, there is yellowish eyes, dryness of the mouth, *epistaxis, pain and swelling in the throat,* pain on the upper arm in front of the shoulder, and an *inability to use the index finger due to pain.* When the Qi is excessive, *heat and swelling occur along the course of the meridian.* When the Qi is deficient, there is *violent shivering and an inability to warm up.*"

Author's Commentary:

The symptoms which appear along the course of the Large Intestine meridian include pain and swelling along the meridian, and an inability to use the index finger, obviously because the meridian originates at its tip. The use of the name tooth meridian in the *Moxibustion Classic* implies that in ancient times the Large Intestine meridian was the primary meridian used for the treatment of toothache. Epistaxis is also associated with the Large Intestine meridian, as are other problems of the nose, such as nasal congestion. Pain and swelling of the throat is often related to Large Intestine imbalance. Shivering violently and being unable to warm up commonly accompanies pain in the throat in cases of tonsillitis. I have no experience seeing yellowish eyes in connection with a Large Intestine imbalance. It is also interesting to note that there are no organ symptoms included in the symptomology of the Large Intestine meridian.

Area	Symptom
General	Violent shivering with an inability to get warm
Head	Toothache
	Nosebleeds and nasal congestion
	Yellowish eyes
	Dry mouth
Throat	Painful and swollen
Upper extremity	Anterior shoulder and arm pain
	Heat and swelling along the course of the meridian
	Pain and loss of function of the index finger

Table 4-2
Symptomology of the Large Intestine Meridian

SYMPTOMOLOGY OF THE STOMACH MERIDIAN

Moxibustion Classic: Yang Brightness Meridian

"When disturbed, disease occurs and there is chills as if one had been doused with water, there is frequent stretching and yawning, the complexion is ashen, and the face is swollen. When the disease reaches a certain level it [affects behavior and] causes an aversion to people and fire, and the sound of wood causes fright and terror. Fear causes one to withdraw alone into a room with the door and windows shut. In extreme cases one climbs up to a high place and begins to sing or throw one's clothes off and run about. This is known as depletion of the thighs. These are diseases that can be treated on the yang brightness meridian. When giving rise to disease, there are the ten diseases of facial pain, nasal congestion, pain in the submandibular and lateral cervical regions, pain in the breasts, heart pain, pain in the flank regions, edema of the upper part of the abdomen, pain in the intestines, rigidity of the knee joint, and ... on the dorsum of the foot."

Vital Axis: Leg Yang Brightness Stomach Meridian

"When disturbed, disease occurs and there is chilling of the body as if one had been doused with water, there is frequent stretching and yawning, and the complexion is ashen. When the disease reaches a certain level it [affects behavior and] causes an aversion to people and fire, the sound of wood causes fright and terror, *and the heart beats wildly.* Fear causes one to withdraw alone into a room with the door and windows shut. In extreme cases one climbs up to a high place and begins to sing or throw one's clothes off and run about. *There is borborygmus and distention of the abdomen.* This is known as depletion of the thighs. When that *which controls the Blood* gives rise to disease, there are *manic malarial disorders, warm diseases, perspiration, epistaxis,* nasal congestion, *distortion of the mouth [facial paralysis], skin lesions around the mouth,* pain and swelling in the throat and cervical region, *ascites, pain and swelling of the knees, pain extending from the anterior thoracic region down to the inguinal region, and down the thigh and the lateral aspect of the shin to the dorsum of the foot. One is unable to use the middle finger. When the Qi is abundant, the anterior aspect of the body becomes hot. When [the Qi is] excessive, digestion is accelerated and there is constant hunger and the urine turns yellow. When the Qi is deficient, the anterior aspect of the body becomes very cold and causes shivering, and when cold invades the stomach, there is fullness and distention."*

Author's Commentary:

Symptoms which appear along the course of the Stomach meridian include epistaxis, nasal congestion, distortion of the mouth due to facial paralysis, cold sores around the mouth, and pain in the breasts and in the knees. Pain and swelling in the throat and neck is also common as the Stomach meridian traverses the anterior aspect of the sternocleidomastoid muscle in the neighborhood of S-9. Symptoms associated

Area	Symptom
General	Mania
	Chilling of the body
	Ashen complexion
	Yawning
	Alternating fevers and chills
	Excessive perspiration
Head	Rash around the mouth
	Nosebleeds and nasal congestion
	Facial paralysis
Throat	Painful and swollen
Neck	Swellings
Breast	Pain
Abdomen	Sensation of either heat or cold
	Accelerated digestion and constant hunger
	Distention
	Pain
	Borborygmus
	Ascites
Genitourinary	Yellow urine
Lower extremities	Anterior thigh pain
	Knee swelling and pain
	Lateral shin pain
	Middle toe dysfunction

Table 4-3
Symptomology of the Stomach Meridian

with the Stomach organ include distention of the abdomen, borborygmus, and ascites. The symptom of accelerated digestion and constant hunger is seen in diabetes; the Stomach Qi is often excessive in diabetic patients, and their urine turns a dark-yellow color.

The psychological symptom of climbing up to a high place, singing, throwing one's clothes off, and running about is a famous passage which stands out from the other symptoms, which are mostly physical in nature. The two extremes of fear and withdrawal and then exhibitionism is typical of severe manic-depressive disorders. The *Moxibustion Classic* also lists facial pain, especially of the forehead. Frontal headache is an important symptom to remember in connection with Stomach imbalances.

SYMPTOMOLOGY OF THE SPLEEN MERIDIAN

Moxibustion Classic: Greater Yin Meridian

> "When disturbed, disease occurs and the Qi rises to reach the Heart, the abdomen becomes distended, and there is much belching. Eating causes nausea, but passing gas or defecating brings great relief. These are diseases that can be treated on the greater yin meridian [of the leg]. When giving rise to disease, there are the ten diseases of ... and irritability in the chest leading to death; heart pain and abdominal distention leading to death; the three symptoms of inability to eat, insomnia, and a constant desire to yawn all leading to death; watery diarrhea leading to death; and edema and oliguria together leading to death."

Vital Axis: Leg Greater Yin Spleen Meridian

> "When disturbed, disease occurs and the *root of the tongue becomes rigid*, eating causes nausea, and there is *stomach pain*. The abdomen also becomes distended and there is much belching. Passing gas or defecating brings great relief. *The whole body feels heavy.* When that which controls the Spleen gives rise to disease, there is *pain at the root of the tongue, inability to move the body, inability to keep food down,* irritability in the chest, *sharp pain in the epigastric region, diarrhea with mucus and blood, oliguria, jaundice,* and insomnia. *Also, when forced to stand, the medial aspect of the thigh and knee swell, there is chilling and numbness, and the big toe cannot be used.*"

Author's Commentary:

Symptoms which appear along the course of the Spleen meridian include pain, swelling, and chilling from the medial aspect of the thigh down to the toes, and pain in the root of the tongue. Symptoms associated with the Spleen organ include nausea after eating, gastric pain, abdominal distention, belching, and the inability to keep food down (esophageal spasm). The symptoms of irritability in the chest and sharp pain in the epigastrium occur both in heart conditions and disorders of the upper gastrointestinal tract. Diarrhea is a common symptom associated with the Spleen, and the relief felt after passing gas or defecating is a classic symptom of Spleen imbalance. Among the non-specific symptoms, there is a feeling of heaviness in the body, which in patients with Spleen meridian imbalances is often accompanied by lassitude and pain in the joints. Insomnia is also quite common in these patients.

Area	Symptom
General	Entire body feels heavy
	Insomnia
	Jaundice
Mouth	Painful and rigid tongue
Chest	Irritability
Abdomen	Epigastric pain (may be acute)
	Difficulty in swallowing food
	Belching
	Nausea and vomiting immediately after eating
	Distention
Bowels	Diarrhea
	Passing of gas brings a sense of relief
Genitourinary	Oliguria
Lower extremities	Medial thigh and knee swelling
	Dysfunction of the big toe

Table 4-4
Symptomology of the Spleen Meridian

SYMPTOMOLOGY OF THE HEART MERIDIAN

Moxibustion Classic: Arm Lesser Yin Meridian

"When disturbed, disease occurs and there is heart pain and thirst with a desire to drink. This is known as depletion of the arms. These are diseases that can be treated on the arm lesser yin meridian. When giving rise to disease, there is the single disease of pain in the flank region."

Vital Axis: Arm Lesser Yin Heart Meridian

"When disturbed, disease occurs and there is dryness of the throat, heart pain, and thirst with a desire to drink. This is known as depletion of the arms. When that which controls the Heart gives rise to disease, there is *yellowish eyes,* pain in the flank region, *pain down the anteromedial aspect of the arm, and heat and pain in the palms.*"

Author's Commentary:

Symptoms along the course of the Heart meridian include pain which extends down the arm, and heat and pain in the palms. Heat in the palms is also associated with Lung imbalances, but in the case of the Heart, this symptom is said to be accompanied by pain. One cannot, however, simply differentiate Lung and Heart imbalances on the basis of this symptom alone. Thirst with a desire to drink is a symptom of heat excess which would suggest that the heat in the palms is caused by an imbalance of the Heart, instead of the Lung. Pain in the flank region probably refers here to pain which occurs between the hypochondriac and axillary regions. Yellowish eyes would seem to indicate a problem with the viscera, and does not necessarily relate to an imbalance of the Heart.

Area	Symptom
General	Thirst with desire to drink
Head	Yellowish eyes
Throat	Dry
Chest	Heart pain
	Hypochondriac pain
Upper extremities	Anteromedial arm pain
	Warm and painful palms

Table 4-5
Symptomology of the Heart Meridian

SYMPTOMOLOGY OF THE SMALL INTESTINE MERIDIAN

Moxibustion Classic: Shoulder Meridian

"When disturbed, disease occurs and there is a sore throat, swelling in submandibular region, an inability to turn the neck to look backward, and intense pain in the shoulder and arm as if it were broken. These are diseases that can be treated on the shoulder meridian. When giving rise to disease, there are the four diseases of pain in the neck, pain and swelling in the throat, pain in the elbow, and pain in the forearm."

Vital Axis: Arm Greater Yang Small Intestine Meridian

"When disturbed, disease occurs and there is a sore throat, swelling in submandibular region, an inability to turn the neck to look backward, and intense pain in the shoulder and arm as if it were broken. When that which controls the thick fluids gives rise to disease, there is hearing loss, yellowish eyes, swelling in the cheeks, pain extending from the submandibular region down the neck and shoulders and along the posteromedial aspect of the upper arm, elbow, and forearm."

Author's Commentary:

Almost all of the symptoms listed above are found along the course of the Small Intestine meridian. (This was also the case for the symptomology of the Large Intestine meridian.) The name shoulder meridian from the *Moxibustion Classic* would there-

Area	Symptom
Head	Yellowish eyes
	Hearing loss
	Swelling of the cheeks
Neck and throat	Swelling below the jaw
	Sore throat
	Difficulty in turning the neck
Upper extremities	Posterior shoulder pain
	Posterolateral arm and forearm pain

Table 4-6
Symptomology of the Small Intestine Meridian

fore seem to be a more appropriate choice than Small Intestine meridian. In any case, hearing disorders, sore throat, and an inability to rotate the head to look backward (pain in the cervical region) are very important symptoms that suggest the involvement of the Small Intestine meridian.

SYMPTOMOLOGY OF THE BLADDER MERIDIAN

Moxibustion Classic: Greater Yang Meridian

> "When disturbed, disease occurs and there is a penetrating headache, ... , pain in the spine, lumbar pain as if the back were broken, an inability to move the hip joint, tightness in the popliteal fossa, and pain in the gastrocnemius muscle as if it were torn. This is known as depletion of the ankle. These are diseases that can be treated on the greater yang meridian. When giving rise to disease, there are the twelve diseases of headache, loss of hearing, a sensation as if the ears were blocked, pain in the occipital region, malarial disorder, pain in the upper back, pain in the lower back, gluteal pain, hemorrhoids, pain in the back of the thigh, pain in the gastrocnemius muscle, and painful obstruction of the little toe."

Vital Axis: Leg Greater Yang Bladder Meridian

> "When disturbed, disease occurs and there is a penetrating headache, *ocular pain as if the eyes were popping out, pain in the nape of the neck as if it were being pulled,* pain in the spine, lumbar pain as if the back were broken, an inability to bend the hip joint, tightness in the popliteal fossa, and pain in the gastrocnemius muscle as if it were torn. This is known as depletion of the ankle. When that *which controls the sinews* gives rise to disease, there is hemorrhoids, *mental derangement with malarial disorder, epilepsy, headache at the vertex, occipital headache, yellowish eyes, excessive tearing of the eyes, epistaxis,* pain in the nape of the neck, upper and lower back, gluteal region, popliteal fossa, shin, and foot. The little toe cannot be used."

Author's Commentary:

All of the symptoms above are associated with the course of the Bladder meridian, with the exception of yellowish eyes, malarial disorders, and epilepsy. Like most of the other yang meridians, the symptoms of the organ are not included. Since the course of the Bladder meridian is so extensive, there are a wide variety of symptoms. The most important of these are occipital headache, pain that extends down the nape of the neck, pain in the spine, lower back pain, hemorrhoids, pain in the buttocks and lower limbs (sciatica), epistaxis, nasal congestion, and excessive tearing of the eyes.

SYMPTOMOLOGY OF THE KIDNEY MERIDIAN

Moxibustion Classic: Lesser Yin Meridian

> "When disturbed, disease occurs and the voice becomes raspy and there is wheezing. When standing up after being seated, the eyes become blurry and are unable to see. There is also restlessness, emaciation, lack of energy, irritability, and there is fear that one is about to be captured. In addition there is anorexia,

Area	Symptom
General	Alternating fever and chills
	Mania-withdrawal
Head and Neck	Vertex headache
	Penetrating headache
	Occipital headache
	Stiff upper neck
	Orbital tension
	Yellowish eyes
	Tears
	Nosebleeds
Back	Vertebral pain
	Thoracic pain
	Lumbar pain
Hips and pelvis	Gluteal pain
	Inability to bend the hip
	Hemorrhoids
Lower extremities	Popliteal tension and pain
	Calf pain
	Dysfunction of the little toe

Table 4-7
Symptomology of the Bladder Meridian

hemoptysis, and the complexion becomes ashen. This is known as depletion of the bones. These are diseases that can be treated on the lesser yin meridian. When giving rise to disease, there are the ten diseases of ... , cracks on the tongue, dryness of the throat, heat in the head, food becoming lodged in the throat, pain in the throat, wasting away, a [constant] desire to lie down, coughing, and loss of voice."

Vital Axis: Leg Lesser Yin Kidney Meridian

"When disturbed, disease occurs and there is hunger but no desire to eat, and *the complexion becomes blackish*. There is coughing and hemoptysis, the voice becomes raspy and there is wheezing, and standing up after being seated causes the eyes to become blurry and blinded. One is restless as if starved. When the Qi is lacking, the patient becomes apprehensive and feels as if he is about to be captured. This is known as depletion of the bones. When that which controls the Kidney gives rise to disease, *there is heat in the mouth, dry tongue, swollen throat,* heat in the head, dryness and pain in the throat, *irritability in the chest, heart pain, jaundice, watery diarrhea, pain in the spine, pain that extends down the posteromedial aspect of the thighs, numbness and chilling [in the lower limbs],* a desire to lie down, *and heat and pain in the soles of the feet.*"

Author's Commentary:

The symptomology of the Kidney meridian includes many symptoms that are associated with other meridians, but there are also some differences. Hunger characterized by a lack of desire to eat is slightly different than the anorexia that accompanies Spleen meridian imbalances, where indigestion is the primary cause. Diarrhea is also common to both Kidney and Spleen imbalances. Wheezing or asthma appears in both

Lung and Kidney meridian imbalances. When there is blood in the sputum, the Kidney meridian should be treated. Heat in the soles of the feet is a sign of internal heat, and contrasts with the cold in the limbs which is also caused by a Kidney meridian imbalance. In severe cases, internal heat and external cold can exist simultaneously. People with a blackish complexion often have a Kidney meridian imbalance. The tendency for blood to rush to the face, the desire to lie down, and dizziness upon standing are all typical of patients with low blood pressure. People with Kidney deficiency tend to have low blood pressure. As for psychological symptoms, paranoia as if one is about to be captured aptly describes the phobia suffered by a patient with Kidney deficiency. Most patients with Kidney deficiency display, to some extent, the psychological symptoms of restlessness, irritability, and apprehensiveness. They also lack assertiveness, have little energy, tend to tire easily, and exhibit a decrease in libido. This is accompanied by a sensation of cold below the waist, tightness in the lower abdomen, a tendency to become dizzy upon standing up, and tinnitus.

In the *Moxibustion Classic,* coughing is listed instead of wheezing. Other symptoms which do not appear in *Vital Axis* include food becoming lodged in the throat (more common in older individuals), and wasting away.

Area	Symptom
General	Dizziness and blurred vision upon standing
	Restlessness
	Paranoia
	Jaundice
	Sensation of hunger without a desire to eat
Head	Flushing
	Dark complexion
Mouth and throat	Dry tongue
	Hot mouth
	Dry and painful throat
	Hoarseness
Chest	Wheezing
	Coughing
	Hemoptysis
	Heart pain
	Irritability
Abdomen	Watery diarrhea
Lower back and hips	Posteromedial thigh pain
	Lumbar spine pain
Lower extremities	Pain and cold in medial thigh and leg
	Pain and heat in the soles

Table 4-8
Symptomology of the Kidney Meridian

SYMPTOMOLOGY OF THE PERICARDIUM MERIDIAN
Vital Axis: Arm Terminal Yin Pericardium Meridian

> "When disturbed, disease occurs and there is heat in the palms, spasms in the elbow and forearm, and swelling in the axilla. In extreme cases there is fullness in the

chest and flank region, and strong palpitations. The complexion is reddish, the eyes turn yellowish, and one laughs incessantly. When that which controls the vessels gives rise to disease, there is irritability in the chest, heart pain, and heat in the palms."

Author's Commentary:

Among the twelve primary meridians, the Pericardium meridian is the only one missing from the *Moxibustion Classic*. This shows that the concept of the meridians developed over time, and that the concept of Qi circulation through the twelve meridians appeared only later in history.

Heat in the palms and swelling in the axilla are symptoms appearing along the course of the meridian. Symptoms associated with the Pericardium organ include irritability in the chest, heart pain, and distention in the chest and flank region. Hiccough is also related to imbalances of the Pericardium meridian, as well as the Spleen meridian. Incessant laughter is generally due to excessive Heart fire, but for some reason it is associated with the Pericardium here.

Area	Symptom
General	Constant laughing
Head	Yellowish eyes
	Reddish complexion
Chest	Heart pain
	Irritability
	Severe palpitations
	Distention of the chest and subcostal regions
Upper extremities	Axillary swelling
	Anterior elbow and forearm pain
	Heat in the palms

Table 4-9
Symptomology of the Pericardium Meridian

SYMPTOMOLOGY OF THE TRIPLE BURNER MERIDIAN

Moxibustion Classic: Ear Meridian

"When disturbed, disease occurs and there is loss of hearing or a sensation of obstruction in the ear, as well as swelling of the throat. These are diseases that can be treated on the ear meridian. When giving rise to disease, there are the three diseases of pain at the outer canthus, pain in the cheeks, and loss of hearing."

Vital Axis: Leg Lesser Yang Triple Burner Meridian

"When disturbed, disease occurs and there is loss of hearing or a sensation of obstruction in the ear, as well as swelling *and soreness of the throat*. When that which controls the Qi gives rise to disease, there is *sweating,* pain at the outer canthus and in the cheeks, *pain that extends from the retroauricular region down the* back of the shoulder and upper arm, as well as the elbow and forearm, and the ring finger cannot be used."

Author's Commentary:

Except for sweating, all the symptoms above are associated with the course of the Triple Burner meridian. The primary symptoms are pain in the ear, tinnitus, loss of hearing, and pain that extends down the posterior aspect of the arm. It is easy to understand how this meridian came to be called the ear meridian.

Area	Symptom
General	Excessive sweating
Head ·	Retroauricular pain
	Outer canthus pain
	Cheek pain
	Hearing loss
	Tinnitus
Throat	Pain and swelling
Upper extremities	Posterior shoulder pain
	Posterior arm, elbow, or forearm pain
	Ring finger dysfunction

Table 4-10
Symptomology of the Triple Burner Meridian

SYMPTOMOLOGY OF THE GALLBLADDER MERIDIAN

Moxibustion Classic: Lesser Yang Meridian

"When disturbed, disease occurs and there is pain in the heart and flank region, and the person cannot turn over in bed. In extreme cases there is lack of oil in the skin, and the foot deviates into eversion. This is known as depletion of yang. These are diseases that can be treated on the lesser yang meridian. When giving rise to disease, there are the twelve diseases of ... , pain in the head, neck, and flank region, malarial disorder, perspiration, pain in all the joints, pain in the lateral aspect of the hip joint, ... , pain, pain along the lateral aspect of the thigh and knee, chills and shivering, and painful obstruction of the middle toe."

Vital Axis: Leg Lesser Yang Gallbladder Meridian

When disturbed, disease occurs and there is *bitterness in the mouth, incessant sighing,* heart pain, and pain in the flank region that makes one unable to turn over in bed. In extreme cases the *complexion becomes dull as if covered by dust,* the body lacks oil in the skin, and *the foot becomes hot* and deforms into eversion. This is known as depletion of yang. When that which controls the bones gives rise to disease, there is headache, *pain in the outer canthus and submaxillary region, pain and swelling in the supraclavicular fossa, swelling in the axilla, scrofula,* perspiration, chills and shivering, malarial disorder, and pain that extends from the flank region down the lateral aspect of the thigh and knee to the *lateral malleolus.* There is also pain in all the joints, *and the fourth toe cannot be used.*

Author's Commentary:

Headache is among the symptoms associated with the course of the Gallbladder meridian. Here it refers to temporal headache along the course of the meridian between G-4 and G-20. When there is pain in the sides, one has difficulty rotating the spine and turning over. Pain and swelling in the neck, axilla, and supraclavicular fossa, as well as scrofula, is related to the course of the Gallbladder meridian. A bitter taste in the mouth is a symptom associated with the Gallbladder organ. The general symptoms include incessant sighing, a dull complexion, and dry skin. These symptoms often appear in patients with disorders of the gallbladder.

Area	Symptom
General	Excessive sweating
	Chills and shivering
	Dull complexion
	Repeated sighing
Skin	Lack of oil
Head	Headache
	Outer canthus pain
	Bitter taste in the mouth
Neck	Submandibular pain
	Scrofula
Chest	Pain and swelling of the supraclavicular fossa
	Axillary swelling
	Chest pain
	Hypochondriac pain
Torso	Difficulty in moving
Lower extremities	Hip pain
	Lateral knee pain
	Anterolateral ankle pain
	Heat in the ankles and feet
	Eversion of the foot
	Dysfunction of the fourth toe

Table 4-11
Symptomology of the Gallbladder Meridian

SYMPTOMOLOGY OF THE LIVER MERIDIAN

Moxibustion Classic: Leg Terminal Yin Meridian

"When disturbed, disease occurs and there is swelling of the scrotum and hernial pain in men, and swelling of the lower abdomen in women. There is also lower back pain and an inability to bend backwards. In extreme cases there is dryness of the throat and wrinkling of the facial skin. These are diseases that can be treated on the foot terminal yin meridian. When giving rise to disease, there is penetration of heat, oliguria, swelling of the scrotum, and one-sided hernial pain. When there is ... and irritability in the chest, death is imminent. No cure is possible. When there is disease of the yang [Gallbladder] meridian together [with these symptoms], treatment is possible."

Vital Axis: Leg Terminal Yin Liver Meridian

> "When disturbed, disease results and there is lower back pain and an inability to *bend forward* or backward. There is also *swelling of the scrotum* and hernial pain in men, and swelling of the lower abdomen in women. In extreme cases there is dryness of the throat and a *poor complexion as if dust is on the face.* When that which controls the Liver gives rise to disease, there is *distention in the chest, vomiting, diarrhea containing undigested matter, inguinal hernia, and oliguria or dribbling urination.*"

Author's Commentary:

Symptoms associated with the course of the Liver meridian include swelling or masses in the lower abdomen or the genitalia accompanied by sharp abdominal pain and dysuria. These are common symptoms of urogenital disorders such as urinary tract infection and prostatitis. Diseases of the urogenital system are often associated with Liver imbalances. Lower back pain with difficulty in flexing or extending the lumbar spine is also related to Liver imbalances. This type of lower back pain arises from sudden muscular strains and spasms in the lumbar region, and is commonly referred to as a "sprained back."

Symptoms of the Liver organ include distention in the chest, vomiting, and diarrhea containing undigested matter. These symptoms were added at a later time, and it is difficult to say whether symptoms from another meridian were included. A dull, lusterless complexion is a general symptom which occurs in both imbalances of the Liver and the Gallbladder meridians. Other important symptoms of Liver imbalance which are not listed above include eye diseases, blurred vision, dizziness, heaviness in the head, knee pain, skin diseases with itching such as urticaria, and fullness and distention in the hypochondriac region. Also missing from the list above are important psychological symptoms of Liver imbalance, such as short temper and apprehensiveness.

Area	Symptom
General	Lack of color in the complexion
Throat	Dry
Chest	Feeling of fullness
Upper abdomen	Vomiting
Lower abdomen	Diarrhea containing undigested food
	Inguinal hernia
	Swelling (in women)
Genitourinary	Oliguria or dribbling urine
Lower back	Pain
	Inability to bend forward

Table 4-12
Symptomology of the Liver Meridian

SYMPTOMOLOGY OF DIFFERENT PARTS OF THE BODY

One way to learn the significance of various symptomatic manifestations is to group the symptoms according to the part of the body affected. Take, for example, the symptoms of the head, among which are headache, heaviness of the head, heat in the head, and dizziness. Focusing on just one of these symptoms — headache — there are several varieties including frontal, vertex, temporal, and occipital. The point is to correlate the symptoms with particular meridians so that each symptom will serve both to indicate the pattern of imbalance, and to identify the meridians to be treated.

The correlation of symptoms with patterns and treatment is a skill which can be acquired through experience, but guidelines are helpful to the beginner. There are many textbooks which offer detailed classifications of symptoms according to the part of the body affected. Studying such texts is a very useful way to learn to differentiate among similar symptoms, and to identify the organs and meridians involved. A concise presentation is provided by Honma in his *Discourse on Meridian Therapy,* which is summarized below.

Symptoms of the Head

The head is known as the meeting place of the yang because all the yang meridians of the hands and feet reach the head. The yang Qi is thus very active in the head region, which is accordingly the part of the body that is most able to withstand cold. When there is an imbalance in the head, it tends to heat up, and in turn is soothed by cooling. The head is also the meeting place of the spirit and the five sensory organs, which are associated with the five yin organs. Through this association, the yin Qi reaches the head to communicate with the yang Qi.

Headaches may be caused by external pathogenic influences, or by deficiency of Qi or Blood. Headaches caused by external pathogenic influences are yang disorders, and those caused by Qi or Blood deficiency are yin disorders. Splitting headaches due to intracranial pathology such as meningitis are known as true headaches, and this type of headache cannot be treated by acupuncture.

Migraine headaches may be caused by external pathogenic influences, as well as by Qi or Blood deficiency. The pulse will usually reflect excess in the Liver, Gallbladder and/or Triple Burner meridians. Frontal headaches often result from excess in the Stomach and/or Large Intestine meridians, while occipital headaches are usually attributed to excess in the Bladder or Gallbladder meridians. One should always consider the pulse and other diagnostic findings in determining the appropriate treatment.

There are many causes and varieties of dizziness and vertigo, but most are related to the Liver meridian. Imbalances in this meridian must therefore be taken into account. Dizziness upon standing is commonly attributed to Kidney deficiency. Blood stasis is another major cause of dizziness, and many meridians may be involved.

Symptoms of the Face

All the yang meridians converge at the face. As part of the head, the face is likewise dominated by the yang Qi. Among the yang meridians, the Stomach meridian is most closely associated with the face. Thus, heat in the face is a sign of heat in the Stomach; conversely, coolness in the face is a sign of Stomach Qi deficiency. Symptoms which manifest on the face are generally associated with the yang brightness (Stomach and Large Intestine) meridians, hence the common use of LI-4 and S-36 for facial skin eruptions. Each of the five sensory organs on the face is associated with, and is the 'opening' for, one of the five yin organs of the body.

Symptoms of the Eyes

It is said that the multitude of the meridians meet at the eyes, which means that all of the meridians are in some manner connected with the eyes. Nevertheless, because the eyes are known as the 'opening' for the Liver, that organ should be considered first whenever there is an eye disease. When the Liver meridian is excessive, there will be eye strain or reddening, or an unusual glare in the patient's eyes. When the Liver meridian is deficient, eyesight tends to deteriorate. Different parts of the eye are said to reflect the condition of each of the yin organs. The iris represents the Liver, the inner and outer canthi the Heart, the upper eyelid the Spleen, the lower eyelid the Stomach, the sclera the Lung, and the pupil the Kidney.

Symptoms of the Ears

The ears are known as the 'opening' for the Kidneys, and the Kidney Qi governs the ears. Owing to their course, the Triple Burner, Small Intestine, and Gallbladder meridians also have a close association with the ears. Since the Kidneys govern the ears, excess and deficiency of the Kidney meridian affects the functioning of the ears. When wind-heat affects the Kidney meridian, the ears may become swollen and painful, and pus may exude from them. If these symptoms are accompanied by high fever, pain in the flanks, and a bitter taste in the mouth, wind-heat in the Gallbladder meridian is likely the cause. Loss of hearing is common in cases of Kidney deficiency, especially in chronic cases. Tinnitus is often caused by deficiency of the Kidney meridian, but deficiency of other meridians together with a general deficiency of Qi or Blood may also account for this symptom. Ear disorders are treated by addressing the deficiency or excess in the associated meridians.

Symptoms of the Nose

The nose is the 'opening' for the Lungs, and the Lung Qi governs the nose. Since the nose is the gateway to the Lungs and provides an opening for breathing, it is natural that imbalances of the Lungs would appear in and around the nose. Aside from the Lungs, the Stomach and Large Intestine meridians are also associated with the nose. When an external pathogenic influence affects the Lungs, there is copious nasal discharge, nasal congestion, and discomfort. Nasal polyps and papillomas are signs of heat in the Lungs. Epistaxis is often caused by stagnation of heat in the Stomach or Large Intestine meridians.

Symptoms of the Mouth, Lips, and Tongue

The mouth is the 'opening' for the Spleen, and the Qi of the Spleen is manifested in the lips. The health of the digestive organs is thus reflected in and around the mouth. In many instances, dryness of the mouth and bad breath are caused by heat in the Spleen and Stomach. Heat in the Liver produces a sour taste in the mouth.

Similarly, heat in the Spleen produces a sweet taste, in the Heart a burnt taste, in the Gallbladder a bitter taste, and in the Lungs a pungent taste. The lips reflect the health of the Spleen and Stomach. Dryness, cracking, or sores around the lips are signs of heat in the Spleen and Stomach meridians.

The tongue is the 'opening' for the Heart. Internal branches of the Heart, Spleen, and Kidney meridians extend upward to the tongue. A swollen tongue is a sign of wind-heat in the Heart and/or the Spleen. Damp-heat in the Spleen produces a thick, greasy coating on the tongue.

Symptoms of the Teeth

The teeth are traditionally thought of as being a product of surplus Kidney Qi. The course of the Large Intestine meridian provides a connection to the lower teeth, and the Stomach meridian to the upper teeth. Conversely, the Stomach meridian is connected to the lower gums, and the Large Intestine meridian to the upper gums. Pain and swelling of the gums is caused by wind-heat in either the Large Intestine or Stomach meridian. Teeth becoming loose and falling out is attributed to deficiency of Kidney Qi.

Symptoms of the Throat

The trachea is governed by the Lung Qi, and any symptom along the respiratory tract is thus associated with the Lung meridian. The symptoms of swelling and pain in the throat (tonsillitis) are usually related to imbalances in the Lungs or Large Intestine, and treating points on these meridians should be very effective.

Symptoms of the Neck and Shoulders

Among the many meridians which pass through the neck and shoulders are the Bladder, Gallbladder, Small Intestine, Large Intestine, and Triple Burner. Neck and shoulder stiffness and pain can result from stagnant Qi in any of these meridians, and treatment should therefore be rendered to facilitate the flow of Qi in the affected meridians. The practitioner who can alleviate all cases of shoulder tension is an expert indeed! Pain which extends downward from the neck to the shoulders and arms is caused by Qi blockage along the meridians. Although the use of strong stimulation (dispersing) at reactive points can be effective in such cases, this technique should be limited to patients with a yang constitution.

Symptoms of the Back

The spine is governed by the Bladder meridian and Governing vessel, but there are points associated with all the other organs and meridians at different levels of the spine. Also the Kidney meridian has a deep connection with the lumbar vertebrae and the sacrum. Lower back pain is a common condition, as is neck and shoulder tension. There are many factors which lead to lower back pain, but the most common cause is fatigue or strain of the musculoskeletal system. Such fatigue or strain is often a result of prolonged exposure to external pathogenic influences (such as wind, cold, and dampness) or deficiency of the Liver and Kidney meridians. The symptomatic manifestations of lower back pain will vary depending on which of the meridians is affected. When the Kidney and Bladder meridians are involved, the pain is dull and chronic and is accompanied by coldness in the lower back, hips, and lower limbs. When the Liver and Gallbladder meridians are involved, the pain (which may be either acute or chronic) extends downward from the flanks to the sides of the thighs. Involvement of the Lung and Large Intestine meridians indicates that the patient has been subjected to wind, and the pain is sudden and changeable. Sometimes lower back pain is caused by heat in the Stomach, which is characterized by fever and an insatiable appetite. The correlation between the pain or abnormality in the back and the affected meridians is made by careful examination of the pulse and abdomen.

Symptoms of the Chest

The chest houses the Heart and Lungs, which are governed by the pectoral Qi. The chest is also the passageway for food, and problems in the upper digestive tract often manifest as symptoms in the chest. Chest pain in traditional Oriental medicine can thus refer to sharp pain either in the epigastrium or in the chest. This includes pain from gastrospasms and ulcers as well as that from angina pectoris, which is traditionally known as 'true' Heart pain. Distention in the chest is a symptom that is common to imbalances of the Pericardium, Lung, Liver, and Gallbladder meridians. Palpitations or 'irritability in the chest' most often occurs with imbalances of the Heart, Pericardium, Spleen, or Kidneys. Palpitations due to yin deficiency are accompanied by dryness of the mouth and a sensation of heat in the chest and palms of the hands.

Symptoms of the Breasts

The yin Qi is dominant in the body of women, and since the yin Qi rises, the chest fills out and the genitals remain retracted. Conversely, in men it is the yang Qi which is dominant, and since the yang Qi descends, the chest remains flat while the genitals fill out. Problems with the mammary organs are viewed as a part of gynecological conditions. The mammary glands are governed by the Spleen and Stomach Qi. Insufficient lactation after childbirth may occur because of Qi and Blood deficiency, or because of an excess of Qi and Blood. In either case, imbalances in the Spleen and Stomach meridians should be treated. Mastitis is often due to external pathogenic influences, and the struggle between the normal and pathogenic Qi generates heat, which causes inflammation. The excess in the Stomach, Large Intestine, or Gallbladder should be dispersed.

Symptoms of the Hypochondria

The hypochondria are governed by the Liver and Gallbladder meridians which pass through this region together with the Spleen meridian. Hypochondriac pain is associated with both yin and yang disorders, but in either case, one should look for Liver and Gallbladder involvement. Pleuritis and intercostal neuralgia often involve both chest and hypochondriac pain. When they are caused by an invasion of an external pathogenic influence, an acute yang disorder arises, and when they are caused by deficiency, there will be a yin-type disorder. In yang-type disorders, there is often an underlying Lung deficiency together with excess of the Gallbladder.

Symptoms of the Abdomen

It is obvious that all the organs and meridians connect with the abdomen since the source of all Qi is in the lower abdomen. As previously noted, the texture of the abdominal wall is very important for diagnostic purposes. Since all the organs and meridians connect with the abdomen, abdominal pain can result from many causes. The location and quality of the pain must be assessed together with the pulse to determine which meridians are imbalanced. Masses or lumps in the abdomen appear when the Qi and Blood stagnate in one of the five yin organs over a long period of time. There are characteristic signs for masses associated with each of the yin organs. Those associated with the Liver are found in the left flank region and are accompanied by flank pain on both sides which extends to the lower abdomen. Masses associated with the Heart appear above the navel and are often accompanied by pain in the chest and a sensation of heat in the upper abdomen. Those associated with the Spleen are found just above the navel, and there is distention in the abdomen and discomfort after eating. Masses associated with the Lungs are found in the right flank region, and the skin is cool and dry. Masses associated with the Kidneys appear below the navel. These are often accompanied by acute attacks of sharp pain which extend upward to the chest. Such attacks generally occur on an empty stomach. Ascites is commonly related to imbalances in the Kidney meridian, and distention due to retention of gas is related to imbalances in the Spleen meridian.

Symptoms of the Extremities

The extremities are traditionally associated with the Triple Burner, and are said to be governed by the Stomach. This is because movement of the extremities generates heat in the body, which in turn promotes digestion. This is a very useful insight because, even if a patient is bedridden, exercising just the hands and feet will increase their appetite and digestion, and thereby facilitate the process of recuperation. Since the arms and legs are primarily responsible for all physical movement, they are subject to a correspondingly wide range of problems. The most common disorder is pain, but numbness and swelling can also cause difficulty in movement, and long-term paralysis can lead to atrophy. Pain as well as numbness and paresthesias result from blockage in the circulation of Qi and Blood. Paralysis may be caused by wind-stroke.

Symptoms of the Genital Region

The Liver meridian, together with the Conception and Governing vessels, are most closely associated with the genitals. Traditionally, the external genitalia are said to be governed by the Liver meridian, and the internal reproductive organs by the Kidney meridian. Problems with the male organs include impotence, priaprism, and lack of sensitivity in the penis. Treating the Liver and Kidney meridians and restoring the circulation of yang Qi is important. The erection of the genital organs is governed by the Liver; the Liver and Gallbladder meridians should therefore be treated for erectile disorders.

The hernial pain which is associated with the Liver meridian refers to a sharp pain in the lower abdomen which extends to the genitals. This includes inguinal hernias, since this disorder is characterized by a sharp, pulling pain that extends to the genitals. However, hernial pain in traditional Oriental medicine is a general term that encompasses prostate problems in men, as well as various gynecological disorders with lower abdominal pain, such as cystitis.

The anus is situated at the end of the Large Intestine, which is related to the Lungs by a yin-yang relationship. The course of the Bladder meridian and Governing vessel also connect with the anus. Anal prolapse is usually attributed to deficiency in the Lung and Kidney meridians. This disorder is best treated by using points on the Lung, Large Intestine, and Kidney meridians, together with points on the Governing vessel. Hemorrhoids are generally attributed to heat in the Small Intestine or Large Intestine, but there are many types of hemorrhoids, and each case must be independently assessed. There is often an imbalance in both the Lung and Large Intestine meridians. When this occurs this imbalance must be treated before providing symptomatic treatment for the hemorrhoids.

USE OF SYMPTOMOLOGY IN DETERMINING THE PATTERN

Each organ and meridian is associated with specific symptoms. When there is pathology in a certain organ or meridian, sometimes the associated symptoms will appear, and sometimes they won't. Moreover, there is no guarantee that only the symptoms associated with one organ or meridian will be present. The patient must be questioned about each of the symptoms to establish which organ or meridian imbalance is indicated. To determine the pattern of imbalance, all the symptoms must be assigned to an organ or meridian. The accuracy of such assignations must then be confirmed by means of other examinations, especially palpation of the pulse and abdomen.

> "When the body shows disease [symptoms] and the pulse is free of disease, [the patient] will live. When the pulse shows disease and the body is free of disease [symptoms], [the patient] will die." *(Classic of Difficulties,* chapter 11)

When the symptoms and the palpatory findings match, there is no problem. For example, if a patient with lower back pain has a Liver deficient pulse, the condition is easy to treat. However, when the symptoms and pulse do not correlate, the palpatory examination must be repeated to see if there is some mistake. If repeated examination still shows a discrepancy, the symptomatic manifestations are deemed to be inconsistent with the pattern of imbalance. Cases with marked discrepancies are difficult to cure. The closer the correlation of symptoms and palpatory findings, the better the patient will respond to treatment.

One way to become more familiar with the relationship between symptoms and patterns of imbalance is to guess what is wrong with the patient. Start by examining a patient without asking about his or her complaint. Then, based primarily on pulse and abdominal diagnosis, make an educated guess as to what complaints the patient has. Finally question the patient to confirm whether the symptoms correspond to what you perceived to be the pattern of imbalance. If you guessed correctly, it will increase your confidence in your diagnostic skills. And if you are mistaken, you will have an opportunity to reflect on the reasons for your mistake. After you become skilled at guessing symptoms based on the pulse and abdomen alone, you can then ask patients whether they have certain symptoms before they even tell you. For example, if you find that a patient has Spleen deficiency, you may ask if they have digestive problems. After awhile, you will be able to say with some confidence, "You have stomach trouble, don't you?" Usually you will be right, but there will be times when you are completely off the mark. Even though the patient may not have digestive problems, there may be other manifestations of a Spleen imbalance such as pain in the knee or big toe, arthritis, or gynecological problems.

There are certain conditions and findings which, through clinical experience, I have come to associate with particular meridian imbalances. These are things I find most frequently with the four basic patterns of yin meridian deficiency. These things cannot be used by themselves to determine a particular pattern, but instead are used to confirm the diagnosis of a pattern based upon examination of the pulse and abdomen.

Liver Meridian Deficiency

▶ History: Liver disease, heaviness of the head, eye problems, lower back pain, pain in the hip or knee joints, pain along the medial aspect of the leg, urogenital disorders

▶ Exam: tenderness or induration along the medial aspect of the knee; pain, tension, or tenderness in the right subcostal region; tenderness or induration at GV-20, GV-22, CV-4, Sp-6, Liv-8

Spleen Meridian Deficiency

▶ History: digestive problems, arthritis, gynecological disorders, insomnia

▶ Exam: thick, greasy tongue coating; discomfort or extreme ticklishness when examining the abdomen; tenderness or induration at CV-12, CV-14, Liv-13, Sp-8

Lung Meridian Deficiency

▶ History: respiratory problems such as wheezing or coughing; sore throat; a feeling of heat in the head, tension in the upper intrascapular region, shoulder pain, numbness in the arms, hemorrhoids, cold hands and feet

▶ Exam: pain, tension, or reduced range of motion in the neck and shoulders; tenderness or induration at G-20, G-21, B-13, B-43, GV-12, L-5

Kidney Meridian Deficiency

▶ History: Kidney disease, low blood pressure, dizziness upon standing, hearing loss, loss of libido, coldness below the waist

▶ Exam: sensitivity to percussion at B-23 and B-52; tenderness or induration at CV-7, CV-9, SI-19, K-7

Although there is no real need to guess a patient's symptoms since one can ask the patient to obtain all the necessary information, guessing nonetheless gives one a chance to test one's palpatory skills and knowledge of symptomology. It also prevents the practitioner from examining a patient with preconceived notions about which imbalance he is most likely to find. Preconceptions tend to bias the outcome of the examination. If the patient has lower back pain, we might suspect Liver or Kidney imbalance and therefore look for imbalances in these meridians. Strong preconceptions influence the findings, which often simply mirror our expectations. Refraining from asking the patient about symptoms until after the examination eliminates this bias. It may seem like a roundabout approach, but it does have its advantages.

So far I have listed the symptoms associated with the organs, meridians, and parts of the body. The assumption is that the correlation of symptoms with imbalances in particular organs or meridians recorded in the classics is basically valid. We can only hope that there is no error in this basic assumption. One of the editors asked me why I had listed coughing, wheezing, and heat in the face as symptoms which are associated with the Lung meridian. I was taken aback by this question. These symptoms are based on chapter 10 of *Vital Axis,* and if someone were to question the validity of what is in that classic, I have no good answer. Recently, however, some scholars have posed just such questions:

> "Symptoms of the organs and symptoms of the meridians are mixed together. [I'm sure] acupuncturists can utilize this information through their own experience, but this [symptomology] is not developed to the point of being explicable as a fully consistent and logical system." (Toyota, 1970)

> "Is chapter 10 of *Vital Axis* really in a completed form? When we reconsider the symptomology of the meridians, the order of Qi circulation through the meridians, the direction of the meridian flow, and their relationship to the organs [presented in this chapter], there seems to be a need to critically reexamine what is presented." (Shimada, 1980)

Based on my own clinical experience, I have found that the symptoms listed in chapter 10 of *Vital Axis* are valid for the most part. I hope that someday a modern version of symptomology will be compiled based on the experience and consensus of prominent contemporary practitioners.

How was the symptomology in the classics originally compiled? According to Fujiki Toshiro, author of *Thoughts on the Origins of Acupuncture Medicine,* the symptoms of the meridians and the symptoms of the organs developed separately and were blended together at the time that the *Vital Axis* was compiled. Perhaps the knowledge which had been orally transmitted in the past was recorded together with the experiences of the practitioners of that era. It can best be understood as a vast accumulation of empirical knowledge. It is certain that many things were added and revised over the course of history, as is reflected in the differences between the symptomologies recorded in the Ma Wang Tui manuscripts and the *Vital Axis.* Although it may be incomplete, the information is nonetheless valuable. The entire system of acupuncture, including the meridians and points, is based on thousands of years of experience. According to Fujiki, however, the symptomology of the meridians has undergone no significant revision or development since the compilation of the *Vital Axis*. If this is true, it would mean that a reexamination of the symptomology of the meridians has only been pursued since the start of the meridian therapy movement just half a century ago.

There are many other assumptions underlying the classical approach upon which meridian therapy is based besides the symptomology of meridians, and these too deserve careful reexamination. Meridian therapy is by no means a perfect system in every respect. Be that as it may, I am aware of no other system whose principles of diagnosis and treatment are as consistent, or is as effective, as meridian therapy. It is, moreover, a therapeutic system that is firmly grounded in the basic principles of Oriental medicine. I can therefore say without reservation that meridian therapy truly captures the essence of classical acupuncture.

DETERMINING THE PATTERN OF IMBALANCE

The primary objective of meridian therapy is to determine the pattern of Qi imbalance in the meridians, and to restore the balance. The pattern of imbalance is based upon the information obtained from the four examinations, including analysis of the etiology and symptomology, and the careful inspection of related acupuncture points.

Before proceeding any further, we should explore what the word 'pattern' means. As used in meridian therapy, it is a unique concept which is not easy to explain. The character for pattern, pronounced *shō* in Japanese and *zhèng* in Mandarin, means proof or evidence. Although this word is found in ancient texts, it does not appear in the earliest works of medicine, such as the *Classic of Difficulties*. The founders of meridian therapy used the word *shō* to denote the pattern of Qi imbalance in the meridians. Let us see how veteran practitioners of meridian therapy explain this term.

> "The signs and symptoms are the manifestations, and the primary pattern is the root. These are not in a cause and effect relationship." (Takeyama, 1965)

> "In terms of origin, I think the patterns were derived from groupings of disorders that were treatable by a particular method. They are therefore 'proof' that performing a certain treatment cures a given condition. I think the pattern is thus proven [by the effectiveness of the treatment]." (Maruyama, 1961)

These explanations are helpful, but still inadequate. There are many therapies other than meridian therapy in which certain treatments are prescribed for particular conditions.

> "The pattern is the main point or objective of a treatment and is deduced from the signs and symptoms." (Honma, 1949)

> "The patterns are neither a specific disease nor a name for a certain syndrome. They represent the essence of a pathological disorder and indicate the objective of treatment." (Fukushima, 1971)

> "The pattern is 'evidence' which means proof or confirmation. It is the evidence which is gathered from the four examinations of looking, listening, questioning, and touching to determine which treatment is indicated for the symptoms presented.

The pattern also denotes a certain grouping of symptoms which is reassembled from the [variety of] symptoms presented, such as headache, fever, chills, diarrhea, constipation, pain, vomiting, insomnia, or stiffness in the shoulders. The symptoms are extrapolated by specific rules and principles to define the objective of treatment. Therefore [the pattern] is something that can immediately be translated into actual treatment." (Okabe, 1974)

These explanations bring us closer to the meaning of pattern as used in meridian therapy, but there is still some room for further clarification. Based on the explanations above, we can say the following things about the term pattern as used in meridian therapy:

▶ It is not merely a group of symptoms or a syndrome.

▶ It is not a name for a specific disease.

▶ It represents the root of a pathological disorder.

▶ It is deduced from the four examinations.

▶ It represents the objective of treatment and indicates specifically what is to be done in treatment.

"Each sign and symptom is correlated one by one with the meridians, and the relationship of the deficiency and excess in the meridians, within [the framework of] the five phases, is determined to capture [the disorder] as a primary pattern. Each and every symptom is related to the meridians, and each one is associated with specific meridian imbalances. Treatment will not succeed if one merely deals with each individual symptom in its own right. One must capture the signs and symptoms in relationship to the meridians. This is why we [practitioners of meridian therapy] say that there is no pathological disorder which lies outside the bounds of the fourteen meridians." (Takeyama, 1944)

Given this perspective, we can add the following characteristics to our definition of the term pattern as used in meridian therapy:

▶ It is based on the association of symptoms to meridian imbalances.

▶ The symptomology of the organs and meridians is applied in determining the pattern.

In discussing patterns, some acupuncture texts mix in the patterns derived from herbal medicine *(kampō),* but these must not be confused with the patterns of meridian therapy. The patterns of herbal medicine were developed in the sixteenth century by the Kohō school of herbalists using a distinct form of abdominal diagnosis. These patterns are used specifically for selecting herbal formulas. The patterns of meridian therapy were developed in this century by applying the five-phase system of acupuncture described in the *Classic of Difficulties.* The patterns we are discussing here are meant to indicate how the meridians should be balanced with acupuncture using the methods of tonification and dispersion.

The four basic patterns in meridian therapy are the simplest expressions of the most common and fundamental types of imbalances in the meridians, all of which involve deficiency of Qi. One or another of these basic patterns can be utilized in every clinical situation. The four basic patterns are Liver deficiency, Spleen deficiency, Lung deficiency, and Kidney deficiency. Each of the four basic patterns represents a deficiency in a yin meridian which is rooted in a deficiency of Qi in the corresponding yin organ. The assumption which underlies meridian therapy is that all imbalances, no matter how complex, initially begin with deficiency in one of the yin organs that is reflected in its corresponding meridian. Thus, Qi deficiency in a yin organ and meridian is considered to lie at the root of all imbalances. The Heart is regarded as the most yang of the five yin organs; it is therefore thought to be predisposed toward excess rather than deficiency. Heart deficiency is accordingly not included among the basic patterns of meridian therapy since Heart deficiency is considered to be untreatable, as it is a stage of disease which precedes death.

In order to perform meridian therapy, it is necessary to determine the basic pattern, i.e., to arrive at a diagnosis of deficiency originating in a single yin organ and meridian. Naturally, one will encounter other patterns of greater complexity which represent imbalances in several organs and meridians. These other patterns, however, can always be viewed in terms of a more fundamental pattern of imbalance, which is one of the four basic deficiency patterns. Even though one of the four basic patterns of deficiency is always presumed to exist at the deepest level or root of the disorder, it is not always the primary focus of treatment. Deficiency of Qi in a yin organ can manifest as either yin meridian deficiency in those suffering from a yin disorder, or as yang meridian excess in those suffering from a yang disorder. Patterns of excess generally predominate in acute disorders, while patterns of deficiency are usually more significant in chronic disorders. Thus, the 'primary pattern' or main imbalance to be addressed at any particular stage of treatment can either be one of excess or deficiency.

> "As to which [meridian imbalance] should be regarded as the primary pattern, as long as there are no signs of deficiency, the yang pattern or excessive yang meridian is, as a rule, regarded as the primary pattern." (Honma, 1949)

In meridian therapy the process of forming a diagnosis is known as establishing the primary pattern. In the course of this process, the most deficient or excessive meridians are identified, and this leads to the selection of points with which to balance the Qi in the abnormal meridians. The points for the root treatment follow almost automatically once the primary pattern is identified. For this reason, meridian therapy is sometimes referred to as "treatment according to the pattern" *(zuishō ryōhō/suí zhèng liǎo fǎ)*. The findings from the four examinations, particularly those derived from palpation of the pulse and abdomen, are carefully evaluated in meridian therapy to determine which pattern is the root of the disorder.

Determining the basic pattern can actually be the most difficult part of meridian therapy. It takes knowledge and experience to sort through the many findings — which are often conflicting — to identify the most fundamental pattern of imbalance. As long as the pattern is correctly identified, the patient will show improvement even if treatment is not performed with optimal skill. If the wrong pattern is chosen, however, the most skillful of needling techniques will fail to bring any improvement. The crucial issue is therefore how to go about determining which is the primary pattern.

Although there may be more complex patterns of imbalance in the meridians involving interrelated excess and deficiency, in the beginning one need only concern oneself with the basic patterns. In meridian therapy, selecting among the four basic patterns of yin meridian deficiency greatly simplifies the matter. I will therefore explain the process of determining the basic pattern with its emphasis on yin meridian deficiency.

STEPS IN DETERMINING THE PATTERN OF IMBALANCE

Deficiency or Excess

The first and most important thing to be determined is whether the patient overall is deficient or excessive. One must therefore decide whether aspects of deficiency or of excess are predominant in a given situation. If the condition is one of general deficiency, the treatment should consist primarily of tonification, and if it is one of general excess, the treatment should consist more of dispersion. Although all the findings from the four examinations must be considered in determining whether a patient is deficient or excessive overall, the most important findings in this respect are those obtained from the looking examination, pulse palpation, and abdominal diagnosis.

▶ Looking: How is the patient's spirit? Does the skin have a healthy tone? In general, does the patient seem to have vitality?

▶ Pulse: The pulse quality is important in determining the overall level of vitality. Check whether the pulse quality in general is deficient or excessive. If the pulse is weak and deficient, emphasize tonification. If the pulse is strong and excessive, emphasize dispersion, but be sure to confirm an excessive condition with other findings.

▶ Abdomen: Check the resiliency of the patient's abdomen, particularly the lower abdomen. Patients who appear robust but have a weak pulse and a mushy lower abdomen should be treated as if deficient, just to be on the safe side. The use of dispersion and strong needle techniques just because a patient has a strong pulse will often exacerbate the problem. Keep the stimulation light, especially during the root treatment.

There are many other aspects to consider in determining whether a patient is deficient or excessive overall, but one should, at the very least, make a habit of checking the above three points.

Acute or Chronic

The second step is to determine whether the disease is new or old. Conditions of recent origin are easier to treat. It is usually sufficient to treat one or two meridians, and in many cases, yang meridians are dispersed. Chronic cases are usually more complicated, as the original imbalance affects other meridians in accordance with the controlling relationships of the five phases. If the problem begins in the Lung meridian, for example, the imbalance will typically spread to the Liver meridian, and from the Liver meridian to the Spleen meridian. It then involves three or more meridians. Such cases are, of course, very difficult to treat. Symptoms are generally more severe in acute cases, and turn milder as the condition becomes chronic. Tonification of the yin meridians is essential in treating chronic disorders.

Etiology

The original cause of the disease, whether internal or external, must be considered in diagnosing the pattern. Among the internal causes are the emotions and irregularities in diet and life-style. Conditions resulting from disharmony of the emotions, irregularities in diet and life-style, or fatigue are yin in nature, and the deficient yin meridian must therefore be treated. Traditionally, all diseases are assumed to have an underlying internal cause, and this is why tonification of the yin meridians is given more emphasis in meridian therapy. The external causes of disease are the external pathogenic influences which originate in the natural environment. Conditions resulting from these influences in the environment are yang in nature, particularly at the onset. An excessive condition due to pathogenic influences will first affect the yang meridians, which must therefore be dispersed. If the appropriate treatment is not rendered during the early stages of a yang condition of external origin, the imbalance will affect the yin meridians and eventually produce a yin disorder.

> "With patients engaged in manual labor, question them carefully about appetite, sleep, and excretions. If there is a problem with any of these three, the illness is due to internal causes. In cases where a laborer has no problems whatever with these three things but does complain of back pain, shoulder pain, or localized pain along a meridian, the illness is due to injury or fatigue. The [treatment of] deficiency is central in those conditions due to internal factors. The [treatment of] excess is central in those conditions due to external factors." (Inoue, 1961)

Meridians Involved

The next step is to evaluate the symptoms in relation to the course of the meridians to determine which meridian each symptom is associated with. Pain in the thumb, for example, is associated with the Lung meridian, and in some cases, with the Large Intestine meridian. Other symptoms have more complex associations. Tinnitus, for example, is associated not only with the Kidney, but also with the Gallbladder, Small Intestine, and Triple Burner meridians, since all of them reach the ear. Meridian involvement must be considered from all possible angles. Knowledge of the internal as well as the external pathways of the meridians is therefore essential. A thorough knowledge of the meridians and points is an obvious prerequisite for all who practice acupuncture.

Organs Involved

The final step is to evaluate the symptoms in accordance with the symptomology of the organs, especially the five yin organs. The symptoms of coughing, wheezing, and heat in the head, for example, are symptoms associated with the Lungs.

EXTENT OF IMBALANCE

Imbalances in One Meridian

If the pattern simply involves deficiency in one meridian, tonification of that meridian should suffice. Similarly, if there is but one excessive meridian, dispersion of that meridian is all that is required. These are the simplest cases, but in practice,

I rarely give such treatments. It is my belief that every patient who comes into the clinic has some constitutional imbalance or internal disharmony. Therefore, even if a patient has only an excessive Large Intestine meridian in the initial stages of a cold, I take the treatment a step further and tonify the Lung meridian (which is coupled with the Large Intestine meridian in a yin-yang pair) as well as the Spleen meridian (which is the mother of the Lung in the five-phase system). In my experience, better results can be obtained in treating excessive patterns by also treating the yin meridians. I think that this is what is meant by treating "incipient diseases" *(mi byō/wéi bìng)* in the *Classic of Difficulties*. I also think that it is more effective to treat a set of meridians as an interrelated group than to treat one meridian alone.

Imbalances in Paired Yin and Yang Meridians

In cases where the yin meridian is deficient and its paired yang meridian is excessive, first tonify the yin meridian and then disperse the yang meridian. For example, if the Lung is deficient and the Large Intestine is excessive, first tonify the Lung and then disperse the Large Intestine. It is very uncommon for a yin meridian to be excessive when its paired yang meridian is deficient.

Imbalances in Meridians in a Controlling Relationship

When two yin meridians in a controlling relationship of the five phases are deficient and excessive respectively, one must decide which of the patterns is primary. For example, if the Lung is deficient and the Liver is excessive, either the deficient Lung or the excessive Liver can be regarded as the primary pattern. It is said that practitioners who prefer aggressive treatment tend to view patterns which are combinations of deficiency and excess primarily as excessive patterns and emphasize dispersion, while practitioners who have a soft touch tend to focus on tonifying the deficiency. Practitioners, being human, are often biased in their evaluation of the relative importance of deficiency or excess as the primary pattern. I personally feel that it is wise to play it safe and treat the deficient meridian as the primary pattern. Even if you are mistaken, there is less harm done when tonification is performed first. One can then disperse the excessive meridian after the deficient meridian has been tonified.

Imbalances in Meridians in a Generating Relationship

When two yin meridians in a generating relationship of the five phases are both deficient, the 'child' meridian is regarded as the primary pattern of deficiency. For example, if both the Kidney and Liver meridians are deficient, the Liver deficiency takes priority, and the Liver meridian is accordingly tonified (Illustration 4-1). This is the most effective approach because to tonify the Liver meridian, the Kidney meridian (which is its 'mother') must also be tonified. Conversely, when two yin meridians in a generating relationship are both excessive, the mother meridian is regarded as the primary pattern of excess. For example, if both the Heart and Liver meridians are excessive, the Liver excess takes priority, and the Liver meridian is dispersed (Illustration 4-2). Here as well, dispersion of the Liver meridian will necessarily involve dispersion of points on the Heart or Pericardium meridian.

LIVER DEFICIENCY

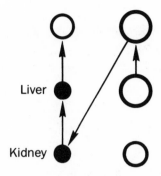

LIVER EXCESS

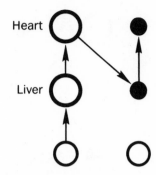

Illustration 4-1
Pulse Findings with Deficiency of Two Yin
Meridians in a Generating Relationship

Illustration 4-2
Pulse Findings with Excess of Two Yin
Meridians in a Generating Relationship

Deficiency of Three Meridians in a Generating Relationship

Theoretically, three meridians in a generating relationship should not all be deficient, but sometimes the pulse shows three deficient meridians and one must then decide which meridian is to be regarded as the primary deficiency. If the symptoms and other findings relate predominantly to one of the deficient meridians, this meridian can be treated as the primary deficiency. When it is not so clear, the most deficient meridian pair should be ascertained. For example, when the Spleen, Lung, and Kidney meridians are all deficient, the primary pattern is determined by closely examining the course of these meridians on the arms and legs to see if the deficiency is more pronounced in the Spleen and Lung (Lung deficiency), or in the Lung and Kidney (Kidney deficiency). The meridian with the most abnormal palpatory findings is considered to be the primary deficiency. In this example, since Lung meridian deficiency may be associated with either Lung or Kidney deficiency, it is appropriate to look for differences along the course of the Spleen and Kidney meridians. If there are more abnormalities along the Spleen meridian, the primary pattern is one of Lung deficiency. If there are more abnormalities along the Kidney meridian, the primary pattern is one of Kidney deficiency.

Another way to determine the basic pattern is to tonify the deficient meridian which is in the middle in accordance with the generating cycle of the five phases. This is done by tonifying the intrinsic point on that meridian, because that is the only one of the five-phase points that has no direct influence on any other meridian. In the above example, it is the Lung meridian that is between the Spleen and Kidney meridians in the generating cycle. Accordingly, this meridian would be tonified by inserting a needle superficially at L-8, the intrinsic point of the Lung meridian. This should strengthen the pulse at either the Spleen or Kidney position. If the Spleen pulse becomes stronger, it may be concluded that Kidney deficiency is more significant since the Kidney and Lung meridians are most deficient. Conversely, if the Kidney pulse becomes stronger, Lung deficiency is regarded as the basic pattern since the Lung and Spleen meridians are most deficient (Illustration 4-3)

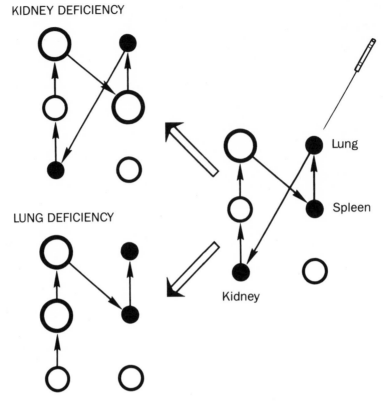

KIDNEY DEFICIENCY

LUNG DEFICIENCY

Lung

Spleen

Kidney

Illustration 4-3
Needling to Determine Which Deficient Meridian to Treat

The diagram below illustrates the factors involved in determining the primary pattern and rendering the root treatment in meridian therapy (Illustration 4-4).

PRACTICAL EXAMPLES OF DETERMINING THE PATTERN OF IMBALANCE

One of the best ways to understand the process of determining the pattern of imbalance is to look at case histories. This will also illustrate how meridian therapy is performed, and prepare the reader for the discussion of treatment which follows in the next chapter.

CASE 1: MALE, 33 YEARS OLD

Chief complaint: For two days the patient had a high fever together with severe diarrhea and slight, recurring abdominal pain. There was also some lower back pain due to staying in bed all day.

Looking: face flushed from fever, a good physique

Pulse: floating, rapid, and slightly wiry

Yin meridians: Spleen and Lung deficient, Liver excessive

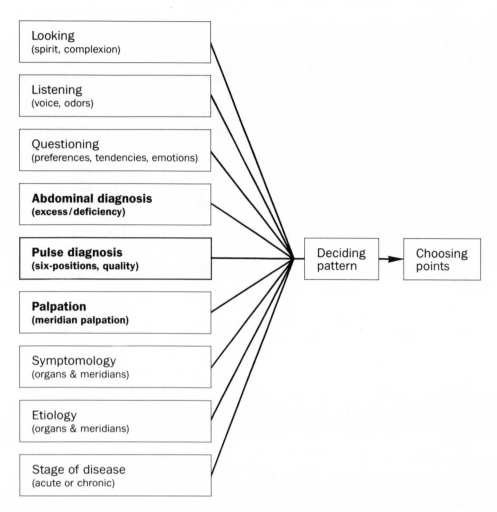

Illustration 4-4
Process of Diagnosis and Treatment

Yang meridians: Large Intestine deficient, Gallbladder excessive

Abdomen: The abdomen was generally firm and resilient. Only the area around CV-6 was a little weak. There was slight tenderness at S-25 and tenderness at L-1.

Palpation: There was a strong reaction along the course of the Lung and Large Intestine meridians, especially between LI-7 and LI-11. There was no reaction along the Small Intestine meridian, but tenderness and induration was found at G-38 on the left side.

Correlation of Symptoms:

▶ The fever was related to the Heart and Lung meridians.

▶ The diarrhea was related to the Lung, Large Intestine, and Spleen meridians.

▶ The lower back pain was related to the Liver and Gallbladder meridians.

▶ The basic pattern was Lung deficiency based on the pulse and other palpatory findings.

Treatment: Because diagnosis is the focus of our discussion, only the outline of the treatment plan will be provided. The Lung and Spleen meridians were tonified. This was followed by tonification of the Large Intestine meridian. Instead of dispersing the Liver and Gallbladder meridians, Small Intestine meridian and abdominal points were slightly dispersed.

Result: The patient's appetite returned after treatment and he was able to eat a full meal. The fever subsided in two hours. The other symptoms also subsequently improved. (Illustration 4-5)

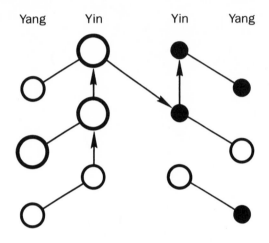

Illustration 4-5
Pulse Findings for Case 1

CASE 2: FEMALE, 77 YEARS OLD

Chief complaint: The patient had pain in the left knee for about a month. Her right knee was also a bit painful due to compensating for the left leg. Pain in the knee was most pronounced when standing up from a seated position, and there was also some pain when walking. The mouth was dry. Bowel movements occurred every day, but with some discomfort. She had tension and stiffness in the neck and shoulders, together with tension in the back (around B-18). She had been diagnosed with cerebral infarction and subsequent necrosis of brain tissue a few years earlier, and had made regular hospital visits since that time.

Looking: The patient's complexion was fair and her skin had luster. Her complexion was a little pale with a slight reddish hue.

Pulse: This patient had a hard pulse typical of arteriosclerosis in the elderly. This quality was especially marked on the left side.

Yin meridians: Initially the Lung position seemed weak, but careful palpation of the pulse at the deep level showed the Kidney and Liver positions to be the weakest.

Yang meridians: The Bladder and Gallbladder positions were excessive, and the excess was particularly marked at the Bladder position.

Abdomen: The abdomen was soft overall. A soft abdomen is not necessarily a sign of ill health among the elderly, for whom a soft abdomen is generally considered to be better than a hard one. The flank region was lacking in resiliency, especially on the left side. There was a pulsation at S-25 on the left side.

Meridian Palpation: Comparing the Lung and Pericardium meridians on the arm, the Pericardium had more tenderness. The lower limbs were unremarkable. Induration and tenderness were found at B-18 and G-20 on the left side.

Local Examination: Tenderness was found just medial to M-LE-16 *(du bi)*. This seemed to be a case of degenerative joint disease.

Correlation of Symptoms:

▶ The knee pain was related to the Liver meridian.

▶ The lower back pain was related to the Liver, Gallbladder, and Bladder meridians.

▶ The shoulder tension was related to the Gallbladder meridian.

▶ The dryness of the mouth and discomfort in bowel movements was related to the Spleen meridian.

▶ The basic pattern was one of Liver deficiency based on the pulse and abdomen.

Treatment: Tonification of the Liver and Kidney meridians followed by dispersion of the Bladder, Gallbladder, and Stomach meridians. (Illustration 4-6)

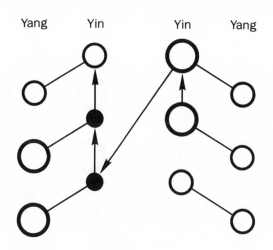

Yang   Yin   Yin   Yang

Illustration 4-6
Pulse Findings for Case 2

CASE 3: MALE, 31 YEARS OLD

Symptoms: Stomach upset and stiffness in the neck and shoulders. There was a lack of appetite, but no diarrhea, and a sensation of heaviness in the head.

Looking: The patient had a thin build, but appeared to have strength.

Pulse: floating, slow, and slightly wiry

Yin meridians: Initially it seemed as if the pulses on the left side were stronger than the right. Careful palpation at the deep level, however, revealed that the Liver and Kidney positions were the weakest.

Yang meridians: The Bladder and Gallbladder positions were strong at the superficial level.

Abdomen: The patient had a typical abdomen for a thin, generally deficient type. The rectus abdominis muscle was tense and rigid, and the flank region and linea alba was depressed. By pressing S-25 on both sides, the left side was found to be more tender.

Correlation of Symptoms:

► The upset stomach and heaviness of the head related to the Liver, Gallbladder, and Bladder meridians.

► The stiffness in the neck and shoulders related to the Gallbladder and Bladder meridians.

► It was difficult to determine whether the basic pattern was one of Liver or Lung deficiency. I therefore inserted needles very superficially at L-9, and left them in place to see the reaction. I then pressed L-1 and Liv-14 and found tenderness at Liv-14 on the right. Pressing the medial aspect of the arms, I found tenderness at P-4 on the left forearm. Reexamining the pulse, the deficiency at the Kidney and Liver positions, as well as the excess at the Gallbladder and Bladder positions, was much clearer. On the back there was also tenderness and induration at B-18. I therefore concluded that Liver deficiency was the basic pattern.

Treatment: Tonification of the Liver and Kidney meridians, followed by dispersion of the Bladder and Gallbladder meridians. (Illustration 4-7)

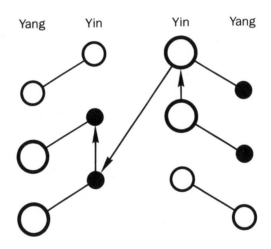

Yang   Yin   Yin   Yang

Illustration 4-7
Pulse Findings for Case 3

Comment: This case is that of a longtime patient who comes in for treatment whenever stress and fatigue cause an upset stomach, loss of appetite, and diarrhea. I usually treat him for Lung deficiency, but sometimes his pattern changes to one of Liver or Kidney deficiency. In this instance he did not have diarrhea, but only the symptoms of an upset stomach and heaviness of the head. The final determination of his pattern was based on the reexamination of the pulse after a test insertion. A comparison of just the deep levels of the pulse can lead to mistakes. A clear difference between the strength of the pulse in one position at the deep and superficial levels (strong at one level and weak at another) is a reliable sign that the imbalance is to be found in that pair of meridians.

The pattern of imbalance is determined for each case in just the manner I have described. Sometimes the patient is thoroughly examined before the pattern is determined, but I generally tend to make a quick decision. The pattern usually becomes apparent after a brief examination of the pulse and a quick look at the abdomen. Although it is not always so easy or quick, I waste little time with the decision when I am busy. It is just simpler to make the determination within a limited time frame. I tend to become indecisive when I am not so busy, or when I take the time to examine the patient meticulously. One must also avoid prejudging the pattern. If you examine a patient thinking that he is Lung deficient, the findings will be biased in favor of this belief. To avoid any preconception, I will occasionally examine a patient before asking him anything about his physical condition. Regardless of how you go about determining the pattern, it is always the most crucial and difficult part of meridian therapy.

More case histories are presented in chapter 6 which further demonstrate how I determine the pattern. The reader should be advised, however, that these cases simply show how I have diagnosed and treated patients in the past. They are by no means ideal examples. Although it is certainly possible to conceive of more complex patterns that involve simultaneous deficiency and excess, I am generally satisfied to determine the basic pattern, and leave the issue of dispersion of excess for later. I find that it is enough in most cases to tonify the deficient meridians first, and then to disperse just those meridians which are still excessive. Leaving the treatment of excessive meridians to the end often reduces the need for dispersion.

Although there is certainly room for improvement in my diagnostic method, there are, as previously noted, different levels of skill in practicing meridian therapy, yet every practitioner can still utilize this approach irrespective of his level of competence. Beginners can expect results at a beginner's level. This book is intended as an introduction to meridian therapy, and I have therefore presented the simplest and most straightforward approach. There are a number of master practitioners of meridian therapy in Japan, and I must admit that I am far from being a master. But I am working diligently to get as close as I can to that level of expertise. And I am confident that my step-by-step approach, which is reflected in the case histories, as well as the personal difficulties which I have experienced in learning meridian therapy, will be instructive to others who wish to learn meridian therapy.

In any event, my approach to diagnosis and treatment should not be viewed as a completely orthodox approach to the practice of meridian therapy. The reader is advised to study the classics and to observe master practitioners for himself. In one important respect, however, my method is always in conformity with the rules set forth by the originators of meridian therapy: determination of the pattern is based primarily on six-position pulse diagnosis. This is the fundamental rule in meridian therapy; all the information drawn from the other methods of examination should be used to confirm or clarify the findings obtained from the pulse.

> "In order to determine the primary pattern, there are the four examinations, but within these there is the root and there are the branches. Pulse diagnosis is the

root and the other examinations are the branches. Even if a certain grouping of symptoms is found through looking, listening, and questioning, it is very difficult to put them together in a uniform pattern [without the pulse findings]. It would be ideal if this could be done, but it is difficult to do so in practice ... In meridian therapy, pulse diagnosis is the foundation and the other findings are secondary. To determine the basic pattern, such as Lung or Kidney deficiency, the pulse is used as the deciding factor. Other findings can be used for selecting points during treatment. ... It is therefore extremely difficult to establish [the existence of] deficiency or excess in certain meridians based on signs and symptoms alone without the pulse findings." (Okabe, 1944)

KEY POINTS

Generalities

- Each organ and meridian is associated with certain symptoms.

- Question the patient about his symptoms and correlate these with imbalances in the meridians.

- When the pulse is consistent with the symptoms, the condition is easy to treat; when it is inconsistent, the condition is difficult to treat.

- Because the pulse is the most important factor in determining the pattern of imbalance, when the pulse and symptoms do not match, treatment is primarily based on the pulse.

- The symptoms are used primarily to confirm the basic pattern, which is discerned from palpation of the pulse and abdomen.

- The pattern of imbalance is not merely a grouping of symptoms, but the essence of a disorder.

- All signs and symptoms can be attributed to specific imbalances in the meridians.

- One way to develop one's diagnostic skills is to conduct a "no-question examination."

- The method of treatment is selected once the pattern of imbalance has been determined.

Specifics

- The most important aspect in determining the pattern of imbalance is whether the patient overall is excessive or deficient, and this is based on the presence of spirit and palpation of the pulse and abdomen.

- Acute disorders are usually associated with excess in the yang meridians, and chronic disorders with deficiency in the yin meridians.

- Disorders attributed to external causes tend to be associated with excess in the yang meridians, while those attributed to internal causes are associated with deficiency in the yin meridians.

- Imbalances between paired yin and yang meridians are generally regarded as excessive yang. In treating such disorders, however, first tonify the yin meridian, then disperse the yang meridian.

- When two yin meridians in a generating relationship are deficient, the 'child' meridian is regarded as the deficient meridian. When two yin meridians in a generating relationship are excessive, the 'mother' meridian is regarded as the excessive meridian.

5

Root Treatment and Symptomatic Treatment

In meridian therapy the terms root treatment and symptomatic treatment are constantly used. What exactly do these terms mean? Let us begin with a careful examination of their meaning and relative importance in meridian therapy.

"Root treatment is performed in accordance with the pattern of the disease, and symptomatic treatment in accordance with the symptoms of the disease. The first priority is to correct the abnormal relationships of deficiency and excess among the meridians. To do this we must determine the overall picture of the disease known as the pattern by identifying and analyzing those relationships of deficiency and excess among the meridians and organs that are abnormal, and those that are not." (Yamashita, 1971)

"Root treatment is the [aspect of] treatment in which the imbalances in the meridians, which are the essence of the disease, are corrected by tonification and dispersion using the five-phase points and the five essential points. Symptomatic treatment is the [aspect of] treatment rendered according to the [manifestations of] disease and the complaints of the patient by treating localized areas." (Fukushima, 1979)

"Root treatment is the correction of imbalances in the meridians by using the essential points on the four limbs in accordance with the primary pattern, which is derived from various [methods of] diagnosis and analysis of the symptomology. Symptomatic treatment is performed simultaneously in accordance with the symptoms by directly tonifying or dispersing reactive points or acupuncture points

151

[resulting] from the imbalances. There are, of course, cases in which the symptoms are relieved by root treatment alone. In such cases, symptomatic treatment is unnecessary. However, in most situations these two [aspects of] treatment are equally important and necessary." (Takeyama, 1944)

These passages reveal the following things about root and symptomatic treatment: **1.** Root treatment is performed in accordance with the pattern, which is determined from the diagnosis. **2.** The five-phase points are used in root treatment. **3.** Imbalances in the meridians are corrected with root treatment. **4.** Symptomatic treatment is performed in accordance with to the symptoms. **5.** Local points and points connected with the symptoms are treated by symptomatic treatment. **6.** The symptoms that are not alleviated by root treatment are treated by symptomatic treatment.

It should be emphasized that both root and symptomatic treatment are necessary and important. No authority on meridian therapy claims that treatment of localized areas is unnecessary. Sometimes local, symptomatic treatment may even have a beneficial effect on the balance of Qi in the body as a whole. The only real difference between meridian therapy and the conventional approaches to acupuncture in Japan is that root treatment is performed to balance the body energetically before the specific symptoms are treated. Symptomatic treatment is of course rendered in practically all approaches to acupuncture. The distinctive feature of meridian therapy is that root treatment comes first. There is a misconception among some in the Japanese acupuncture community that practitioners of meridian therapy believe that root treatment is *all* that is necessary, but the truth is that symptomatic treatment is by no means neglected in meridian therapy.

Be that as it may, in the absence of root treatment, the use of symptomatic or local treatment will be less effective. There are considerable differences of opinion among practitioners of meridian therapy regarding just how important root treatment is relative to symptomatic treatment. Some believe that root treatment takes care of 70-80% of the symptoms, and that the remaining 20-30% are dealt with by symptomatic treatment. Others believe that while root treatment corrects imbalances of Qi in the meridians, it is not immediately effective in ameliorating the symptoms. For this reason they believe that specific symptoms must be treated separately with symptomatic treatment. Finally, some practitioners believe that root and symptomatic treatment are of equal value.

Some question the distinction between root and symptomatic treatment on the basis that some practitioners of meridian therapy actually spend more time on symptomatic treatment. These critics say that symptomatic treatment is necessary because practitioners of meridian therapy lack confidence in the effectiveness of root treatment. This is a sore point, especially for those who are new to meridian therapy. Nevertheless, based on my own experience I can say with certainty the following about the relationship between root and symptomatic treatment: **1.** When the proper root treatment is administered, functional abnormalities of the visceral organs and discomfort in the head often disappear with just a few needles. **2.** When root treatment is totally ineffective, either the pattern has been misdiagnosed, or the needling technique is incorrect. One should therefore reexamine the pulse and the abdomen, or repeat the same treatment with much shallower needle insertion. **3.** When the condition is caused by simple imbalances in one meridian without any internal cause, such as a sprain of the lower back, sometimes root treatment alone is completely effective, and at other times it is totally useless in reducing the pain. I have had cases in which root treatment alone alleviated lower back pain only to have it return with a vengeance as soon as the patient stepped out of my office. When localized structural damage reaches a certain order of magnitude, it is unlikely that root treatment can cure the problem instantly. Even if this were possible, it goes against the spirit of meridian therapy to aim for quick cures. **4.** Although root treatment alone may be sufficient to relieve the symptoms, it does not go over so well in Japan to use only a few needles. This is because most Japanese patients equate a larger number of needles with a more thorough treatment.

When it comes to symptomatic treatment, there is practically no limit to the variety of approaches and techniques that can be employed. Symptomatic treatment is an area in which every practitioner can display his own talent and unique skills. Each of us must spend a lifetime developing our own treatment style. Although this may sound a bit nebulous, there are a few important considerations to keep in mind in providing symptomatic treatment: **1.** The overall deficient or excessive condition of the patient must be considered, and care must be exercised not to exceed the optimal amount of stimulation (discussed at greater length later in this chapter). **2.** The depth of insertion must be kept shallow for those patients with a floating pulse. **3.** The deficient or excessive nature of the area being treated must be noted, and tonified or dispersed accordingly. Generally speaking, tonification techniques are applied first and then followed, when necessary, by dispersion. **4.** Treatment should be confined to a few key areas associated with the chief complaint, palpatory findings, and the pattern so that the patient is not overtreated. After a certain point, the more a person is treated, the less effective it becomes.

The concepts of root and symptomatic treatment were redefined with the advent of meridian therapy. The classics mention treatment of the root (*honji/běn zhì*) and treatment of the manifestation or branch (*hyōji/biāo zhì*), but this is generally just a matter of emphasis, rather than two distinct aspects of treatment. Root treatment is emphasized so much in meridian therapy because the majority of practitioners in Japan are only concerned with symptoms and the stimulation of tender points. Since root treatment in acupuncture is a unique approach introduced with meridian therapy, it is naturally presented as the more important aspect of treatment. All practitioners of meridian therapy agree that root treatment comes first, and symptomatic treatment second. With this understanding, the principal feature of meridian therapy — root treatment — will now be discussed.

A SIMPLIFIED APPROACH TO MERIDIAN THERAPY

As noted in the last chapter, the most difficult part of meridian therapy is to determine the primary pattern. Once the pattern has been identified, there is no need to be overly concerned about the quality of treatment. Even if the needling technique is somewhat poor, as long as the correct pattern is treated, the patient will eventually improve. Mastery of technique merely accelerates this process. Looking back on my own experience with meridian therapy, I recall there was a great deal of trial and error, and at times I had my doubts about this approach based on the classics. However, as I persevered in mastering this system, it became clear to me that there were simply a few secrets to effective needling technique and point location. It took me some time to reach this conclusion, but today I am convinced of the validity of this approach based on the classics. I may have arrived at this conclusion in a roundabout way, but I am thankful for all the detours since all of them, in one way or another, contributed to my learning. I have always had a rather simple mind and therefore never could master all the levels and complexities of meridian therapy in a short time. As I explained in an earlier chapter in connection with my approach to pulse diagnosis, I mastered the different components of meridian therapy one step at a time. Some people may think that this approach oversimplifies meridian therapy. But in all fields of learning, beginner's texts must be simple and understandable. If the textbook is too difficult from the start, most people will not be able to follow it.

When I learned German on my own, I bought a good, standard beginner's text. The book was fun to read, and reading the stories and jokes gradually increased my vocabulary. I became enthusiastic and bought an intermediate German text that looked interesting. But to my dismay, I found this text to be way over my head. Through this experience I learned that it is important to progress slowly and surely in small steps when learning something new. The best way to attain a goal is to start small and to keep building on small accomplishments. The most distant goal is attainable if small steps are taken patiently over a long period. The time it takes to reach the goal of mastering meridian therapy may vary according to an individual's innate ability and past experience. Be that as it may, I think everyone can master the basics in about five years. Those who are fast should be able to do it in three, and slower people may take up to ten years. But no matter how long it takes, the benefits of meridian therapy can still be appreciated at each stage.

I explained how to find the most deficient meridian in chapter 3, and how to determine the primary pattern in chapter 4. The problem now is how to deal with the yin meridian deficiency that has been identified. This is the essence of meridian therapy. It has already been noted that once the pattern becomes evident, the method of treatment will be clear. That is, the primary pattern leads directly to the treatment principle, which in turn leads to specific points for producing the desired effect. Each meridian has key points with special functions known as the five-phase points. To perform meridian therapy, it is essential that one have a clear understanding of these points. I will therefore explain the theory and rationale for selecting specific five phase-points in meridian therapy.

FIVE-PHASE POINTS AND THEIR APPLICATION

In *Discourse on Meridian Therapy* acupuncture points are divided into four categories: **1.** essential points that exist for all meridians; **2.** essential points that are not specific to any particular meridian; **3.** meridian points other than the essential points; and **4.** miscellaneous points and Ahshi points known through experience.

The first category includes the five-phase points[1] *(go gyō ketsu/wǔ shū xüe)* and the five essential points *(go yō ketsu/wǔ yào xüe)*. The points in this category are the most important in meridian therapy for performing root treatment. The second category includes points that have specific effects on certain tissues or aspects of the body, such as the eight influential points and the eight confluent points of the extraordinary vessels. The third and fourth categories of points should require no explanation.

The five-phase points and the five essential points are ten important points that are found in common on each of the twelve meridians. The five essential points are the source *(gen/yuán)*, connecting *(raku/luò)*, accumulating *(geki/xì)*, alarm *(bo/mù)*, and associated *(yu/shù)* points (Table 5-1). These points primarily affect only the meridian with which they are associated. For example, needling L-6, the accumulating point of the Lung, primarily affects the Lung meridian. Therefore, tonification of L-6 tonifies only the Lung meridian, and dispersion of L-6 only disperses the Lung meridian.

	Source	Connecting	Accumulating	Alarm	Associated
Liver	Liv-3	Liv-5	Liv-6	Liv-14	B-18
Heart	H-7	H-5	H-6	CV-14	B-15
Pericardium	P-7	P-6	P-4	CV-17	B-14
Spleen	Sp-3	Sp-4, Sp-21	Sp-8	Liv-13	B-20
Lung	L-9	L-7	L-6	L-1	B-13
Kidney	K-3	K-4	K-5	G-25	B-23
Gallbladder	G-40	G-37	G-36	G-24	B-19
Small Intestine	SI-4	SI-7	SI-6	CV-4	B-27
Triple Burner	TB-4	TB-5	TB-7	CV-5	B-22
Stomach	S-42	S-40	S-34	CV-12	B-21
Large Intestine	LI-4	LI-6	LI-7	S-25	B-25
Bladder	B-64	B-58	B-63	CV-3	B-28

Table 5-1 Five Essential Points

The five-phase points are the well *(sei/jǐng)*, spring or gushing *(ei/yíng)*, stream or transporting *(yu/shū)*, river or traversing *(kei/jīng)*, and the sea or uniting *(gō/hé)* points (Table 5-2). In meridian therapy the five-phase points are the most important for tonification and dispersion. Just as there is yang within yin and yin within yang, all of the five phases exist within each of the five phases. Accordingly, the five-phase points on a meridian connect or resonate with the Qi in those meridians associated with the other phases. Taking the Liver meridian as an example, the Heart Qi connects with Liv-2, the Spleen Qi with Liv-3, the Lung Qi with Liv-4, and the Kidney Qi with Liv-8. This is a fascinating concept by which all of the meridian have points where the Qi from other meridians can be accessed.

In *Discourse on Meridian Therapy* the analogy of embassies is used to illustrate the five-phase points. This is a brilliant idea by Honma that clearly demonstrates the role of the five-phase points in each meridian. The five major governmental

[1]Here, as elsewhere in the book, the transliteration of the term in Japanese is followed by that in Mandarin.

	Well (Wood)	Spring (Fire)	Stream (Earth)	River (Metal)	Sea (Water)
Liver	Liv-1	Liv-2	Liv-3	Liv-4	Liv-8
Heart	H-9	H-8	H-7	H-4	H-3
Pericardium	P-9	P-8	P-7	P-5	P-3
Spleen	Sp-1	Sp-2	Sp-3	Sp-5	Sp-9
Lung	L-11	L-10	L-9	L-8	L-5
Kidney	K-1	K-2	K-3	K-7	K-10
	Well (Metal)	Spring (Water)	Stream (Wood)	River (Fire)	Sea (Earth)
Gallbladder	G-44	G-43	G-41	G-38	G-34
Small Intestine	SI-1	SI-2	SI-3	SI-5	SI-8
Triple Burner	TB-1	TB-2	TB-3	TB-6	TB-10
Stomach	S-45	S-44	S-43	S-41	S-36
Large Intestine	LI-1	LI-2	LI-3	LI-5	LI-11
Bladder	B-67	B-66	B-65	B-60	B-40

Table 5-2   Five-Phase Points

units of the world at this time are the United States, the Soviet Union, the People's Republic of China, the European Economic Community, and Japan. This is just an analogy so there is no need to bicker over the choice of these particular governments. Let us suppose that Japan represents the Liver meridian, the United States the Heart meridian, the Soviet Union the Spleen meridian, the People's Republic of China the Lung meridian, and the European Economic Community the Kidney meridian. These governments can be placed in the five-phase pentagram and correlated with each of the five-phase points (Illustration 5-1). Considering Japan only, or just the Liver meridian, Liv-1 is the Japanese government, Liv-2 is the embassy of the United States, Liv-3 the embassy of the Soviet Union, Liv-4 the embassy of the People's Republic of China, and Liv-8 the embassy of the European Economic Community. In other words,

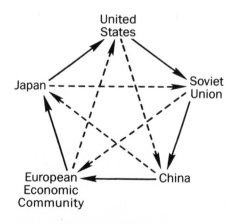

Illustration 5-1
Government Relationships as an Analogue of the Five-Phase Relationships

in the single country of Japan there are representatives from other governments that exert significant influence in terms of supporting or controlling the Japanese government.

Using the Liver meridian as an example, Liv-1, the wood point, accesses the Liver Qi circulating in the Liver meridian. In this sense, among all the Liver meridian points, Liv-1 has the strongest connection to Liver meridian Qi. For this reason, needling Liv-1 strongly affects just the Liver meridian. Liv-2, the fire point, accesses the Heart Qi in the Liver meridian. Therefore, needling Liv-2 affects both the Heart meridian as well as the Liver meridian. Liv-3, the earth point, accesses the Spleen Qi in the Liver meridian. Tonifying Liv-3 automatically tonifies the Spleen meridian as well as the Liver meridian. Liv-4, the metal point, accesses the Lung Qi in the Liver meridian. Needling Liv-4 influences the Lung meridian as well as the Liver meridian. This is why Liv-4 is effective in treating symptoms associated with the Lung such as coughing, wheezing, and fever. The functions of Liv-4 also relate to the indications of the five-phase points as noted in chapter 68 of the *Classic of Difficulties*. I will explain this notion in more detail later, but the idea is that all the five-phase points have special properties besides their association with the meridians. Liv-8, the water point, accesses the Kidney Qi in the Liver meridian. Tonifying Liv-8 means that both the Liver and Kidney meridian are tonified simultaneously. This relationship of the five-phase points on the Liver meridian to other organs and meridians can be illustrated in a simple diagram. (Illustration 5-2)

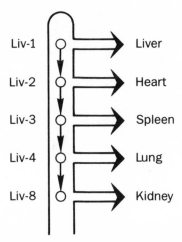

Illustration 5-2
Five-Phase Points of the Liver Meridian

In this manner each meridian, in addition to the Qi of that particular meridian, contains Qi from the four other phases or their associated organs and meridians. The Qi of the other meridians within a particular meridian is most accessible at the respective five-phase points. This is one of the basic postulates underlying meridian therapy and is the reason the five-phase points are by far the most important among all the essential points. But does it really work this way in practice? It may be fine as a theoretical construct, but how are we to know that there is such a clear difference in the function of the five-phase points? If we do no more than question the plausibility of such classical concepts and theories and never apply these principles, their validity would remain forever in doubt. On the other hand, if we put these principles to work and give it some time, we can prove their worth. Applying these principles sometimes even produces astonishing results when everything works right. At the very least, after repeated treatment, you should begin to notice progressive improvement at a core level in your patients.

SELECTION OF POINTS FOR TONIFICATION AND DISPERSION

The method of selecting acupuncture points for root treatment in meridian therapy is based on the principles of tonification and dispersion outlined in chapter 69 of the *Classic of Difficulties*. Simply put, to tonify a meridian, points corresponding to its 'mother' phase are needled, and to disperse the meridian, points corresponding to its 'child' phase are needled. This means that the appropriate five-phase point on that meridian, as well as the intrinsic point on its corresponding meridian, are both needled. The intrinsic point of a meridian is the five-phase point that corresponds to the same phase as the meridian itself. Needling the intrinsic point only affects the meridian it is on, as previously noted.

For example, when tonification is required in treating Liver deficiency, water, the mother phase of wood which is associated with the Liver, is treated. In terms of the yin meridians, water corresponds to the Kidney meridian, thus the Kidney meridian is treated. Of course, the point associated with the Kidney on the Liver meridian also must be tonified. Therefore, in cases of Liver deficiency, both the water point of the Liver meridian, and the water or intrinsic point of the Kidney meridian, are tonified. A table of correspondences among the five-phase points of the yin meridians can be used to find the appropriate tonification and dispersion points. (Table 5-3)

	Wood	**Fire**	**Earth**	**Metal**	**Water**
Liver	Liv-1	Liv-2	Liv-3	Liv-4	Liv-8
Heart	H-9	H-8	H-7	H-4	H-3
Pericardium	P-9	P-8	P-7	P-5	P-3
Spleen	Sp-1	Sp-2	Sp-3	Sp-5	Sp-9
Lung	L-11	L-10	L-9	L-8	L-5
Kidney	K-1	K-2	K-3	K-7	K-10

Table 5-3 Five-Phase Points of the Yin Meridians

As shown above, the tonification and dispersion points of each meridian precede and follow the intrinsic point. This fundamental principle of point selection is applied rather consistently in the treatment of basic yin meridian deficiency patterns. The five-phase points of the yang meridians, however, are not used as often for tonification and dispersion in meridian therapy. Instead, other important points (e.g., the source, connecting, or accumulating points) are used in treating the yang meridians. The treatment of yang meridians will be discussed later in greater detail. To practice meridian therapy, one must memorize the tonification and dispersion points of the yin meridians. It is helpful in the beginning to keep a list of these points close at hand for quick reference. The *Five Element Acupoint Chart* by Honma is an ideal tool for this purpose. Having this chart on the wall greatly simplifies the process of learning and using the five-phase points. (See fold-out at back of book for smaller version of this chart.)

To explain briefly how this chart works, it consists of a pentagram with one phase or pair of yin and yang meridians at each corner. All the five-phase points are shown in relationship to the other phases. For example, looking at just the wood section of this diagram (Illustration 5-3), the following points are used for basic treatments: For Liver (wood) deficiency, the points listed in the direction of the mother phase are used. These are Liv-8 and G-43. The tonification point for the Liver meridian is Liv-8. For Liver excess, the points listed in the direction of the child phase are used. Thus, Liv-2 is the dispersion point for the Liver meridian. The points in the center of the circles are the intrinsic points. These are the wood points on the wood meridians (Liver and Gallbladder). The intrinsic point for the Liver meridian, Liv-1, is used when there is an imbalance in the Liver meridian that cannot be identified as either excessive or deficient. This is in accord with the principle of simply using a point on the involved meridian if it is neither deficient nor excessive.

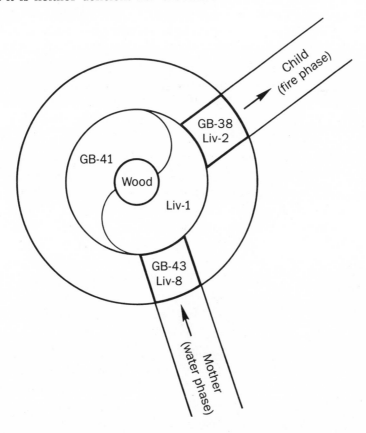

Illustration 5-3
Wood Section of *Five Element Acupoint Chart*

SIMPLE TREATMENT FOR THE BASIC PATTERNS

Meridian therapy can be performed on many levels with varying degrees of complexity, but it is best to keep things simple at first and gradually build on a basic approach. Let us first begin with the simplest treatment for the basic patterns. It is more important to master the basics of treatment than to learn about complicated theories. I will therefore explain in detail how to locate and needle the most important tonification point for each type of yin meridian deficiency. Since we have been using the example of Liver meridian imbalances, I will begin by explaining the treatment for Liver deficiency.

Liver Deficiency

There are several points used for tonification of Liver deficiency, but the most important one on the Liver meridian is Liv-8. The Liver meridian is associated with the wood phase, and Liv-8 is the water point that tonifies wood. When the Liver is deficient, no matter what else you do, be sure to tonify Liv-8. Even when only the Liver meridian is deficient, this imbalance may tend to cause excess in the Spleen, and then Kidney deficiency. Thus, needling the water point to influence Kidney Qi from the Liver meridian is also meaningful from the standpoint of preventing further complications. Needle Liv-8 on the side that seems more deficient by meridian palpation, or needle both sides if this is not clear.

It is important to become proficient at needling this point, and to use it often. If one were to see five patients a day with Liver deficiency, that would mean Liv-8 would be needled as many as ten times. If one works twenty-five days a month, that would mean Liv-8 could be needled as many as two hundred and fifty times. Over the course of a year, this point would be needled three thousand times, over five years it would be fifteen thousand times, and over ten years it would be thirty thousand times! This is what it takes to become really good at needling a point. The secret to needling proficiency is to practice over and over. Some teachers say that the only way to become proficient at acupuncture is to insert needles into the abdomen fifty thousand times. The idea is to become thoroughly accustomed to inserting needles at specific points. With familiarity the acupuncture needle, just like the brush of an artist, can be used with greater precision and refinement. The temptation for the beginner is to try more points. When I first started practicing meridian therapy, I also felt that needling Liv-8 alone was not enough. I also would needle K-9 and K-10, and sometimes Liv-3 and Liv-4. But I have recently come to appreciate Liv-8 more, and often find that needling just this point is sufficient. It may seem improbable that needling just one or two points can replenish the Qi in a depleted meridian, but as long as the diagnosis is correct, using just a few points is actually far more effective than using too many points.

HOW TO LOCATE LIV-8

> "It is on the medial aspect of the knee, below the [corner] of the tibia, in the depression above the large tendon and below the little tendon. Bend the knee and locate it on the head of the crease." *(Gatherings of Eminent Acupuncturists)*

"In the depression on the medial aspect of the knee joint. Look for a small, movable nodule at the medial head of the crease in the knee joint." (Yanagiya, 1979)

The keys to locating Liv-8 are as follows: **1.** The knee should be in the flexed position. **2.** Look near the medial end of the skin fold of the knee. **3.** Find the depression between the large tendon (sartorius muscle) and the small tendon (semimembranosus muscle). (Illustration 5-4)

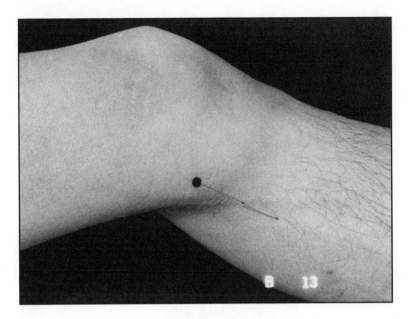

Illustration 5-4
Location of Liv-8

Beginners should ask the patient to flex the knee to find the end point of the crease, and thereby accurately locate the point. After some practice, you can locate Liv-8 without flexing the knee. Sometimes Liv-8 is tender, and sometimes it is not. The tenderness usually appears more toward the insertion of the sartorius than in the depression. When there is tenderness very close to Liv-8, the best results are obtained by needling the tender point.

HOW TO NEEDLE LIV-8

This point can be needled in either the supine or prone positions; I personally prefer the supine position. To locate the point, the knee should be flexed, except for those practitioners who are very proficient at point location. Before inserting the needle, the knee should be at least partially extended. For those patients who have discomfort or other difficulty in keeping the knees straight, or in those with delicate skin (indicating greater sensitivity), the knees can be kept relaxed and slightly bent. If the knee is to be bent, a firm pillow should be used to keep the leg relaxed and in position.

When I needle this point on myself, I lie supine and bend both knees at a right angle, then cross the leg to be needled over the top of the other. With my head propped up with a pillow, I can needle both Liv-8 and K-10 comfortably (Illustration 5-5). This works better than when I sit up with my legs straight and needle the points, and then lay back down. Perhaps this method works well for me because I am thin. Although the knees may be bent while needling points in this area, is best to keep the knee as straight as possible and the leg relaxed.

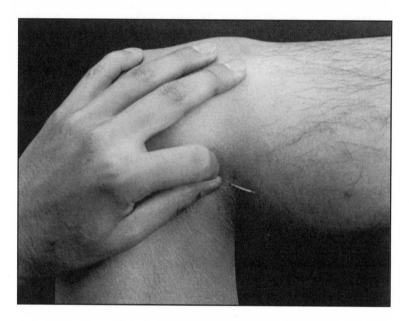

Illustration 5-5
Self-Needling of Liv-8

Some practitioners say that tenderness and induration do not appear at the five-phase points, but quite often I find such reactions at these points. Of course the difference is not as marked as on back or abdominal points, but reactions may still be found. To feel for slight differences, you must use the very tips of your fingers and palpate very carefully. It is difficult to say which is more effective, using the point location provided in the textbooks or the tender point in the same area, but in my experience, the tender point has proven to be more effective. Each point should be located with care so that every point counts.

Spleen Deficiency

There is some controversy in meridian therapy about the main tonification point for Spleen deficiency. According to the basic principle of point selection, since the Spleen is associated with the earth phase, points associated with the fire phase must be needled to tonify the Spleen. The tonification point on the Spleen meridian is therefore said to be the fire point, Sp-2. Despite this, many practitioners use Sp-3, the earth and source point, as the main tonification point for the Spleen. Some consider it unwise to tonify the fire phase, even indirectly. The theory is that the Heart, being the most yang of the yin meridians, is predisposed toward excess and should therefore not be tonified. This theory is based on the absence of a Heart deficiency pattern in meridian therapy. Be that as it may, there is no real problem in tonifying the fire point. One of the reasons Sp-3 is preferred over Sp-2 is because it is easier to insert a needle at Sp-3 without causing pain. In my own experience, Sp-3 is more effective for tonifying the Spleen, but when there is abdominal pain, I have found that Sp-2 works better. The question of which point is more important for tonification requires that other clinical considerations be taken into account, but based on my own experience, I would recommend Sp-3 as the main tonification point for Spleen deficiency.

HOW TO LOCATE SP-3

"It is in the depression on the medial side of the foot just behind the joint."
(Elaboration of the Fourteen Meridians)

"It is in the depression proximal to the mound behind the first joint, which is like a plum pit. To locate this point, look for a small, movable nodule [in the depression]." (Yanagiya, 1979)

"It is proximal to the mound and at the border of the red and white skin. It is located where the finger comes to a stop when lightly stroking the medial aspect of the first metatarsal in the distal direction." (Inoue, 1977)

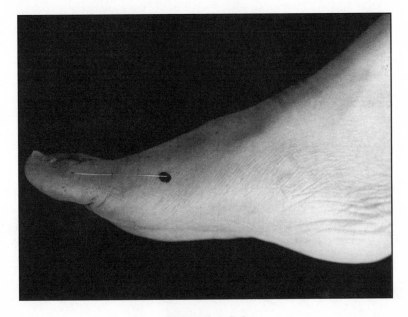

Illustration 5-6
Location of Sp-3

Locating Sp-3 at the point where the finger stops is a good method, but this point varies (Illustration 5-6). It could either be more toward the sole or toward the dorsum of the foot (the border of the red and white skin). When the point is located close to the sole, the needle can be inserted deeply. Locating the point higher up toward the back of the foot means that the needle can only be inserted superficially, but this spot is more likely to be tender. In some patients a depression can be felt over the entire area between Sp-3 and Sp-4. This is usually caused by chronic Spleen deficiency. Sometimes this depression is plainly visible, but otherwise it becomes apparent with light palpation. In such cases, inserting the needle at the deepest depression between Sp-3 and Sp-4 is effective. According to Yanagiya and Honma, the actual location of Sp-2 is between the textbook locations of Sp-2 and Sp-3, right on the joint. This alternative location for Sp-2 is also very effective as a Spleen tonification point when it is tender (Illustrations 5-7 & 5-8).

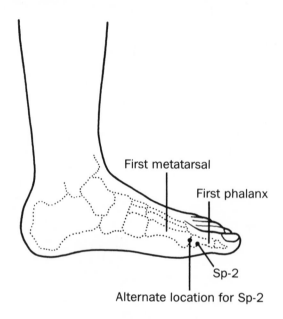

First metatarsal

First phalanx

Sp-2

Alternate location for Sp-2

Illustration 5-7
Alternate Location of Sp-2

The skin is usually soft around Sp-3 in patients with Spleen deficiency, which makes needle insertion easy, but occasionally a patient will have thick skin, which makes it difficult to insert the needle without pain. Care must be taken during tapping insertion to avoid pain. (How to insert a needle without pain is discussed later in this chapter.) Patients with Spleen deficiency tend to have a depression in the neighborhood of Sp-3, and inserting a needle obliquely with the tip pointing in the direction of the meridian is difficult in such cases. Quite often the needle ends up in a vertical position, or even angled in the wrong direction. There is nothing to worry about as far as the angle of the needle is concerned. Effective tonification is possible irrespective of the direction of the needle tip. I have found that when tonifying by superficial insertion, the angle of needle has no effect on the outcome. Sp-3 can be a very sensitive point, and sometimes just touching the tip of the needle to the skin will induce the arrival of Qi, which is often accompanied by abdominal sounds.

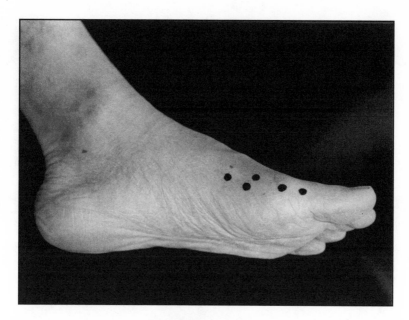

Illustration 5-8
Location and Alternate Locations of Sp-2 & Sp-3

Lung Deficiency

The principal tonification point for Lung deficiency is L-9. The Lung meridian is associated with the metal phase. According to the basic principle, earth, the mother of metal, is tonified when metal is deficient. Thus, L-9, the earth and source point, is needled. L-9 is also the influential point for the pulse, and is very useful for raising the level of Qi to make the pulse easier to discern.

HOW TO LOCATE L-9

"It is at the anterior distal border of the styloid process of the radius on the radial side of the wrist joint. The way to locate this point is to look for a small, movable nodule just medial to the tendon of the brachioradialis muscle." (Yanagiya, 1979)

Other texts explain the location of L-9 as follows: **1.** "One unit proximal to the thenar eminence in the middle of the depression." *(Vital Axis)* **2.** "In the depression just proximal to the palm." *(Elaboration of the Fourteen Meridians)* **3.** "On the radial side of the radial artery." (Okabe, 1974)

When locating L-9 the first thing to look for is the depression on the wrist between the tendons of the flexor carpi radialis and the brachioradialis muscles. Then palpate the pulsation of the radial artery in this depression, and finally palpate the radial side of the artery. When the Lung meridian is chronically deficient, there is a large depression around L-9. One must locate a point with some difference within this depression. Besides tenderness and induration, which seldom appear here, there is often a spot that feels to be the deepest or weakest point within the depression. When there is tenderness, it usually appears on the corner of the trapezium. (Illustration 5-9)

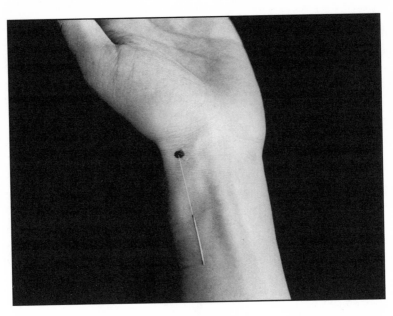

Illustration 5-9
Location of L-9

HOW TO NEEDLE L-9

Although it is accessible, L-9 can be very difficult to needle properly for toni-fication. Poor insertion technique can cause pain, and pain is not conducive to toni-fication. There are also bones and tendons very close to L-9, not to mention the radial artery, which makes it difficult to needle, especially in thin people. Some practitioners say that, since Lung Qi is the most superficial of all the Qi circulating in the meridians (due to its association with the protective Qi), placing the tip of the needle on this point is sufficient; the needle need not actually be inserted. In my experience, there is no harm in inserting the needle as long as it is kept very superficial. To prevent the needle from going too deep, one must be careful when breaking the skin with tap-ping insertion. A depth of no more than two millimeters is usually enough to induce the desired result. Care must be taken to keep the insertion shallow for the sake of tonification during root treatment. The precise location of the point is the greatest determinant of effect, and it is unnecessary to insert the needle more than a few millimeters.

Kidney Deficiency

The principal tonification point for Kidney deficiency is K-7. The Kidney meridian is associated with the water phase. Metal, which is the mother of water, must therefore be tonified when water is deficient. K-7 is the metal point on the Kidney meridian, and is accordingly the most important tonification point.

HOW TO LOCATE K-7

"It is two units above the medial malleolus in the depression with a pulsation."
(Elaboration of the Fourteen Meridians)

"It is two units above the medial malleolus. Locate it on the anterior margin of the Achilles tendon just above the point where there is a small, movable nodule or fibrous induration." (Yanagiya, 1979)

As described, K-7 can be found two units above the medial malleolus just in front of the Achilles tendon. This point is on the flexor digitorum longus muscle. In practice, K-7 is sometimes found more anteriorly midway between the Achilles tendon and the tibia. In locating the point it is important to look for differences from the surrounding area, such as tenderness or induration. (Illustration 5-10)

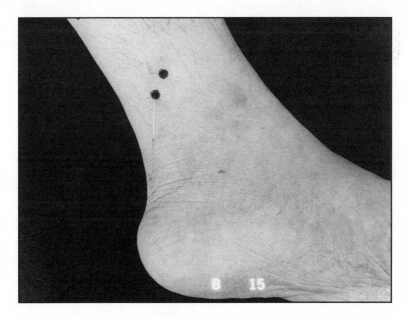

Illustration 5-10
Location of K-7

HOW TO NEEDLE K-7

Among the principal tonification points for the four basic patterns of deficiency, K-7 is the only point that is not directly above a bone. Because of this, there is a tendency to insert the needle too deeply. A deep insertion can cause a strong, electric-like sensation to shoot downward toward the sole of the foot. This strong sensation is not desirable for purposes of tonification, and care must be taken to insert the needle very shallowly when using this point for root treatment.

The area surrounding K-7 is sometimes depressed in Kidney deficient patients, but just as often the area is swollen. Any abnormality in this area is a sign of Kidney imbalance. Such changes in the tissues surrounding the principal tonification point often appear with the other basic patterns as well, and it is therefore important to inspect and palpate these points carefully.

LOCATING THE EXACT POINT
(INDURATIONS AND TENDER POINTS)

Some practitioners locate points by rote and thereby fail to take the time to examine the area around the points carefully. My teacher practiced the Sawada style of acupuncture which puts great emphasis on locating acupuncture points where there is some palpable reaction. He was very particular about point location, and at certain points would press the skin with the head of a match or the end of a blunt pencil to find a tender spot. When he examined an acupuncture point carefully, he literally looked for reactions one square millimeter at a time. As a result, I learned to locate points with special care. When I am looking for a point, my fingertips are constantly on the move feeling for differences. Instead of pressing straight down, I tend to make a minute, circular motion with my fingertip. I find it easier to detect differences in the skin and subcutaneous tissues in this manner.

Generally speaking, the skin surface at acupuncture points on meridians with imbalances is less resilient than the surrounding area. Sometimes a tight band of tension or a knot-like induration can be palpated in the subcutaneous tissues with the fingertips. In other cases, the patient may feel tenderness when these points are pressed. The following passage from the *Guide to the Secrets of Acupuncture* should be helpful to the beginner in understanding the nature of these points:

> "Locate the point by measuring the units and press the point with the hand. When there is a hollow area that is painful, but penetrating and indescribably satisfying, this is truly a sign of an acupuncture point." (Wada, 1728)

Among the many points we use in acupuncture, however, there are those for which the reaction is not so clear. When searching for such points, it is better to follow the advice in the *Clarification of Acupuncture Points:*

> "Acupuncture points are located in the clefts of muscles, in the joints, sutures, and depressions. It is thus said that they are in the center of bowl-like hollows, or in depressions, or otherwise in areas where a pulsation can be felt by the hand. One must therefore probe for a [small] depression like a bowl or seek the pulsation to find the point. It should be known that the unit measurements do not always apply. Even though the ancients spoke of the unit measurements, many also mentioned this feature [of acupuncture points]. One therefore need not always be bound by these [measurements]." (Hara, 1807)

One of the most detailed studies of indurations in relation to acupuncture points is an essay by Okabe Sodo entitled, "The Study of Indurations in Relation to the Meridians." The value of this essay lies in its view of indurations not only as localized reactions, but as changes within the meridian system itself. Indurations thus serve as an aid in the assessment of meridian imbalances. When a practitioner becomes absorbed in finding and treating individual indurations or tender points, as is true in Japan, he tends to overlook their true significance. The following passage from Okabe's essay on indurations provides some valuable information on the types of indurations and palpation techniques:

"There are five types of changes associated with acupuncture points.

1. Induration — A small, movable nodule that can be felt under the fingers. Pressing the nodule firmly causes a dull sensation or pain that radiates in both directions along the meridian.

2. Tenderness — When stroking along a meridian with the tips of the four fingers, a slightly hard spot may be found. Pressing this spot causes a strong reaction of tenderness or pain.

3. Hyperesthesia — Certain areas along the course of a meridian that are more sensitive when stroked and lightly pinched.

4. Depression — When stroking along a meridian, a small depression may be found that the fingertip falls into. Depressions often appear at source points, such as L-9 and P-7.

5. Congestion — This change appears most often on the abdomen, and it mainly results from Qi stagnation. It is a slightly bloated area that feels like an inflatable pillow when pressed. This type of change (being very superficial) is quite hard to detect, and requires great skill.

The method of palpating along the meridians is to use the pads of the four fingers or thumb to stroke along their course. The meridians also can be stroked in a diagonal direction or at right angles to probe specific areas, and pressure can be applied with the fingertips. One can learn to feel subtle changes and become skilled at palpation by concentrating totally on what is felt at the fingertips.

Indurations are hardenings of muscle tissue that appear as tight nodules. They vary in size from that of a soy bean to the tip of the thumb, and come in many shapes. Indurations are mainly found along the course of meridians, and appear when there are imbalances in the meridians or when there is pathology in the internal organs. Pressing and kneading a point with an induration reveals a difference from the surrounding healthy skin surface in that one has a peculiar sensation of a small nodule moving back and forth.

Indurations can roughly be divided into three levels or types. The first type is a spongy mass. The third type is extremely constricted and forms a hardened mass. The second type of induration is somewhere between the first and third types; it is softer than the third type, but is readily palpated. When inserting needles into indurations, very little resistance is encountered when penetrating the first type, though there is more compared to normal tissue. There is obvious resistance when penetrating the second type of induration. This resistance feels almost the same as that felt when penetrating the outer portion of the third type of induration. There is considerable resistance when the third type of induration is needled, and insertion becomes even more difficult when the core of the induration is reached. The first and second type of indurations can be reduced easily by inserting a needle, but the third type is extremely difficult to alleviate. The first and second types tend to occur on the limbs, while the third type appears mostly on the back." (Okabe, 1940)

It is said that experience with massage is very useful in learning to detect changes associated with acupuncture points such as indurations and tenderness. One must always search for the point of greatest difference when locating an acupuncture point. It is also important to develop sensitivity in the fingertips. However, some practitioners of meridian therapy beliveve that changes such as indurations and tenderness cannot be found at the five-phase points used for root treatment.

"Indurations and tender points are abnormal changes related to Blood. Indurations and tender points tend not to appear among the five-phase points used in meridian therapy, particularly those on the yin meridians. This is because these points are associated with changes in Qi. Needling, especially in connection with root treatment, is meant to move the Qi and bring about changes in [the balance of] Qi, and only indirectly to effect changes in the Blood. (Inoue, 1962 A)

The notion that gross changes at acupuncture points are related to Blood and subtle changes to Qi is a concept that was advanced by the founders of meridian therapy. In practice, however, the differences palpated along the meridians often cannot be clearly assigned to either Qi or Blood, as there seem to be many gradations in between. Nevertheless, it is true that tenderness and induration appear less often and are less marked at distal points, which are more closely related to the Qi. It is therefore important to pay close attention to subtle differences on the skin surface of acupuncture points related to Qi. To detect the more subtle changes associated with Qi, the skin along the course of the meridian must be stroked very gently. For example, if Liver deficiency is apparent, one should start by lightly stroking along the Liver meridian for about five centimeters on either side of Liv-8. The strength of the meridian Qi is thereby assessed. Then the range of stroking is reduced to about one centimeter to determine where the greatest difference lies. It does not matter which finger is used, but when the point is being located while the needle is held in the right hand ready to insert, the left index, middle, or ring finger should be used. The changes that can be detected around the point include differences in temperature (warm or cool), texture (smooth or rough), and resiliency (slightly protruding or depressed). Needless to say, it is more difficult to detect these subtle changes than it is to find indurations and tender points.

Careful location of an acupuncture point for insertion necessarily implies that the area is being prepared in advance. Before the needle is inserted, the skin over the point must be stroked, flicked, and pressed to gather Qi. This is an important step that should not be missed when inserting needles into five-phase points during root treatment. It requires more attention than just the careful location of a point.

GATHERING QI: PREPARING THE POINT FOR INSERTION

Using the same example as in the previous section, let us say we determine that a patient has Liver deficiency. We have chosen Liv-8 as the primary tonification point, and have carefully stroked the skin in the vicinity of the point to find the spot of greatest difference. The next step is to insert the needle. But before doing so, we must draw Qi to that point to maximize the effect of the insertion. The temptation, when we are busy or a little tired, is to locate the point quickly and insert the needle right away, but this is not good technique. Paying close attention and preparing the point thoroughly is very important for tonification in root treatment, which is intended to balance the Qi in the meridians.

"The statement, 'When it is apparent, then insert' means that as soon as the arrival of Qi is [felt] with one's left hand, insert the needle." *(Classic of Difficulties,* chapter 80)

In needling a point for tonification during root treatment, before inserting the needle one should feel a sensation like a slight pulsation with the fingertips of the supporting hand. This sensation is considered to be a sign of the arrival of Qi. To obtain this sensation, it is often necessary to gather the Qi at the point. Gathering Qi or preparing the point is simply a matter of lightly stroking or pressing the area. How exactly is this done? Let us see what other authorities have to say about this subject:

> "When tonifying, the point to be needled is massaged and pressed with the supporting hand before inserting the needle. The massaging and pressing should be done either in the direction of flow of the meridian, or toward the center of the body. The finger should be held vertical to the skin to apply force. The needle is inserted once the point becomes slightly reddened and there is greater tension across the skin." (Ikeda, 1977)

> "To tonify the needle is warmed, the course of the meridian is stroked, and the point is massaged and pressed, and then the point is pressed with the nail (of the thumb or index finger of the left hand). One must wait for the appearance of Qi and then place the needle on the point, slanting it in the direction of [the flow in] the meridian. The needle is then inserted as the patient exhales." (Yanagiya, 1948 A)

> "It does not matter whether the thumb, index, or middle finger is used (but the point must be prepared for insertion as follows: **1.** Press the point in a manner that is comfortable for the patient without using too much or too little force. **2.** Press gently, but make the pressure penetrate deeply. **3.** Press with the feeling of slowly drawing small circles. **4.** Apply between 10-30 small rotations. **5.** When making the small rotational movements with pressure, they should be slow and deliberate. One should not massage superficially or just move over the skin surface. The movements must be soft, slow, and deep." (Yanagiya, 1948 B)

From these descriptions it is apparent that there are several steps involved in preparing the point for insertion. In my experience, the steps of stroking and pressing are very important. In doing these things, one must pay attention to the following items: **1.** Stroke over the point in the direction of the meridian flow. Never stroke back and forth. **2.** Use the pads of the index, middle, and ring fingers of the left hand, or the ball of the thumb. **3.** Stroke at least 5-6 times. **4.** Press and massage the acupuncture point to be needled. Continue until some change is felt at the point. Either the skin over the point will protrude very slightly, or it will tense up just a bit.

When a needle is inserted without preparation, there is a greater potential for pain. According to the *Sugiyama Style of Treatment in Three Parts* (the original text for needle techniques using the insertion tube), pain upon insertion causes dispersion. This means that when pain is caused at the tonification point, the meridian is dispersed so that an already deficient meridian will become even more deficient. This would naturally lead to poor results.

According to Yanagiya Sorei, forcing the needle is akin to rape, and if all we do is stick the needles in people, we are nothing but needle-stickers. These words are really to the point. The secrets of acupuncture are no different from those of life itself. We need to take care and pay attention to all we do. Qi is gathered around the point by stroking, brushing, and pressing the point. When the preparation is good, the area becomes slightly reddened. When the skin is ready to receive the needle, all one has to do is place the needle tip on the point and the needle practically goes in by itself. Forcing the needle into the skin without adequate preparation makes it difficult both for the needle and the skin that is being penetrated. As long as the preparation is thorough, there is plenty of time for Qi to gather around the point. In addition, the stimulation reduces sensitivity during insertion.

In Japan acupuncture licensure examinations are conducted in every prefecture and on occasion I have served as an examiner. In the practical portion of the examination, the examinee inserts needles into the examiner. When you tell students to insert a needle into any point on the leg, they almost always choose S-36. This point lies over the tibialis anterior muscle which is usually quite tense, so it is rather hard for a beginner to insert a needle here without causing pain. The points on the medial aspect of the leg are much easier to insert a needle into, but since the students are most familiar with S-36, they usually choose this point. Quite a few students fail the examination because they cause too much pain when inserting the needle. I recall one particular examinee who, like everyone else, chose to insert a needle on my leg at S-36. He began by thoroughly kneading the point with his thumb. He kept massaging for the longest time until I began to wonder how long this was going to continue. It almost seemed as if he were massaging my leg rather than preparing to insert a needle. Finally he began to insert the needle with great care, and to my surprise, it went in without any pain at all. He got the highest score of any examinee that day. Later I happened to talk with a teacher from this student's school and was surprised to learn that this student was the one they were most worried about.

INSERTING THE NEEDLE

Let us assume that a patient has Liver deficiency and that we are going to needle Liv-8 as the principal tonification point. We have located the point, and have stroked and pressed the point to prepare it for insertion. The greatest concern in inserting the needle is the initial step of breaking the skin. The concern is to avoid causing any pain as the needle penetrates the skin. First the needle is loaded in the tube and readied for insertion. Then the tube and the needle are placed on Liv-8 at an angle so that the tip of the needle is inclined proximally following the direction of flow in the meridian. The angle should be between 20-40 degrees off the vertical. Approximately 30 degrees is best. The needle can be slanted much more easily when it is inserted without a tube, but it takes a great deal of practice to insert a needle painlessly at an angle using a tube. The needle is least likely to cause pain when it is inserted at right angles to the skin.

Since I am most accustomed to inserting needles with a tube, I do not point the needle in the direction of the meridian for tonification as much as one might expect. At times, when the patient is very sensitive, I just insert the needle vertically. The rule for tonification dictates that the needle be pointed in the direction of the flow of the meridian. Is the effect of tonification then reduced when the needle is inserted vertically? In my experience it does not make that much difference. Be that as it may, it is best to follow the basic rules of tonification as closely as possible, especially as a beginner, to obtain the best results. Therefore, whenever you can, angle the tube and needle at the beginning of insertion so that the point of the needle is inclined in the direction of meridian flow.

Inserting with an Insertion Tube

The whole idea behind using an insertion tube is to reduce the pain felt at insertion. This is very good for tonification, but there is one problem in using an insertion tube for inserting a needle for tonification of a five-phase point. Since it is so easy to get the needle started with a few quick taps on the handle of the needle, the temptation is to get the insertion over in a hurry. The insertion may be painless this way, but the needle often penetrates too deeply. Root treatment in meridian therapy is intended to balance Qi, and I feel that the effective range for accessing Qi is between the very surface of the skin to one or two millimeters below the skin. I say that I feel this to be the case, not because I have any research or evidence to support this view, but because it is what I have found in my own experience. Insertions deeper than a few millimeters are often ineffective for root treatment. Therefore when insertion tubes are used, care must be taken not to tap the needle in too far, or else the effect will be drastically reduced.

This explains why the Sugiyama style of acupuncture involves so many refined techniques for inserting a needle with the tube. It should be enough just to tap the needle in and get on with the rest of the insertion, but instead there is an incredible variety of methods designed just for getting the needle started. For root treatment, the needle should not be more than three millimeters longer than the tube. The insertion tubes available today are a little too short for our purposes. I advise that you shop around and find just the right tube which has the right length, thickness, and bore. If the handle of the needle protrudes more than three millimeters when the needle and tube are placed on the skin, the force used to tap the needle in must be moderated to keep the needle from penetrating too far.

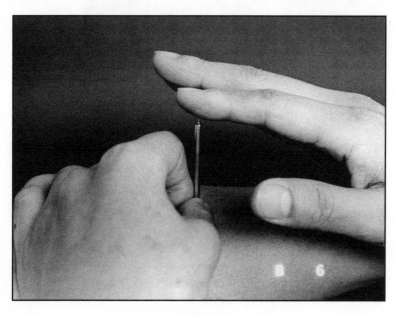

Illustration 5-11
Tube Insertion: Tapping with Finger Pad

The tapping insertion, or breaking of the skin using an insertion tube, is usually accomplished with the tip of the right index finger. In this case the pad of the index finger is used to lightly tap the very end of the handle in a few relaxed motions (Illustration 5-11). It is important not to hit the handle with excessive force as this will cause the needle to penetrate much deeper than necessary.

The method of tapping insertion must be modified somewhat for insertion into tonification points. There are several possibilities: **1.** Slow the descent of the index finger before it reaches the needle handle. **2.** Tap the needle in with a more proximal portion of the index finger. The distal interphalangeal joint can be brought over the handle of the needle. Instead of hitting, the weight of the finger can simply be brought over the needle (Illustration 5-12). **3.** The needle can also be tapped in with the proximal interphalangeal joint (Illustration 5-13). **4.** Instead of tapping the needle in, the handle can be lightly pressed in with the fingertip. **5.** The needle can be placed on the skin with the insertion tube, and then the tube is removed without doing any tapping. This essentially amounts to the same thing as a tubeless insertion technique.

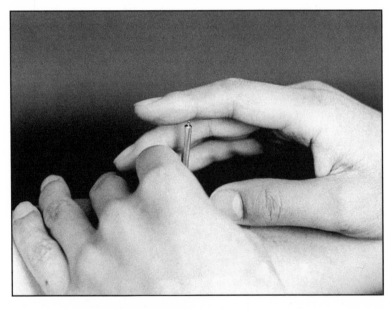

Illustration 5-12
Tube Insertion: Tapping with Distal Interphalangeal Joint

Since some type of tapping motion is generally used to get the needle started, the manner of tapping is also an important consideration. Japanese practitioners usually tap the head of the needle several times to get the needle started. This can be done in several ways. Among the more common methods: **1.** The needle can be tapped slowly about five times. **2.** The needle can be tapped in quickly about five times. **3.** The needle can be tapped by alternating the force applied between light and heavy. **4.** My favorite method is two quick taps followed by three light taps. It goes tap-tap, tap, tap, tap. My teacher used old-fashioned steel needles, and his insertion technique

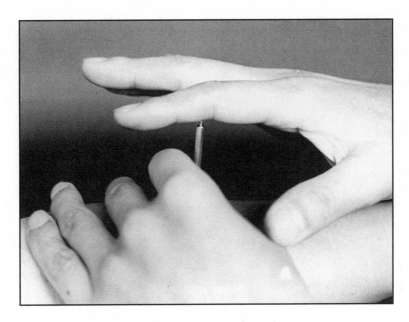

Illustration 5-13
Tube Insertion: Tapping with Proximal Interphalangeal Joint

was also quite unique. He would hold the tip of his index finger with his thumb and flick the needle in (Illustrations 5-14 & 5-15). This is a good method for painless insertion, but when the needle is flicked in this way with force, it shoots in 1-2 millimeters deeper than the top of the tube. If this technique is used for tonifying five-phase points,

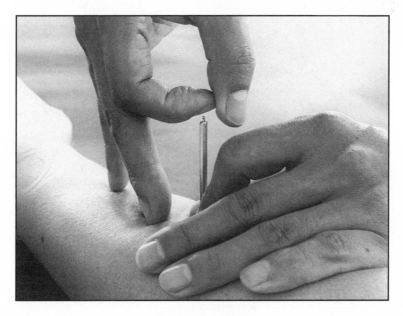

Illustration 5-14
Tube Insertion: Flicking (positioning)

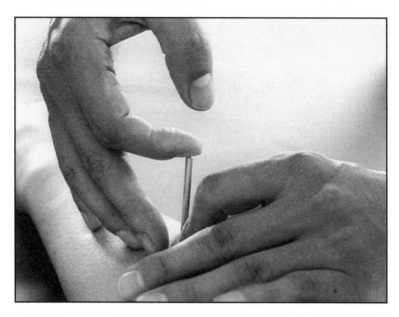

Illustration 5-15
Tube Insertion: Flicking (flicking)

the head of the needle before insertion cannot stick out of the tube more than a couple of millimeters. Also, since a sudden force is brought to bear on the body of the needle, gold or silver needles cannot be used because they are likely to bend. This insertion technique was very useful when I first started practicing acupuncture, since without

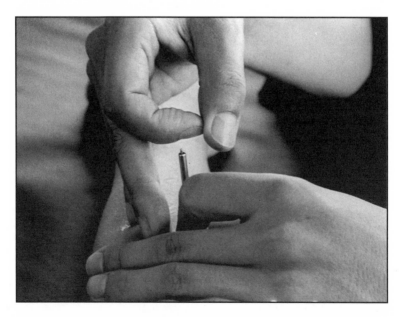

Illustration 5-16
Tube Insertion: Flicking from Side (positioning)

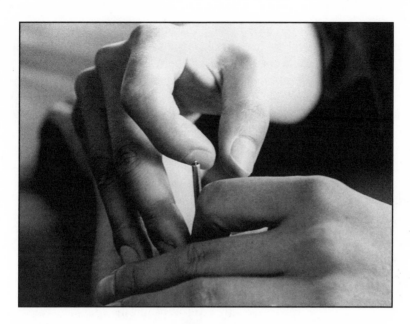

Illustration 5-17
Tube Insertion: Flicking from Side (flicking)

having developed much skill, I was still able to insert the needles painlessly.

Be that as it may, this method is inappropriate for the tonification of the five-phase points. It is possible, however, to modify the flicking technique slightly so that it works for tonification. Instead of hitting the head of the needle on the very top, it

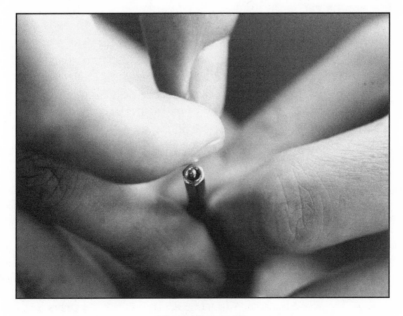

Illustration 5-18
Tube Insertion: Flicking from Side (view from above)

can be flicked more from the side in such a manner that both the top corner of the tube and the head of the needle are struck at the same instant (Illustrations 5-16, 5-17, 5-18). The force of the flick not only drives the needle in, but also strikes the tube and thereby offsets any sensation of pain. The force of the flick can actually be softened considerably. With this modified flicking method it is easier to painlessly insert softer needles made of gold or silver. While it is thus a useful variation on tapping insertion, for the reasons mentioned above, it is still not ideal for tonification. It should be used for that purpose only when there seems to be no other way to insert the needle painlessly.

Inserting without an Insertion Tube

Although it is rare for Japanese practitioners to insert needles without an insertion tube, the tubeless insertion technique is very good for tonifying five-phase points with superficial insertion. The only problem is that it is difficult for a beginner to insert the needle painlessly. Yanagiya Sorei, who inspired the development of meridian therapy, was among a handful of Japanese practitioners who inserted needles directly without using an insertion tube. He explains his technique as follows:

"Press the point to be needled with your left thumbnail, and then press the tips of your middle finger and thumb together and place them over the point. Bring the tip of the needle against the skin (between these fingers) and press on the point with the middle finger. Hold the [handle of the] needle between the right thumb and index finger and gently twist the needle down into the point." (Yanagiya, 1948 B)

This explanation seems a bit inadequate. The crucial moment in needling without an insertion tube is when the tip of the needle is brought into contact with the skin. With practice anyone can learn to insert needles painlessly without a tube, but it is not easy at first. The key seems to be in checking whether there is any pain when the needle is first brought into contact with the skin. If there is any pain at all, the whole process of pressing the point and bringing the tip into contact with the skin should be repeated. It is useless to attempt to insert the needle when there is pain at the very surface. The aim of tonification will not be achieved if there is pain.

Keiri Inoue, another of the founders of meridian therapy, gave a more thorough explanation about methods of tubeless insertion in an article entitled, "On Needling Techniques Used for Meridian Therapy," which appeared in a journal of Japanese acupuncture called *The Oriental Medical Journal:*

"The following is a list of a few techniques I use regularly: **1.** Press the point with the [left] thumb and then place the needle [on the point] against the thumb. Then bring the index finger over the opposite side [of the needle] and insert the needle. **2.** Press the point with the [left] index finger, and in the same manner place the needle [on the point] against the index finger. Then bring the tip of the thumb over the tip of the index finger and insert the needle. **3.** Press the point with the thumbnail and then place the needle vertically up against the thumbnail. Then bring the index finger over this and insert the needle. This technique is useful for inserting long needles. **4.** The simplest method which can be used even by beginners is to press the point and put the needle down horizontally on the skin following the course of the meridian. Then the thumb or index finger of the left hand is brought up against the needle to support the body of the needle and it is raised (making the needle more vertical in relation to the skin). At the same time, the thumb or index finger is brought over the needle on the opposite side of the finger supporting the needle. The needle is then inserted.

It becomes clear when one considers the technique of inserting a needle without a tube that the most important thing just prior to insertion is to ensure that there is no space between the tip of the needle and the skin." (Inoue, 1941)

Regardless of how the needle is inserted, with or without an insertion tube, the two basic conditions for tonification during root treatment are the same — to insert the needle without pain, and to insert it very superficially.

NEEDLING TECHNIQUES FOR TONIFICATION

There are many aspects to needling for tonification, and so far we have looked at some important factors up through the insertion of the needle. We should now examine the essential elements of needling for tonification once the needle has been inserted. Before we do so, we must consider the breathing of the patient in relation to the insertion of the needle:

"This is known as the law of exhalation and inhalation (for tonification and dispersion) in which the insertion and withdrawal of the needle is coordinated with the patient's breathing. For tonification the needle is inserted during exhalation and withdrawn during inhalation. Conversely, for dispersion the needle is inserted during inhalation and withdrawn during exhalation." (Honma, 1949)

The analogy of a balloon serves to explain why insertion and withdrawal of the needle is timed in this manner with the patient's breathing (Illustration 5-19). Air can

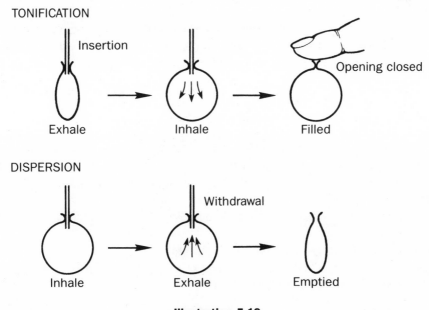

Illustration 5-19
Tonification and Dispersion

best be added to a balloon when it is deflated. Thus the needle is inserted in the body while the patient is emptying the lungs and in a relaxed state. Once the body or meridian becomes filled with Qi, the needle is quickly withdrawn while the patient inhales, and the hole left by the needle is tightly sealed. To disperse excessive Qi, it is best if the patient is full of air, like an inflated balloon. Then the needle is inserted to cause the Qi to drain out of the body. The hole left by the needle after withdrawing the needle is left alone to allow the Qi to continue leaking out. Although the principle of tonification and dispersion by inserting and withdrawing the needle in conformance with the patient's breathing may be based on a very simple notion like the balloon, it still seems to have clinical validity. Since causing pain during insertion is counterproductive to tonification, inserting the needle while the patient exhales and relaxes is a very useful idea.

The consensus about inserting the needle for tonification once the skin has been penetrated is that it should be done slowly. It is best to proceed very slowly since the needle need not penetrate much deeper. Instead of really inserting the needle, it is usually just a matter of gently twisting the needle back and forth to let the needle go in by itself. Once the desired depth is reached, how long is the needle retained? It is difficult for a beginner to know the right amount of time. Just keep twisting the needle a little bit back and forth. Eventually the needle will begin to feel heavier, and will become harder to manipulate. This is known as the arrival of Qi *(ki itaru/qì dào)*. Some important passages describing the arrival of Qi can be found in the very first chapter of the *Vital Axis:*

> "The essence of acupuncture is that the effect comes with the arrival of Qi. The sign of this is like the wind blowing the clouds away. It becomes clear and bright as if looking into the blue sky. This means the purpose of acupuncture has been fulfilled."

There is thus a pronounced effect when Qi arrives at the point. The result is very clear because symptoms are cleared away like the clouds by wind. There is no doubt when the needle has done its work.

> "If the needle is inserted but the Qi does not arrive, do not question how many needles are used or how much they are manipulated. If a needle is inserted and the Qi arrives, remove it and do not needle again."

This passage suggests that if the Qi does not arrive, one should needle as many times as necessary until it does, and when the Qi does arrive, to remove the needle right away and desist from further needling. These are famous passages relating to the arrival of Qi. When the seasoned practitioner feels a sudden change at the site of needle insertion which indicates that the needling is having an effect, this is known as the arrival of Qi.

These days we hear a lot about a similar term known as obtaining Qi *(tokki/dé qì)*. The literal meaning of the terms arrival of Qi and obtaining Qi seem to differ very little, but there is actually a great difference.

> "Obtaining Qi is generally known as needle sensation *(zhēn gǎn)*." (Shanghai College of Traditional Chinese Medicine)

"In our country [Japan] obtaining Qi is known as needle echo *(hibiki)*." *(Concise Dictionary of Acupuncture Medicine,* 1981)

"In contrast to obtaining Qi, which is felt by the patient, the arrival of Qi is something that the practitioner feels. The extremely delicate changes that an experienced practitioner learns to sense are known as needle subtleness *(shin myo/zhēn miào)*." (Yanagiya, 1948 B)

It is therefore obvious that, even though the words are similar, the arrival of Qi and the obtaining of Qi are completely different notions. Even when the patient feels no needle sensation, as long as the practitioner feels some response, the treatment will be effective. Sometimes the arrival of Qi is accompanied by a mild and pleasant needle sensation, but a needle sensation felt by the patient is by no means a prerequisite for effective tonification.

Although the arrival of Qi is felt by the practitioner, different people experience it in different ways. There are those who feel it in the index finger and thumb of the right (inserting) hand, and there are those who feel it in the left (supporting) hand. I think, however, that most people feel it in the left (supporting) hand. This no doubt relates to the following passages from the *Classic of Difficulties:*

"He who knows how to needle relies on his left hand, and he who does not know how to needle relies on his right. When inserting the needle, first use the left hand to press the acupuncture point, then flick it to encourage [Qi], and then depress it with the nail. The coming of Qi is like a pulsation, and the needle is oriented to follow [the meridian] and is inserted here." (Chapter 78)

"To enter after the appearance means that the needle is inserted after the arrival of Qi is felt in the left hand. After inserting the needle, when it is apparent that the Qi has completely left, the needle is removed." (Chapter 80)"

The arrival of Qi is felt as a pulsation or sensation of warmth in the thumb of the left hand which is supporting the needle. The right hand is busy inserting the needle; thus the left hand, which is relaxed and in contact with the needle and surrounding skin, is the first to feel the arrival of Qi.

"When there is sinking, heaviness, dullness, tightness, and fullness after the needle is inserted, and it feels as if a fish has swallowed the hook, and there is movement which seems sinking at one moment and floating at another, it means that the Qi has come ... When there is floating, lightness, slipperiness, emptiness, and smoothness, and it feels like being alone in a quiet room where there is stillness with no sound to be heard, it means that the Qi has yet to arrive." (Sugiyama, 1682)

The sensation felt during the arrival of Qi is compared to the movement felt while holding a fishing pole just as a fish bites. This analogy seems a little exaggerated, but there is a similarity on a subtle level. The resistance in the skin increases, the needle seems heavier, and there is also a feeling of movement. Conversely, when the needle moves freely back and forth as if it were in a piece of tofu, and there is no feeling of movement, Qi has yet to arrive.

Gold and silver needles are better for attracting Qi than stainless steel needles. Since stainless steel needles are more rigid and their polished surface penetrates the tissues with less resistance, they tend to attract less Qi. Gold and silver needles are softer and less smooth so that more resistance is encountered in the tissues during insertion. This makes them better for attracting Qi. However, gold and silver needles are more difficult to insert because their tips tend to dull easier and it takes skill to insert them without pain. Pain disperses Qi, and the ability of the needle to attract Qi is of no use unless the needle is inserted painlessly. Therefore, very fine gauge stainless steel needles are best for tonification, especially for beginners. Thin stainless steel needles can be inserted painlessly, and yet they are quite flexible and require gentle manipulation.

> "In the case of acupuncture, one must sense whether or not Qi has been collected under the tip of the needle by the feeling in the inserting and supporting hands. What at first felt soft, weak, and empty at the tip of the needle will gradually tighten up as Qi gathers, and it will feel as if the tissue is contracting, with resistance felt at the tip of the needle. The phenomenon of Qi gathering will be felt by the patient as warmth, slight heaviness, or a mild needle sensation." (Yamashita, 1971)

> "[With the arrival of Qi] a sensation is felt at the fingertips, there is a sticky feeling as if stepping into deep mud and being sucked in, or as if one were trying to pick up an upside down umbrella with the handle, and otherwise there is a sensation of warmth or coolness." (Yanagiya, 1979)

How do you know when the needle you inserted is effective?

> "Okabe: In practical terms one often knows from the sensation in the inserting and supporting hands. This [sensation] can especially be felt when you insert the needle by holding it very lightly and the pressing hand is placed very gently. When you use force, I think it is hard to tell when you have achieved the desired effect.

> "Inoue: The right amount of pressure on the supporting hand. I think this is a very difficult thing to know. In the beginning, people tend to press too hard. An acupuncturist of an earlier era wrote in some text that the supporting hand should press against the skin but not the flesh. Looking at it from this perspective, I think the amount of pressure from the supporting hand is a very important issue." *(The Oriental Medical Journal,* 1961)

The arrival of Qi does not always happen at once. In fact, sometimes it seems to take forever. In such cases there are things that can be done to facilitate the arrival of Qi.

> "When the Qi has not arrived, if you rub around with your fingers, press and flick with your nail, vibrate the needle, or stroke and massage, the Qi will surely arrive." (Sugiyama, 1682)

> "[One must] slowly rotate the needle, withdraw it, insert it, or just stop and feel for the Qi. At times the handle of the needle is flicked or vibrated." (Fukushima, 1971)

> "To gain the skill of regulating Qi, one must constantly strive to establish mental composure. Attention should be concentrated at the tip of the needle. One must practice by using opposing techniques such as holding the needle firmly and holding it softly, using a thick needle and using a thin needle, or inserting it swiftly or very slowly. This must be repeated hundreds and thousands of times to accumulate experience." (Fukushima, 1979)

When I encountered trouble in sensing the arrival of Qi at first, I intentionally tried to relax my hands and shoulders. I followed the above advice and held the needle very, very lightly. I even relaxed my abdomen and breathed diaphragmatically. In sum, I did everything I could to relax my whole body. This seemed to help in sensing the Qi. But I still had some difficulty. I found that inhaling caused me to tense up slightly, so I began to breathe with my mouth open and emphasize the exhalation. This really worked. I was able to sense the arrival of Qi. I thought I had really discovered something important here with breathing through the mouth. But one day I happened to read the round table discussion quoted above, and discovered that it was there all along. I suppose that people pursuing the same goal all arrive at the same place by one route or another.

> "Okabe: The most important thing is one's attitude when tonifying and dispersing. I think this is the key. When dispersing I feel as if gritting my teeth and putting strength in my abdomen somehow makes it dispersion. Conversely, when I keep my mouth partly open and relax my body, it becomes tonification."

No matter how good one becomes at gathering the Qi and sensing the arrival of Qi, there are inherent differences in the time it takes depending on the patient. Naturally, if there is an abundance of Qi, the arrival of Qi will be felt quickly. When there is not as much Qi available, the arrival of Qi will accordingly take much longer.

> "The effect is rapid in those for whom the arrival of Qi is rapid, and the disease will be cured easily. The effect is slow in those for whom the arrival of Qi is slow, and the disease will be difficult to cure. Those who live will have resistance [in the tissues], and those who die will be flaccid. When Qi does not arrive after seeking it, there is no doubt that the patient will die." (Sugiyama, 1682)

> "If Qi cannot be obtained this is called incurable, and [there will be] death in ten out of ten." *(Classic of Difficulties,* chapter 78)

Once the arrival of Qi is clearly felt, it is unnecessary to leave the needle in place any longer. For tonification, the needle is removed as the patient inhales. The rationale for this was explained above with the analogy of the balloon. The needle should be removed while the patient is in a full state. Some practitioners ask the patient to take a breath and then swiftly remove the needle. I just wait until the patient begins to inhale and then quietly withdraw the needle. There are two different approaches to tonification as far as the speed of withdrawing the needle is concerned. Some practitioners remove the needle very quickly, while others remove the needle slowly and carefully. In both cases, a fingertip is placed over the point immediately after the needle is withdrawn. I myself remove the needle as gently and smoothly as possible, but not quickly.

The idea behind withdrawing the needle quickly is to prevent the leakage of Qi as the needle is withdrawn. But the purpose behind withdrawing the needle gently is also to keep the Qi from leaking. Both approaches find support in the classics. During tonification the insertion of the needle should be emphasized, and it is therefore inadvisable to spend too much time removing the needle. Care must also be taken to avoid removing the needle in a rough manner, as this can cause the Qi to leak out. Thus, the main points to keep in mind when withdrawing the needle for tonification are to do it smoothly so that the Qi does not leak out, and immediately to close the point with the fingertip after the needle is removed. Some practitioners apply very light pressure to close the point, while others lightly massage the point with the fingertip. I feel it is beneficial to massage the point briefly with a small, circular motion.

Thus far I have detailed all the needling techniques related to tonification, from preparing the point to closing the point. It may be useful to conclude with a list that contrasts the techniques of tonification with those of dispersion (Table 5-4).

Tonification	
Breathing:	Insert during exhalation, withdraw during inhalation
Stroking:	With the direction of flow in the meridian
Pressing:	Flick and press the point before insertion
Needle Thickness:	Thin needle
Angle:	Angle the tip of the needle toward the end of the meridian
Insertion & Withdrawal:	Insert slowly and withdraw quickly
Depth of Insertion:	Insert superficially
Vibration:	Support the skin around the point and vibrate the needle with the inserting hand
Pain:	Insert without pain
Conclusion:	Gently press the point after removing the needle
Dispersion	
Breathing:	Insert during inhalation, withdraw during exhalation
Stroking:	Against the direction of flow in the meridian
Pressing:	Do not prepare the point for insertion
Needle Thickness:	Thick needle
Angle:	Angle the tip of the needle toward the beginning of the meridian
Insertion & Withdrawal:	Insert quickly and withdraw quickly
Depth of Insertion:	Insert deeply
Vibration:	Relax the supporting hand and vibrate the needle
Pain:	Some pain is acceptable
Conclusion:	Either leave the point alone after removing the needle, or spread the skin surrounding point to open it

Table 5-4   Needling Techniques for Tonification and Dispersion

As I noted at the beginning, the most crucial part of treatment is to make the right diagnosis; needling technique is of secondary importance. With Liver deficiency, for example, needling Liv-8 is the most effective approach. If the wrong point is selected, even if the technique is perfect, no positive result can be expected. As long as the right point is selected and located with a fair amount of accuracy, the treatment will be effective to some degree. This is true even if the angle is wrong, there is pain during insertion, or the needle is inserted too deeply. Properly determining the pattern is more important than needling technique.

JUDGING THE RESULTS OF TREATMENT

Meridian therapy has many unique features, and dividing the treatment into root and symptomatic phases is certainly one of them. After the root treatment, which consists of tonification and dispersion to correct Qi imbalances in the meridians, is completed, there must be some way to determine if the desired effect has been achieved. In root treatment, unlike symptomatic treatment, relief from symptoms is not the primary indicator of success. Nonetheless, after tonifying a point, one still needs to know if the needling accomplished its objective.

There are many ways to judge, or rather to deduce, the effect of tonifying a point or points. Following is a list of indications that the needling has had the desired effect:

► The pulse strength at different positions becomes more balanced. For example, if the Liver was deficient, the pulse at the Liver position should become stronger.

► Marked differences in strength between the deep and superficial positions disappear. In the case of Liver deficiency, the excess felt at the Gallbladder position should normalize.

► The pulse quality changes. For example, floating pulses should become less superficial and submerged pulses less deep. Slow pulses should become faster and rapid pulses slower. Deficient pulses should become more firm and excessive pulses softer. In other words, the quality of the pulse should become closer to a healthy quality.

► There are changes in the abdomen. Abdominal symptoms such as tension or tenderness diminish, and color and luster return to pale and dry areas.

► Abnormal palpatory findings such as tenderness or hypersensitivity along the affected meridians are reduced.

► Cold hands and feet warm up.

► There is a general increase in skin luster.

► The arrival of Qi is clearly felt during needling.

► Abdominal sounds are audible during needling.

► There is improvement in the subjective symptoms of the patient.

I doubt if a beginner will be able to recognize these differences at first, particularly the first item. It is unlikely that a beginner could cause a weak pulse in the Liver position to strengthen substantially just by treating a few points. The following passage from chapter 79 of the *Classic of Difficulties* describes how to judge changes in the strength of the pulse: "[To become] deficient and excessive is as if [the pulse were] gaining or as if [it were] losing." Thus, the pulse for the deficient meridian may gain in strength after tonifying its principal tonification point, but there is seldom more than a hint of improvement. In his *Discourse on Meridian Therapy,* Honma notes, "It is not as simple as feeling a marked increase [in the strength of the pulse] after tonifying the deficiency. After tonification, there is a sense that some gain has been made. Just a small increase in strength is sufficient."

Before treatment the pulse positions at the deep level are carefully evaluated to determine if any of them are particularly deficient. After treatment the deficient position is checked again to see how much it has improved. One is looking for an increase in pulse strength. Although it is possible, it is simply too much to expect of a beginner that he will be able to recognize such a subtle change.

The second indicator is also quite difficult for a beginner to discern. It is unlikely that a floating pulse will suddenly become much deeper. As with pulse strength, the change is subtle. Sometimes the degree of change is within the range of one's imagination. Also, if one disregards the pulse quality in the beginning (as I have recommended in the chapter on diagnosis), this indicator would be of little use. Once one gains experience in palpating the pulse, however, the change in pulse quality after treatment becomes easier to detect.

All the other indicators of effect listed above, except abdominal sounds and improvement in the symptoms, are generally very subtle changes. This means that it is difficult for the beginner to tell if treatment has actually been effective. The immediate, subtle response of the body to needling sends a very important message to the practitioner about the correctness of the treatment. Unfortunately one is unable to take advantage of this valuable aspect of meridian therapy without a fair measure of clinical experience.

RETAINING THE NEEDLE FOR ROOT TREATMENT

When I first began learning meridian therapy, I gave up on looking for the various subtle changes that one was supposed to feel after inserting a needle, and instead adopted a simple, three-step treatment system. This greatly simplified the process of performing root treatment, and permitted me to integrate this with my standard symptomatic treatment. The three steps are as follows: **1.** Perform root treatment by retaining the needles superficially in the principal tonification points on the deficient meridian after Qi has arrived at the points. In most cases, the needles will lie horizontally on the skin because they are not inserted deeply enough to stand up. **2.** Perform symptomatic treatment with the needles still retained in the tonification points. Also retain the needles inserted for symptomatic treatment. **3.** Retain all needles for 10-20 minutes. Examine the pulse for any change in strength or quality, but do not be concerned about the change or lack of it. Final judgment about the effectiveness of the treatment is based on whether the patient experiences any improvement in symptoms over the next few days.

This system was very convenient for me since I already had a busy practice and my own approach to treatment. Just adding the root treatment aspect of retaining the needles in the principal tonification points proved to be quite useful. My long-time patients began to comment on how my acupuncture treatments were becoming more effective. Perhaps it is because I am a conservative person, but I do not like sudden or drastic change. Even when I decide to change, I take my time in doing so. Some patients who I had treated for over twenty years didn't realize that I had changed my treatment style. My transition from the Sawada style to meridian therapy was a very gradual process, and I think my experience will be of value to those who wish to incorporate meridian therapy into their own practice.

There are some special considerations in retaining the needles instead of rendering tonification and dispersion techniques individually at key points, as is usually done in meridian therapy. When the needles are retained, a physiological response of either inhibition or excitation is possible, and the body usually reacts to the stimulus in a way which brings about a beneficial adjustment. In other words, even without complicated needle techniques, the body will make the most of the needle stimulation as long as the right points are needled. That is why we can retain the needles and leave the rest to the body. Some teachers say that it is not good for beginners to rely too much on the simple technique of retaining needles. Beginners should supposedly make an effort to feel the various changes associated with needle insertion, and attempt to master the delicate needling techniques. However, this criticism of retaining needles during root treatment is not necessarily warranted because it all depends on the expertise and judgment of the individual practitioner.

In any case, the following things should be noted about retaining needles during root treatment: **1.** As already mentioned, retaining the needles is a simple and convenient approach for beginners. **2.** Sometimes retaining the needles is more effective than manipulating the needles for purposes of tonification. **3.** Retaining the needles after superficial insertion is very effective for hypersensitive patients, who cannot tolerate much needle stimulation. This is a good way to prevent the adverse effects of excessive stimulation. **4.** The needles should not be retained when a patient has a rapid pulse. Also, when a patient who is extremely deficient has a floating pulse, the stimulation can prove to be too much if the needles are retained, even when they are inserted very superficially. **5.** One should know how to do more than just retain needles for tonification. Any self-respecting acupuncturist should master a variety of needling techniques. One skill that by all means must be learned is the ability to feel the arrival of Qi.

The important thing in retaining needles during root treatment in meridian therapy is to experiment on different patients and find out what works best. There are a variety of needling techniques, just as there are a variety of needles. No one technique or approach is correct in every situation. The point is to find a method that works best for you and to continually refine it. When it comes to the effectiveness of different approaches, so many methods are effective that no one can claim that his or her method is best.

NEEDLES USED FOR ROOT TREATMENT

The needles used for root treatment in meridian therapy are generally very fine and relatively short. There is, however, no particular thickness or length that is perfect for everyone. Try several varieties of needles yourself to find the one that is easiest to use. Generally speaking, the ideal thickness is between the Japanese no. 1 and no. 3 needles (0.16-0.20mm, or 34-36 gauge), and the best length is between 25-40mm (for the body of the needle). The needles can be gold, silver, or stainless steel. Stainless steel needles can be extremely fine since they are stronger and easier to insert than the gold or silver varieties. Slightly thicker needles are required when gold and silver are used since they are weaker and more flexible. Silver needles are softer and provide milder stimulation than stainless steel needles; they are ideal if one can insert them without causing pain. The problem with silver needles is that they do not hold up well to repeated autoclaving, and the tips tend to dull faster than stainless steel needles. For this reason, I find it most practical to use 40mm no. 2 (approximately 36 gauge) stainless steel needles for the majority of my patients.

If, as is commonly the case in Japan, reusable needles are used, another issue that must be addressed is the care and management of needles. If one intends to use a needle repeatedly, and to insert the needle painlessly each time, the needle tip must be regularly inspected and sharpened when necessary. Inoue Keiri, one of the founders of meridian therapy, stated that as long as a needle was inserted without forcing, the act of inserting the needle itself would serve to sharpen the needle. In this way a 40mm gold needle could be used until it wore down to 30mm. This implies that the needle is always inserted very gently, and is never forced in. Perhaps using the same needles repeatedly without sharpening works under ideal conditions, but I myself recommend regular inspection and care. By taking good care of the needles, one can use them with confidence and provide the best treatment. Good treatment is not only a product of skillful needling, but is also the result of daily practice, which includes care and upkeep of one's instruments. The only difficulty with this is being disciplined enough to do it every day without fail.

AMOUNT OF STIMULATION

The question of how much needle stimulation is appropriate in each situation is a difficult one to answer. It takes many years of experience to truly understand the problem. Experienced practitioners have a sense of how much stimulation is enough, but there should be some general rules of thumb that a beginner can follow to determine the right amount of stimulation in any given case. Many teachers have actually written about this matter. I gathered all the information concerning the quantity of stimulation, great or small, from various sources in preparing the following table (Table 5-5).

	Weak Stimulation	Strong Stimulation
Pulse Strength:	Weak	Strong
Pulse Level:	Floating	Submerged
Abdomen:	Soft	Hard
Thickness of Skin:	Soft & Thin	Firm & Thick
Moistness of Skin:	Moist	Dry
Texture of Skin:	Fine	Coarse
Sex:	Female	Male
Age:	Young	Old
Speech:	Talkative	Laconic
Weight:	Underweight	Overweight
Occupation:	Mental Work	Physical Work
Environment:	Urban	Rural
Experience:	New to Acupuncture	Used to Acupuncture
Stage of Disease:	Acute	Chronic

Table 5-5   Factors in Determining the Amount of Stimulation

Obviously, the factors listed in the table are general guidelines for determining the amount of stimulation, and none of them is absolute in any sense. Among all the factors listed, the three relating to the condition of the skin are of greatest relevance.

I use the condition of the skin as the foremost measure of how much stimulation to apply. This is recommended in Yamashita's *Introductory Text of Acupuncture for Meridian Therapy*. Although Honma's *Discourse on Meridian Therapy* also mentions the condition of the skin as an important factor, Yamashita takes this one step further by adding the factor of moistness or dryness of the skin.

> "[Patients who have] skin that is soft, smooth, and oily should be given acupuncture treatment with utmost care. Practitioners make the greatest mistakes [in treatment] with this body type." (Yamashita, 1971)

The factors which are of secondary importance, but important nonetheless, are the quality of the pulse and the condition of the abdomen. If either the pulse or the abdomen indicates a major deficiency, special care should be taken in treating that patient with acupuncture. The other factors in the table are useful as general indicators, but are of less significance since there are so many variables. The main thing to remember is to avoid too much stimulation. As the saying goes, too much of a good thing is good for nothing.

SIDE OF THE BODY TO BE TREATED

There is one matter that has yet to be discussed, and that is the order of using the tonification points, which are bilateral. Which side should be needled first, and should only one or both sides be treated? The traditional approach in treating men is to start on the left side and finish on the right side. The reason for this approach is that men are yang, and the left side is the yang side. By the same reasoning, for women needling is begun on the right side and finished on the left side. In either case, both sides are used, and only the order is reversed. It is questionable whether beginning on the left side for men and the right side for women is absolutely necessary, and there are great differences of opinion among practitioners of meridian therapy regarding this issue. Among them are the following: **1.** Always needle both sides. **2.** Needle the asymptomatic (stronger) side. The circulation of Qi and Blood is better on the stronger side. **3.** First compare the strength of the pulse on the right and left sides, and then needle the side with the stronger pulse since there is greater circulation of Qi and Blood on the stronger side. **4.** Needle the symptomatic (weaker) side because needling this side seems more effective in many cases. **5.** Needle the yin meridians on one side, and then the yang meridians on the other.

In *Basic Questions* (chapter 63) a needling technique called contralateral insertion is discussed. In contralateral insertion, when the pathology or symptom is located on one side of the body, points on the opposite side of the body are needled. It is therefore mistaken to believe that only needling the symptomatic side can be effective. As long as one is aware that using points on the asymptomatic side can also be effective, one can apply whichever approach seems appropriate.

I once treated a patient with strong gastric pain localized around S-19 on the left side. When I needled K-9 on the left, the needle sensation radiated upward to the area of pain. When I needled the same point on the right side, however, not only did the sensation radiate upward to the same area, but it was much stronger and more effective. I have had similar experiences with many other patients in treating various types of pain. I do not have a hard and fast rule concerning which side to treat, but I generally treat the affected side first, and then, if the effect is incomplete, I also treat the opposite side. In my experience, it matters very little which side is treated first. It is the nature of the meridians to circulate bilaterally, and to influence both sides of the body. I therefore usually treat both sides as long as the patient is not overly sensitive to needle stimulation.

When needling the principal tonification points on very sensitive patients, I usually start with the affected side and check the pulse after inserting the needles. If there is a significant change in the pulse, I do not needle the same points on the other side; if there is no clear improvement, however, I do so. It is best to proceed carefully when a patient seems very sensitive, and to avoid using too many points. Nevertheless, during root treatment the amount of stimulation is quite small, and most patients can therefore tolerate needling the same points on both sides, even if one side would be enough. As long as the patient is not overly sensitive, needling both sides will not diminish the effect.

STANDARD APPLICATIONS OF MERIDIAN THERAPY

Thus far I have discussed the principles and procedures involved in needling the tonification points to treat the four basic patterns. It should be obvious by now how much skill and experience is required to properly locate, insert, manipulate, and remove the needles. In the beginning, I recommend that just one pair of tonification points be used during root treatment, and that special attention be given to locating the points and inserting the needles. One may remove the needle after the arrival of Qi, or retain it in place for about ten minutes. Even when the needle is removed after the arrival of Qi, one should spend a few minutes on each point, especially the principal tonification points. Taking your time and giving careful attention to the insertion of the needles is essential for effective tonification during root treatment. The important thing in the beginning is to use the principal tonification points over and over to gain experience in point location and tonification.

After you have practiced this simplified approach for some time, it will become less and less satisfying, and you will no doubt start to search for a method that offers more of a challenge. It will begin to feel as if you have reached a plateau and that nothing new is being learned. At this point you will naturally start to look for greater variety and flexibility in your treatment. Once you have learned to identify the deficient meridian with some accuracy using six-position pulse diagnosis, and the excessive meridians become easier to detect at both the deep and superficial levels, you are ready to move on to the next stage. There are many levels at which meridian therapy can be practiced, but the purpose of this book is to explain the basic approach and practical applications of meridian therapy. The patterns derived from the four basic patterns of deficiency will be discussed in greater detail to give the reader an idea of how root treatment is performed for more complex patterns of imbalance. Once one has a clear understanding of the basic principles governing the occurrence of imbalances in relation to the five phases, one is free to apply the appropriate root treatment as the situation demands.

Treatment of Liver Deficiency Patterns

The typical pulse associated with Liver deficiency is weakness at the Liver and Kidney positions, and strength at the superficial levels of the Gallbladder and Bladder positions. The Spleen and Lung positions are also strong, and the superficial levels of the Stomach and Large Intestine positions are weak (Illustration 5-20). Thus the Kidney, which is in a generating relationship with the Liver, is also deficient, and the Spleen and Lung, which are respectively controlled by the Liver and Kidney, are excessive. The paired yang meridians often reflect a tendency which is opposite that of the yin meridians. The pulse findings mentioned above are only hypothetical, since there is usually some discrepancy in the clinic. It would be ideal if the pulses associated with the basic patterns were always true to the five-phase correspondences, such that the meridian controlling the deficient meridian would always be excessive, but in reality there are many variations in pulse findings. The simplest indication of Liver deficiency is that the pulse at the Liver position is weaker than that at the Spleen position.

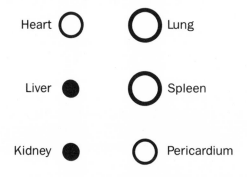

Illustration 5-20
Typical Pulse Associated with Liver Deficiency

"With deficiency of wood ... the first condition is to reduce the strength of metal, and in accordance with the principle of tonifying the mother for deficiency, water, the mother of Liver wood, is tonified." (Honma, 1941)

There are a number of things that can be done to treat a pattern of Liver deficiency, but in every case, tonification must come first. The following steps should be taken to correct this imbalance: **1.** Tonify Liv-8 and K-10 (Kidney water point). **2.** Check the pulse to see if excess exists in the Lung, Spleen, Gallbladder, or Bladder meridian. Lung excess is unusual, even as a reactive excess. The reasoning for this is that the Lung controls Qi, and the majority of patients tend to be deficient in Qi. Excess in the Gallbladder or Bladder meridian, however, is common. **3.** One way to weaken metal is to disperse Liv-4, the metal point of the Liver meridian. Personally, I am against the idea of first tonifying, and then turning around and dispersing points on the same meridian, especially on the most deficient meridian. **4.** If the Spleen meridian is excessive, it can be dispersed by needling Sp-3 or Sp-5. Some practitioners of meridian therapy refrain from direct dispersion of yin meridians in the belief that the yin aspect always tends to be deficient. Instead, they tonify points on the corresponding yang meridian, reasoning that drawing Qi into the yang meridian will reduce the level of Qi in the paired yin meridian. Thus, Large Intestine and Stomach points can be tonified instead of dispersing the Lung or Spleen points, but deficiency must be found at the Large Intestine and/or Stomach position for this method to be effective. **5.** If the Gallbladder meridian is excessive, disperse G-37 (the connecting point). If the Bladder meridian is excessive, disperse B-58 (the connecting point).

As a rule, it is best to treat only two or three meridians during root treatment. Therefore, first the Liver and Kidney should be tonified, and then the pulse should be checked again to find and treat the most excessive meridian that remains. When more than three meridians are treated during root treatment, this increases the number of points used, and the treatment becomes diffuse and less effective. It is best to focus treatment on the meridians with the greatest imbalance. There are many points that may be used in root treatment of Liver deficiency. When you are unsure of which point to use, choose the one with the greatest reaction (tenderness, induration, etc.) Points recommended in the *Gathering of Eminent Acupuncturists,* and those used by the founders of meridian therapy, are listed below for each basic pattern (Table 5-6).

	Tonify	Disperse
Gatherings	Liv-8	
Yanagiya	Liv-8, K-10	L-8, Liv-4
Inoue	Liv-8, K-1	S-1, LI-4, LI-11
Okabe	Liv-8, K-10	L-5

Table 5-6   Points For Treating Liver Deficiency

Treatment of Spleen Deficiency Patterns

The typical pulse associated with Spleen deficiency is weakness at the Spleen and Heart positions, and strength at the superficial levels of the Stomach and Small Intestine positions. The Liver and Kidney positions are also strong, and the superficial levels of the Gallbladder and Bladder positions are weak (Illustration 5-21). Thus the Heart is deficient along with the Spleen, and the Liver and Kidney tend to show a reactive excess. As with Liver deficiency, however, the pulse findings are rarely so

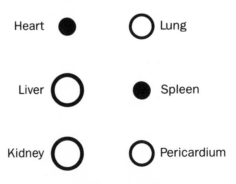

Illustration 5-21
Typical Pulse Associated with Spleen Deficiency

clear-cut. The simplest indication of Spleen deficiency is a weak pulse at the Spleen position, and secondarily at the Heart position.

"With deficiency of the earth meridian ... the principle of point selection is to weaken the control of wood and tonify fire, the mother phase." (Honma, 1941)

During the root treatment phase in meridian therapy, the deficiency must be tonified first in every case. The following steps should be taken to correct the imbalance when the basic pattern is one of Spleen deficiency: **1.** Tonify Sp-3 and P-7 (the Pericardium's earth point). Although it might seem better to follow the basic principle of point selection and tonify H-2 or H-3 (the Heart's fire and earth points), in meridian therapy, points on the Pericardium meridian are used instead of those on the Heart meridian. The Pericardium, as the ministerial fire, is thought to act for the Heart. Because the Heart meridian is considered to have a tendency toward excess, it is never tonified directly. **2.** Check the pulse to see if there is any excess in the Liver or Kidney. If the Liver pulse is excessive, disperse the Liver meridian. Do not disperse the Kidney meridian even if it is excessive. This is because in meridian therapy the Kidney is always considered to be verging on deficiency, thus the Kidney meridian is seldom dispersed. **3.** To disperse excess in the Liver meridian, disperse Liv-1 (intrinsic point). As an alternative to dispersing the Liver meridian, it is also possible to tonify or disperse points on the Gallbladder meridian, such as G-37, G-40, and G-43, depending on whether it is deficient or excessive (Table 5-7).

	Tonify	Disperse
Gatherings	Sp-2	
Yanagiya	Sp-2, H-8	Liv-1, Sp-1
Inoue	Sp-2, P-7	B-65, G-40, G-43
Okabe	Sp-2, Sp-6, H-7, S-36, S-41	Liv-1

Table 5-7 Points for Treating Spleen Deficiency

Treatment of Lung Deficiency Patterns

The typical pulse associated with Lung deficiency is weakness at the Lung and Spleen positions, and strength at the Large Intestine and Stomach positions. The pulse at the Liver and Heart positions is also strong, and there is weakness at the superficial levels of the Gallbladder and Small Intestine (Illustration 5-22). The Liver pulse is not always particularly strong when there is Lung deficiency, and sometimes it is normal. The simplest indication of Lung deficiency is weakness at the Lung position, and secondarily at the Spleen position.

"With deficiency of metal, it is important to reduce the strength of fire and to tonify earth, the mother phase." (Honma, 1941)

During root treatment, the deficient yin meridian must always be tonified first. The following steps should be taken to correct the imbalance when the basic pattern

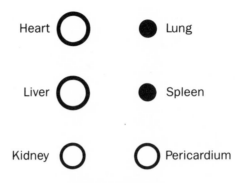

Illustration 5-22
Typical Pulse Associated with Lung Deficiency

is one of Lung deficiency: **1.** Tonify L-9 and Sp-3. **2.** Check the pulse to determine if the excess in the Liver and/or Heart has been reduced. **3.** If it has not, disperse either the Liver or the Heart, whichever is stronger. **4.** The Liver meridian can be dispersed at Liv-1 or Liv-2. When the Gallbladder meridian is deficient, points such as G-43 (water point) can be used to tonify the Gallbladder and thereby control the excess in the Liver meridian. If both the Gallbladder and Liver meridians are excessive, G-38 (fire point) and G-37 (connecting point) should be dispersed. **5.** To disperse excess in the Heart, P-8 (fire point) or H-7 (earth point) can be used. Otherwise, when the Small Intestine is deficient, SI-3 (wood point) can be tonified. When the Small intestine is excessive, SI-4 (source point), SI-6 (accumulating point), or SI-7 (connecting point) should be dispersed. The presence of tenderness or sensitivity is particularly important in choosing points on yang meridians. **6.** If the Large Intestine meridian needs to be dispersed, needle LI-4 (source point). **7.** If the Stomach meridian needs to be dispersed, needle S-40 (connecting point) or S-43 (metal point) (Table 5-8).

	Tonify	**Disperse**
Gatherings	L-9	
Yanagiya	L-9, Sp-3	SI-8, L-8
Inoue	L-9, Sp-5 (L-7, Sp-4)	G-38, SI-3, TB-4 (G-37, TB-5)
Okabe	L-9, Sp-3, S-36, LI-11	H-7

Table 5-8   Points for Treating Lung Deficiency

Treatment of Kidney Deficiency Patterns

The typical pulse for Kidney deficiency is weakness at the Kidney and Lung positions, and strength at the superficial levels of the Bladder and Large Intestine positions. The Heart and Spleen positions are strong, and the superficial levels of the Small Intestine and Stomach positions are weak (Illustration 5-23). Thus both the Lung and Kidney are deficient, and the Heart and Spleen tend to show a reactive excess to this imbalance. The simplest indication of Kidney deficiency is weakness at the

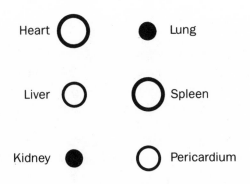

Illustration 5-23
Typical Pulse Associated with Kidney Deficiency

Kidney position, and secondarily at the Lung position.

> "With deficiency of the water meridian, the basic principle [of treatment] is to reduce the earth meridian which controls water, and to tonify metal, its mother phase." (Honma, 1941)

The following steps should be taken to correct the imbalance when the basic pattern is one of Kidney deficiency: **1.** Tonify K-7 and L-5. Alternatively, the intrinsic point of the Lung meridian, L-8, may be tonified instead of L-5. **2.** Check the pulse again to see if the Spleen meridian, which is in a controlling relationship with the Kidney meridian, is excessive. If it is, disperse the Spleen by needling Sp-3 or Sp-4; or tonify the Stomach at S-41 or S-42. While it may also be possible to disperse K-3 (earth point), it is imprudent to disperse the Kidney meridian directly. **3.** Sometimes both the Spleen and Kidney meridians are deficient. In this case, tonify the Spleen meridian after tonifying the Kidney. The term Kidney-Spleen deficiency pattern can be found in some texts. The concept that both the Kidney and Spleen may be deficient together seems to have come from herbal medicine. In any case, as with other patterns, the pulse serves as the main indicator for this variation (Table 5-9).

	Tonify	**Disperse**
Gatherings	K-7	
Yanagiya	K-7, L-8	Sp-3, K-3
Inoue	K-7, L-5 (L-7, K-4)	SI-8, S-41, S-42 (S-40, SI-7)
Okabe	K-7, L-5, L-8	Sp-4, K-3

Table 5-9 Points For Treating Kidney Deficiency

Regardless of the basic pattern, usually two or more meridians are treated during root treatment. Typically, both the deficient meridian and its mother meridian are tonified. If excess remains in any of the yin or yang meridians after tonification, then the excess meridian is dispersed. The discussion above describes the treatment for standard patterns, but the pulse, abdomen, and symptomology should always be taken into account in determining which meridians and points to tonify and disperse. There are no strict rules regarding point selection, and once you become proficient at treating the principal tonification points you may begin to experiment on your own to see which points are most effective. Once the basic principles are learned, I think it is most practical for each practitioner to develop his or her own system as far as point selection is concerned. It is problematic when the points are all decided in advance, such as listing all the points to be treated for a certain pattern. However it is also confusing if point selection is left entirely to the discretion of each practitioner.

Finally there remains the issue of why Heart deficiency is not included among the basic patterns. Among practitioners of meridian therapy, the consensus is that Heart deficiency implies imminent death and that treatment is dangerous. The Heart, as the most yang of all the organs and meridians and the core of all the yang Qi in the body, is thought to never be deficient unless life is about to end. The Heart also houses the spirit *(shin/shén)* and is regarded as the sovereign organ in that it coordinates the activities of the other organs. Thus, in meridian therapy, the Heart meridian is more closely associated with the yang functions of consciousness, and the Pericardium with the circulatory functions. The Pericardium is thought to act for the Heart as it is the first organ to be affected when there is an imbalance of Qi, or when pathogenic influences reach the Heart. A basic deficiency or absence of spirit is analogous to a terminal diagnosis.

In my clinical experience, the absence of a Heart deficiency pattern presents no obstacle to effective treatment. The four basic patterns essentially enable us to treat all our patients, and there seems to be no particular need to treat for Heart deficiency. Although the Heart may sometimes appear to be deficient, as the diagnosis and treatment progress, it often becomes clear that the problem is really one of Liver or Spleen deficiency.

TREATMENT OF YIN MERIDIAN EXCESS PATTERNS

I have never treated anyone primarily for a pattern of yin meridian excess, although theoretically such a pattern is possible. The emphasis in meridian therapy is always on tonifying the yin meridians. I do not use the yin meridian excess patterns in my practice because I share the opinion that the vast majority of diseases originate from deficiency, i.e., from internal causes. As long as the normal Qi is properly circulating, no external pathogenic influence can disturb a person's health. Internal disturbances due to emotional imbalances or irregular life style may cause deficiency of Qi in a particular organ and meridian. This in turn causes susceptibility to disease. Thus, when there is disease, a preexisting deficiency of Qi or deterioration in the function of a yin organ and meridian is assumed.

The main objective in root treatment is to rectify this fundamental imbalance. Excess in one yin meridian occurs largely in reaction to deficiency in another yin meridian. An excess of this type can be corrected by tonifying the deficient meridian. The excesses that should be treated as part of root treatment are by and large those of the yang meridians, which are caused by external pathogenic influences. In the acute stage of a disease, yang meridian excess does often become the focus of treatment.

Nevertheless, some practitioners of meridian therapy do use the patterns of yin meridian excess, and there is a formula for their treatment based on the *Classic of Difficulties*. The standard treatment regimens for patterns of yin meridian excess are as follows:

Liver excess—Tonify metal and disperse fire. Tonify L-8 and disperse Liv-2.
Heart excess—Tonify water and disperse earth. Tonify K-10 and disperse H-7.
Spleen excess—Tonify wood and disperse metal. Tonify Liv-1 and disperse Sp-5.
Lung excess—Tonify fire and disperse water. Tonify P-8 and disperse L-5.
Kidney excess—Tonify earth and disperse wood. Tonify Sp-3 and disperse K-1.

It is said that the Heart is never deficient and that the Kidney is never excessive, so one must avoid diagnosing a patient as having Heart deficiency or Kidney excess. While the table above includes a treatment for Kidney excess derived from the principles of the *Classic of Difficulties,* this is not used in meridian therapy. According to Honma,

> "The Kidney is an organ that easily becomes deficient, but it rarely receives pathogenic Qi directly. It either gets the pathogenic Qi from its paired yang (Bladder) meridian, or from its mother (Liver) meridian, or otherwise becomes excessive in reaction to deficiency of the Spleen. No matter how excessive the Kidney becomes, the duration is short, and it usually becomes deficient soon after that." (Honma, 1949)

TREATMENT OF YANG MERIDIAN EXCESS

Even though correcting deficiency in the yin meridians is the primary objective of root treatment in meridian therapy, treating imbalances in the yang meridians is also important. Root treatment of the yang meridians consists primarily of dispersing excess, especially for the beginner. Treating yang meridian excess is very effective in the early stages of a disease, or when only the meridian, and not the organ, is affected. Even in cases of chronic disease affecting the organs, treating excess in the yang meridians greatly enhances the effect of the treatment as a whole.

Deciding which of the yang meridians to treat during root treatment is based on six-position pulse diagnosis. Once this determination is made, however, there is more flexibility in the selection of points than in the treatment of yin meridians. For example, if the Gallbladder meridian is to be dispersed, aside from G-38, which is the five-phase dispersion point of the Gallbladder meridian, points such as G-31, G-34, G-36 (accumulating point), G-37 (connecting point), and G-40 (source point) can be used.

Reactions such as tenderness, depression, or induration appear along the yang meridians far more often than along the yin meridians, and treating these points is usually more effective. While one may use only the five-phase points during the root treatment of yang meridians, in my experience tonifying depressed points or dispersing indurated points achieves the same result faster. Thus, the selection of points for dispersion should be based more on palpatory findings such as tenderness and indurations than on the principles of the five phases. Below is a list of points on the yang meridians that I use most often during root treatment.

Gallbladder meridian: G-31, G-38
Small Intestine meridian: SI-3, SI-4
Stomach meridian: S-36, S-40, S-43
Large Intestine meridian: LI-4, LI-11
Bladder meridian: B-58, B-59, B-60
Triple Burner meridian: TB-3, TB-4

POINT SELECTION BASED ON CHAPTER 68
OF THE *CLASSIC OF DIFFICULTIES*

Chapter 68 of the *Classic of Difficulties* presents a method for selecting five-phase points based on the patient's symptoms. This adds another dimension to the selection of points during root treatment.

> "All five yin organs and six yang organs have a well, spring, stream, river, and sea [point]. What do these [points] control?
>
> It is thus: the well [points] control fullness in the epigastrium. The spring [points] control heat in the body. The stream [points] control heaviness in the body and pains in the joints. The river [points] control wheezing, coughing, and alternating chills and fever. The sea [points] control rebellious Qi and loss of fluids. These are the conditions controlled by the well, spring, stream, river, and sea [points] of the five yin organs and six yang organs."

In this way, each the five-phase points has specific symptoms for which it is indicated. This is a useful thing to keep in mind, even though every five-phase point is not always effective for the conditions it is supposed to control. Let us examine in more detail the symptoms associated with each type of point.

1. "The well [points] control fullness in the epigastrium."

Fullness (or distention) in the epigastrium seems to be a fairly specific symptom, but let us see what practitioners of meridian therapy have to say about it.

> "[This is] a symptom in which the epigastric region is tight and distended." (Honma, 1949)

> "[This is] when tension collects in the epigastric region in reaction to dizziness, extreme agony, stabbing pain in the chest and abdomen, or any other form of excruciating pain." (Fukushima, 1971)

> "[This is] a subjective sensation of distention in the epigastric and gastric regions." (Ikeda, 1977)

My own definition of fullness in the epigastrium is tension in the epigastric region between CV-12 and CV-14, which can either be felt subjectively, or palpated objectively. In some cases this tension is due to disease in the heart or a visceral organ. The discomfort in the epigastric region associated with hangovers, dizziness, motion sickness, and increased intracanial pressure may all be related to distention in the epigastrium.

Once when I had a bad hangover with nausea, dizziness, and distention in the epigastrium, another young practitioner who had come to observe my practice gave me a treatment for Liver deficiency. The symptoms of nausea and dizziness disappeared completely, but a few days later I came down with an excruciating headache. It was not localized in the occiput or vertex, but instead was a throbbing headache that seemed to originate from the core of the cranium and covered my entire head. To treat this headache myself, I placed a needle in Liv-1 and gently twisted it around for awhile. My headache subsided like a wave retreating from a beach, and by the time I was ready to remove the needle, it had penetrated about one millimeter. In this manner, Liv-1 can be very effective in treating other symptoms associated with fullness in the epigastrium such as hypertensive headaches in patients with Liver imbalances.

2. "The spring [points] control heat in the body."
What exactly is meant by heat in the body?

> "[This is] heat that can be felt objectively, or that which is felt by the individual." (Honma, 1949)

> "[This includes] all manifestations of heat whether felt subjectively or objectively, including localized [sensations of] heat. The pulse is generally rapid." (Fukushima, 1971)

When a patient has a temperature the pulse is often rapid, but there are times when the patient feels feverish despite the fact that the temperature measures normal. I suffered from pulmonary tuberculosis in my youth, and I am very familiar with this type of heat. It is commonly known as heat in the body, and otherwise as heat in the core or the Heart. Sometimes the pulse is rapid, and other times it is not. The main thing is that the patient himself feels hot or feverish. The spring points are very useful for relieving this symptom of heat in the body. It goes without saying that they are also effective in treating fevers.

3. "The stream [points] control heaviness in the body and pain in the joints."

> "The body feels tired and heavy, and the joints ache." (Honma, 1949)

> "[This is] fatigue, edema, joint pain, lassitude, obesity, or conversely a loss of weight." (Fukushima, 1971)

A sensation of heaviness in the body is felt when one is tired, or when there is edema. Sometimes only the legs feel heavy. Some people describe it as sensation of the whole body being weighed down with lead. Pain in the joints of course refers to arthralgia, but it also implies nonspecific pain and soreness all over the body. The stream points can be used instead of the standard tonification points when such symptoms are present. Thus, if a person with arthritis has Liver deficiency, Liv-3 can be tonified instead of the standard tonification point, Liv-8.

4. "The river [points] control wheezing, coughing, and alternating chills and fever."

> "There is tidal fever with chills in between. This is accompanied by asthmatic breathing or coughing." (Honma, 1949)

> "Wheezing, coughing, and alternating chills and fever refer to all respiratory conditions, such as asthma, which involve respiratory difficulties like wheezing and coughing." (Fukushima, 1979)

It is unclear whether the river points are appropriate only when all three symptoms of wheezing, coughing, and alternating chills and fever are present, or whether just one of these symptoms is enough. I consider the presence of any one of the symptoms to be sufficient cause to use the river points. The river points are very effective in cases of asthma or the common cold when there is wheezing or coughing. If the basic pattern is one of Lung deficiency, instead of using the standard tonification points L-9 and Sp-3, one can use L-8 and Sp-5. For Kidney deficiency, one can use K-7 and L-8, and for Liver deficiency, Liv-4 and K-7.

5. "The sea [points] control rebellious Qi and loss of fluids."

> "Qi rises to the head, and there is incontinence of urine and feces. There is also the symptom of excessive perspiration." (Honma, 1949)

> "The fluids in the abdominal cavity become disturbed and leak out of all the openings. [This is] a condition in which all types of excretions leak out." (Honma, 1965)

The symptoms associated with the sea points thus include blood rushing to the head (heat in the head) and excessive excretions. All types of abnormal excretions are implied, including nasal discharge, epistaxis, perspiration, hemorrhoids, functional uterine bleeding, hemoptysis, hematemisis, and diarrhea. The sea points are effective in treating all of these conditions.

To apply the principles of chapter 68 of the *Classic of Difficulties* in the clinic, first the symptoms of the patient must be analyzed to see if they fit into one of the five categories. If none of them do, these principles of point selection should not be used. If there is some correspondence, the basic pattern must be determined to use the appropriate five-phase points on the deficient meridian and its mother meridian. One may question how all symptoms can be divided into five simple categories, and indeed there is some debate among practitioners of meridian therapy concerning the extent to which this approach is applicable:

> "It is doubtful whether point selection according to [the symptoms of] the well, spring, stream, river, and sea points is applicable to all the five-phase points. For example, among the well points that are supposed to control distention in the epigastrium, only those of the Liver and Spleen have a significant effect. It is also questionable whether the symptom of distention in the epigastrium appears for [imbalances in] all the meridians." (Kamichi, 1978)

There are obviously questions here that require further study, but in general, the approach presented in chapter 68 of the *Classic of Difficulties* is very useful. The thing to remember in the clinic is that the pattern must always be considered first, and some abnormality should be found through palpation at the points chosen for treatment.

MOXIBUSTION AND ROOT TREATMENT

As a practitioner who turned to meridian therapy after practicing the Sawada style of acupuncture for a long time, I have a great interest in moxibustion. Sawada Ken (1877-1938) stands out in recent history as one of the most skilled and famous practitioners of acupuncture and moxibustion. Few know that he used moxibustion almost exclusively, never having acquired an acupuncture license. Nevertheless, Sawada's approach to treatment has been widely emulated by Japanese acupuncturists. My teacher, who used Sawada's approach, taught these techniques to me. In addition to these techniques, I also like to use the moxibustion techniques developed by Fukaya Isaburo (1900-1974), another widely-respected practitioner of moxibustion in modern Japan. I like Fukaya's approach because it is very effective without using many points, as is done in Sawada's approach.

Since moxibustion is such an important part of my treatment, it once occurred to me that perhaps I could perform root treatment using moxibustion instead of acupuncture. I was always extremely interested in how practitioners of meridian therapy used moxibustion in their treatment, and whenever I had a chance, I watched closely to see what points they used. What I found was that only rarely did they use moxibustion on the five-phase points, which are routinely used for root treatment. I wondered why, and eventually decided to experiment with moxibustion during root treatment.

The patient on which I chose to experiment was an asthmatic who lived far away and could come for treatment only infrequently. He was willing to do the moxibustion on himself at home. The distal points used for root treatment are on the limbs, where it is easy to apply moxibustion on oneself. I taught this patient how to apply moxibustion at Sp-3 and L-9, or otherwise at Sp-4 and L-8. Although he faithfully followed my instructions, the results were not very good. He seemed to do much better when I performed the standard root treatment with needles, and then applied moxibustion at tender points such as L-5 or GV-14 as part of the symptomatic treatment.

After this experience, I paid close attention once again to the points at which moxibustion was applied in meridian therapy. I found that most points used for moxibustion were associated, connecting, and source points. For example, for a patient with Liver deficiency, points such as B-18, B-23, Liv-3, and K-3 were used. In my practice, I try to limit the number of points used for direct moxibustion. When, therefore, a patient is Liver deficient, after finishing the root treatment with needles, I apply moxibustion at the point showing the greatest reaction along the Liver meridian. There are, however, moxibustion points with special indications, such as GV-14 for colds, so a reaction of tenderness or induration along the affected meridian is not the only basis for selecting a point for moxibustion. Honma Shohaku, the author of *Discourse on Meridian Therapy*, made the following observations about the role of moxibustion in meridian therapy:

> "Needles adjust the Qi. In moxibustion, the Qi is adjusted by moving the Blood. Even if moxibustion is part of meridian therapy, it is a mistake to burn moxa at L-9 and Sp-3 in the case of Lung deficiency. In the first place, tenderness and indurations are rarely found at L-9 or Sp-3. Tenderness appears at associated points, connecting points, and some source points, or otherwise along the yang meridians. Moxibustion is indicated for tender points." (Honma, 1949)

I do have some questions regarding the view that acupuncture affects the Qi and moxibustion affects the Blood. In meridian therapy, tenderness and indurations are generally attributed to changes in the Blood. Although I agree that moxibustion is more effective when applied at points showing a reaction, I am not convinced that its effects are on the Blood rather than the Qi. There is really no way to confirm whether Qi or Blood is being affected more by a particular form of treatment. In meridian therapy, Qi and Blood are associated with function and form respectively, and the primary aim of treatment is to correct imbalances of Qi. Acupuncture is considered to be the most effective means of influencing the Qi, and therefore only acupuncture is used during the root treatment phase. Since the pulse closely reflects the condition of Qi in the meridians, it is used to determine the root treatment and to confirm its effectiveness.

Nevertheless, I do not agree with those who maintain that meridian therapy is somehow unique in being able to balance the Qi. There are many ways to improve the balance of Qi and the pulse. My reasoning is as follows: **1.** There are other ways of curing disease besides meridian therapy. **2.** Disease can be cured by other means than acupuncture and moxibustion. **3.** It is one's innate healing potential that cures disease. Treatment is thus a means to assist the body in activating its innate healing potential. **4.** One sign of health is that the pulse is normal, or that the strength in the six positions is balanced. **5.** When one recovers from disease, it means imbalances in the pulse have become more evenly balanced. **6.** Therefore all effective treatment can be considered to bring the pulse closer to a normal, balanced state.

It is thus assumed that, even without root treatment using needles, if moxibustion is applied at B-20 and B-13 for a patient with Spleen deficiency, his pulse will become balanced, if not right away, in the course of a few days. I say this can be assumed because unfortunately, I do not have hard evidence to back up this argument. Sawada Ken relied solely on moxibustion with tremendous success. In my treatment, I rely too heavily on acupuncture, so I cannot make any definitive statement about the effect of moxibustion by itself. The direct moxibustion I do use is only meant to augment the effects of my acupuncture treatment. Nevertheless, I feel that this question about the role of moxibustion and other approaches within meridian therapy is an important one that requires more in-depth study.

When Root Treatment is Ineffective

I was fortunate in my first experience with meridian therapy because the root treatment I performed on myself had an immediate, beneficial effect. In all methods of treatment, one becomes motivated to pursue the method further after good results are obtained. If there are no results after repeated attempts, one is naturally inclined to give up on that method. It is therefore important that you be able to confirm the effects of root treatment either on yourself or with your patients. I hope that you will be as fortunate as I in getting good results. If for some reason the effect of root treatment does not appear after a few treatments, one must reexamine the treatment:

1. The wrong pattern could have been chosen. The pulse and abdominal diagnosis must be repeated to see if there was something that was missed. The symptoms and pattern must correlate.

2. One must spend more time and take greater care in needling the principal tonification points, as explained in the simple treatment for basic patterns section above.

3. Be sure to sense the arrival of Qi when needling the tonification points. To feel the arrival of Qi, relax your body and breathe with your mouth. Insert the needles very superficially, or try contact needling instead of tapping the needle in with a tube. Try using silver needles if you do not succeed with ones made of stainless steel, since it is easier to sense the arrival of Qi with this type of needle.

Always examine the pulse after performing root treatment to see if there is any noticeable change. The abdomen and tender points can also be checked for changes. Even when there is no immediate symptomatic relief, if there is a marked change in any of the palpatory findings, the root treatment has had a significant effect and the symptoms will soon be likely to show improvement (Illustration 5-24).

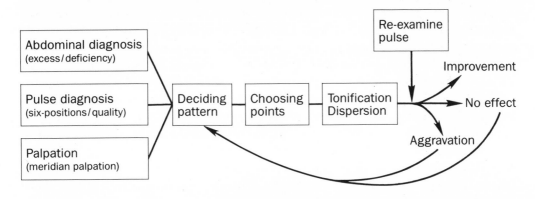

Illustration 5-24
Relationship Between Diagnosis and Treatment

IMPROPER TREATMENT

"It is difficult to render each treatment perfectly, and at times the expected results cannot be obtained. This is called improper treatment." (Fukushima, 1971)

In his *Compendium of Meridian Therapy*, Fukushima Kodo lists four aspects of improper treatment: **1.** misdiagnosis of the basic pattern; **2.** inaccurate location of the points; **3.** inadequate or excessive stimulation; and **4.** inappropriate symptomatic treatment.

Except for the first item, all of these things relate to the skill involved in performing acupuncture. I would like to limit the discussion here to mistakes in choosing the basic pattern, since it takes a great deal of time and practice to improve one's skill. The question then is, what happens if the wrong basic pattern is chosen? For example, when a patient with Liver deficiency is treated for Spleen or Lung deficiency, sometimes there is no adverse reaction at all. In some instances not only is there no negative result, but the patient begins to improve. Let us say a patient with Spleen deficiency and Liver excess is mistakenly diagnosed with Liver deficiency, and that Liv-8 is therefore tonified. If the patient shows improvement despite the erroneous treatment, it might be construed to mean that the needle placed in Liv-8 to tonify the Liver meridian acted instead to disperse. It may also be possible that the symptomatic treatment was performed skillfully, and that the good results where obtained that way.

Whatever the reasons, improper treatment sometimes brings unexpected results, but the outcome is not always positive. Now and then, a patient will have a strong adverse reaction that can put you on edge. Common adverse reactions include the following: **1.** nausea, headache, chills, coughing, and gastric pain (Maruyama, 1974); **2.** dizziness, headache, coughing, skin eruptions, and anal prolapse in those with such a tendency (Fukushima, 1971).

Whatever the symptoms, there are two possibilities with adverse reactions. Either the existing symptoms are aggravated, or new symptoms begin to appear. It is conceivable that lack of skill in needling could cause existing symptoms to worsen, but when new symptoms start to appear, it is obvious that improper treatment has been applied. I have caused a variety of adverse reactions with acupuncture in my years of practice. These include palpitations, nausea and cold sweats, dizziness, a feeling as if falling into a pit, and a sensation of heat in the head or face.

I think that some of these adverse reactions were due in part to the large number of needles I chose to retain during my years as a beginner, and in part because I inserted the needles too deeply. Retaining needles in patients with a rapid pulse is generally contraindicated. The reason for this is that patients who have a rapid pulse even without a temperature tend to be nervous types who are afraid of needling. When such patients have little or no experience with acupuncture, they are tense for about half an hour before the needles are actually inserted. If this tension due to fear of needles is sustained by retaining the needles, it is easy to understand how the stress alone could give rise to a host of symptoms. The treatment may even be basically correct, but retaining the needles in such patients is risky. Adverse reactions can largely be prevented by not retaining the needles, or by retaining only a few needles (3-5) and inserting them very superficially.

I recall one occasion many years ago when, during treatment, an old woman suddenly spoke out in a loud voice that she was feeling very dizzy. She never returned for treatment again. These side-effects are, after all, very unpleasant. For this reason, we must do everything in our power to avoid causing such adverse reactions.

I recently treated a patient for whom the treatment was obviously improper. The patient was a middle-aged woman who was not particularly afraid of needles, since she had received acupuncture treatment before. Her chief complaint was stiffness in the neck and shoulders. She was slightly plump, and her pulse seemed to show Liver deficiency. But the moment I tapped a needle in Liv-8, the woman said there was something wrong. I asked her what was the matter, and she said she felt dizzy. I could not believe this was happening because treating the Liver meridian is usually good for dizziness. So I continued placing needles carefully in Liv-8 on the other side, and in K-10 on both sides. I went on to treat another patient when this woman spoke up again and said her dizziness was getting worse, and that she felt a sensation as if she were falling down into a pit. I checked her pulse and, to my surprise, it clearly showed Spleen deficiency. I quickly removed the needles and pressed Sp-3 on both sides, then asked her how she felt. She said she felt much better, so I put needles in Sp-3 and retained them, and was then able to proceed with the rest of the treatment as usual.

Occasionally, patients who are very sensitive react this way to improper treatment. If adverse reactions should occur during root treatment, apply finger pressure on the source point of the yin meridian that is controlled by the meridian being tonified. The idea behind this is tonification can cause one meridian to overcontrol another, leading to the adverse reaction. When this is the case, tonifying the overcontrolled meridian will alleviate the adverse reaction. For example, if tonification of the metal phase causes an adverse reaction, the source point of the wood phase is pressed. If the finger pressure serves to reduce the adverse reaction, needles are retained to consolidate the effect.

It is my experience that even when treatment is given for the wrong pattern, the adverse reactions are only noticeable when the meridian in a controlling relationship with the meridian that is actually deficient is mistakenly tonified. When a meridian in a generating relationship is treated, the adverse reactions are minimal or nonexistent. In other words, if the patient has Liver deficiency and is treated for Kidney deficiency, a negative outcome is not so likely, but if the same patient is treated for Spleen or Lung deficiency, an adverse reaction is more likely to occur. Mistaken identification of the pattern and adverse reactions to acupuncture are things that beginners cannot easily avoid. It is therefore very important that, before encountering such problems, every practitioner must study and practice techniques that can remedy the possibly adverse effects of acupuncture. This is not only a matter of personal integrity and professional competence, but also has to do with the credibility of our profession as a whole.

The standard method for reviving a patient from needle shock due to excessive stimulation is to needle S-36 or LI-10. When the adverse reaction comes from needling the lower half of the body, S-36 is used; if it occurs after needling the upper half, LI-10 is used. These points, when used to counteract the adverse effects of acupuncture, are needled on the opposite side of that in which the needles were originally inserted. Thus, if a needle at G-21 on the right side causes an adverse reaction, LI-10 on the left side should be needled.

My teacher once had a bitter experience with adverse reactions. It was not caused by misdiagnosis of the pattern. Rather, he caused a patient to become very dizzy and nauseous by needling S-9. He then tried to remedy the situation by needling S-36 and other points known to alleviate adverse reactions, but to no avail. The symptoms only got worse. There happened to be a general practitioner of medicine right next door, and he called on him for help. The doctor took one look at the patient and firmly pressed the lower abdomen with his fingertips. This relieved the dizziness and nausea, but the loss of face for my teacher was too much to bear, and he was compelled to move his practice elsewhere. What he learned from this was that deep pressure in the lower abdomen is a very useful method for alleviating adverse reactions to acupuncture. I have had patients fall forward in a dead faint while needling them in the seated position, and successfully used this method to revive them.

"To tonify yin when yang is exhausted, to tonify yang when yin is exhausted, this is [to impose] excess on excess and deficiency on deficiency. It is known as taking away from that which is lacking, and adding to that which is replete. Death in this manner is death caused by the physician." *(Classic of Difficulties,* chapter 12)

KEY POINTS

Generalities of Treatment

- Root treatment is performed in relation to the pattern, and symptomatic treatment is performed in relation to the symptoms.

- Both root and symptomatic treatment are of equal importance.

- Every meridian has not only its own Qi, but the Qi of the other four yin organs circulating through it. The Qi of the five yin organs is most readily accessed through the five-phase points, which are also known as the well, spring, stream, river, and sea points.

Mechanics of Needling

- The principal tonification points must be located very carefully. Time must be taken to find a point with some difference from the surrounding area.

- Before inserting a needle to tonify, Qi must be gathered to the area by stroking, brushing, and pressing the point.

- Tapping insertion with a tube should be kept very shallow. There are many ways to keep the initial insertion shallow, including striking the tube from the side, but the most important thing is to insert the needle painlessly.

- The arrival of Qi must be felt at each point tonified during root treatment. The arrival of Qi is a subtle change that is felt primarily by the acupuncturist. It is a feeling of increasing tension around the needle, which is sometimes felt as a slight pulsation.

- When the arrival of Qi cannot be felt, relax your whole body and breathe through your mouth.

- The most important indication of how much needle stimulation is appropriate is the condition of the skin. Patients with fair and delicate skin require special care so that the optimum amount of stimulation is not exceeded. Another important indication is the deficient or excessive state of the pulse and abdomen.

- As a rule, points on both sides of the body should be needled.

Tonification and Dispersion

- For tonification, insert the needle while the patient is exhaling, and withdraw the needle while the patient is inhaling. For dispersion, insert the needle while the patient is inhaling, and withdraw the needle while the patient is exhaling.

- For tonification, insert the needle with the tip pointed toward the end of the meridian, and for dispersion, insert the needle with the tip pointed toward the origin of the meridian.

- For tonification, insert the needle slowly and withdraw the needle carefully, and close the point afterward. For dispersion, insert and withdraw the needle quickly, then leave the point alone.

Root and Symptomatic Treatments

- When a yin meridian is deficient, first the five-phase point on that meridian that corresponds to the mother phase is tonified. These are Liv-8 for Liver deficiency, Sp-3 for Spleen deficiency, L-9 for Lung deficiency, and K-7 for Kidney deficiency. This should be your first step in applying meridian therapy to your own practice.

- To evaluate the results of root treatment, examine the pulse and abdomen again for changes, and otherwise note any differences in the luster of the patient's skin, and the warmth in their hands and feet.

- When unable to detect any changes, retain the needles in the tonification points for 10-20 minutes.

- Thin needles between no. 1 and no. 3 should be used for tonification during root treatment.

- The standard tonification point combinations are Liv-8 and K-10 for Liver deficiency; Sp-3 and P-7 for Spleen deficiency; L-9 and Sp-3 for Lung deficiency; K-7 and L-5 for Kidney deficiency.

- Excess in the yang meridians is usually dispersed by needling the source, connecting, or accumulating points. When needling points on the yang meridians, it is more important to use points where there is tenderness or induration than to use five-phase points.

- To apply the principles of point selection from chapter 68 of the *Classic of Difficulties,* the well point is needled for distention in the epigastric region, the spring point for heat in the body, the stream point for heaviness and pain all over the body, the river point for wheezing, coughing, and alternating chills and fever, and the sea point for heat in the head and excessive excretions.

- Root treatment must be performed with needles, since needles are thought to affect the Qi most. Moxibustion is used mostly for symptomatic treatment because it is thought most to affect the Blood or the structural aspects of the body. Moxibustion is best applied at source, connecting, and associated points that are tender or indurated.

Adverse Reactions

- Dizziness, nausea, and palpitations are the most common adverse reactions. These can occur as a result of performing improper root treatment, or by exceeding the optimal amount of stimulation. If an adverse reaction should occur during root treatment, press or needle the source point of the yin meridian that is controlled by the meridian being tonified. Otherwise, firmly press the patient's lower abdomen with your fingertips.

6

Case Histories

The case histories presented in this chapter are representative of my practice. They are intended to show how I have integrated meridian therapy into the practice of acupuncture. However, it should be understood that my approach, be it the root or symptomatic treatment, does not reflect the most orthodox style of meridian therapy. My approach combines a simple root treatment in meridian therapy with a fairly standard symptomatic treatment in accordance with the principles of Japanese acupuncture. I was originally trained in the methods of the Sawada school, which emphasizes the treatment of tender and indurated points. In this distinctively Japanese school of acupuncture, points are selected less because of their general functions or effects in relation to the diagnosis, than on the basis of differences palpated at the site of the points. Because of my background in the Sawada school, I tend to search for and use tender and local points more often than do those acupuncturists who have been trained from the beginning in meridian therapy. Given this difference, the case histories below may be inadequate in some respects as true examples of meridian therapy. The purpose of presenting them here is to illustrate how the principles of meridian therapy can be successfully integrated with other approaches.

In studying these case histories, the reader should thus be aware that I am always looking for differences on the skin surface in locating acupuncture points. I generally prefer to needle the point where these differences occur, rather than relying on the textbook locations. The acupuncture points I list as having treated were those that were closest to the points I actually needled. In other words, the location of a particular point varies according to the situation. I have found through many years of experience that treating points that exhibit differences in sensitivity or texture brings the best results. This is particularly true for symptomatic treatment.

There are several different types of changes that can be detected on or just below the skin surface. Sensitivity to pinching, which reflects an imbalance in the related meridians, is the most subtle change, and I use these findings to confirm my diagnosis. When I choose to treat such points directly, superficial needling is generally enough to normalize the sensitivity. Depressed points or areas indicate deficiency in the related meridians, and I usually retain the needles superficially at these points. Tenderness means sensitivity to pressure, the extent of which can vary considerably, but I always search for and treat the most tender points during symptomatic treatment. When needle stimulation is ineffective in relieving the tenderness to any appreciable extent, I often follow it up with a few small cones of direct moxibustion.

Indurations vary in size and shape from small nodules to cord-like bands of tension, but all indurations indicate a more chronic reaction than does tenderness. Points of tension on the abdominal wall can sometimes be quickly relieved by needling alone, but indurations on the back often require repeated treatment. Direct moxibustion is particularly useful in treating stubborn indurations. Sensitivity to striking or hitting with the knuckles in the vicinity of the vertebral column indicates that there is some injury to the deep tissues, such as intervertebral discs or ligaments; there is also a possibility of nerve impingement. Moxibustion is very effective in increasing circulation, and in promoting the healing of injuries once the acute phase has passed. I therefore prefer to use moxibustion at points that are sensitive to striking.

The needling techniques and methods I use in my practice are those that are commonly used by practitioners of Japanese acupuncture, except that I do not use any electrical devices or infrared lamps. The needling techniques I use include contact needling, simple insertion, retaining the needles, and bleeding distal points; I also use intradermal needles and direct moxibustion. In contact needling, instead of inserting the needle, its tip is held against the skin surface. This method can be quite effective when stimulation must be kept to a minimum because the patient is very sensitive or depleted. With the simple insertion technique, the needle is inserted to a certain depth and then withdrawn, without any manipulation. I prefer to use simple insertion when the pulse is rapid or the patient is very deficient overall.

On the other hand, I like to retain the needles when the patient is not so deficient, and is accustomed to acupuncture. Retaining the needles gives the body more time to respond to needle stimulation. At most points I obtain good results with superficial insertion to a depth of less than 5mm. The needles are usually retained from 10-15 minutes. I use the bleeding technique in cases of acute upper respiratory infection and chest pain. I prick distal points on the fingers such as L-11 and H-9 to squeeze out a drop or two of blood. This is an effective technique for dispersing excess and alleviating pain.

I use intradermal needles mostly to increase and prolong the effect of my treatments. I prefer the pin-type intradermal needle, which is inserted horizontally so that the needle remains within the epidermal layer. Intradermal needles are very good when there is tenderness or induration which shows little improvement after treatment with acupuncture or moxibustion. They are also effective for acute, inflamed areas where acupuncture is contraindicated. I sometimes use intradermal needles at auricular points as well.

Direct moxibustion is a traditional method of treatment that is widely used in Japan. It increases circulation, and has a general relaxing effect. It thus provides a perfect complement to acupuncture. Acupuncture has always been coupled with moxibustion, as the Chinese term for acupuncture indicates, and moxibustion is an indispensable part of my treatment regimen. However, even for people in Japan, where moxibustion has been practiced for many centuries, direct moxibustion takes some getting used to. Nevertheless, most patients come to like it once they recognize its benefits, and I encourage patients with chronic disorders to get moxibustion at home between treatments. Direct moxibustion should only be attempted with the best quality moxa. It burns faster and cooler so that, when properly applied, the sensation of heat lasts only an instant.

The key to successful application of direct moxibustion is to make the size of the cones small enough so that the pain is tolerable and no burn is left. This takes practice, but it is possible to get the optimal amount of heat stimulation without causing any burn at all. The size of the moxa cone I use most frequently for direct moxibustion is the small size, which is known in Japan as the half-rice grain size. The largest size cone I use for direct moxibustion is the rice grain size, which is the size of a cooked grain of rice. For sensitive patients, I use small cones that are about the size of a sesame seed. For extremely sensitive patients or sensitive locations, I also use the very small size cones, otherwise known as string-like moxa. It takes skill to form and apply thin strands of moxa, but the application of such minuscule pieces of moxa is very useful when the amount of stimulation must be kept to a minimum.

The methods I use are typical of those used by many Japanese acupuncturists, but over the years the importance I attach to root treatment in my practice has grown steadily. Effective symptomatic treatment is also important, but I am convinced that in acupuncture it is essential that the patient's innate healing powers be strengthened by balancing the meridians. The purpose of presenting these case histories is not to describe the symptomatic approaches of Japanese acupuncture, but rather to demonstrate how simple root treatment can enhance the effect of any style of treatment. The reader will note in these case histories that the application of root treatment varies according to the situation. There is no hard and fast rules in the practice of meridian therapy, and each practitioner can apply it flexibly according to his or her own abilities. In summary, it is hoped that the reader will find clues in these case histories for putting the basic principles of meridian therapy to work in his or her own practice.

Case 1

FEMALE, 53 YEARS OLD

Chief Complaint: Slight pain in the left shoulder joint for one week. She had been examined at a hospital the day before, and was told that the tendons were injured. She was given an injection of cortisone in the shoulder around LI-15. The pain suddenly intensified after returning home, and she was unable to sleep all night due to the pain. She could not move her fingers without causing pain. She returned to the hospital today and was given an intravenous injection of an analgesic. The pain stopped for an hour, but then returned. She phoned the hospital but was told they could not give her an injection twice in one day.

Looking: The entire left shoulder is inflamed and swollen, with LI-15 as the focal point.

Pulse: The pulse was examined with the patient in the right lateral recumbent position, since she was unable to lie supine. The Lung position was deficient, and the Large Intestine position was excessive. The quality of the pulse was slightly submerged.

Abdomen: Unable to examine the abdomen because the patient could not lie supine.

Palpation: Searched for particularly tender points on the shoulder by very lightly stroking over the affected area. There were about five points within a one-inch radius, located around and anterior to LI-15. On the back there was induration at B-13 and B-14 on the left side. Only slight tenderness was found at B-12, bilaterally.

Pattern: Lung deficiency and Large Intestine excess.

First Treatment (November 18): This was an acute condition in which the shoulder pain had been aggravated by an injection. Symptomatic treatment was given precedence over root treatment. Direct moxibustion with ten small cones was applied on the indurations at B-13 and B-14 with the patient in a seated position. Needles were retained superficially at L-9 bilaterally with the patient in a lateral recumbent position. Simple insertion was performed at SI-11, G-20, and LI-4 on the left, and B-12 bilaterally. A few drops of blood were drawn from L-11. Two intradermal needles were placed at tender points on the shoulder. The patient was instructed not to bathe, nor to use her injured arm.

    The use of many cones of direct moxibustion at indurations on the associated points of the upper back (B-13 to B-17) has proven effective in the treatment of shoulder joint inflammation. Such indurations usually appear on the affected side, but sometimes also appear on the opposite side. Wherever they appear, at least six cones of direct moxibustion should be applied in succession at these indurations. No appreciable effect can be obtained when fewer cones are used, or when needles are inserted. L-9 is the principal tonification point for Lung deficiency. Retaining needles superficially at these points enhances the effect of the symptomatic treatment. SI-11 is known to react in people with shoulder problems, and is an effective point in treating such problems. G-20 is useful for dispersing excess in the neck and shoulder area. LI-4 is the source point of the Large Intestine meridian and is often used for problems of the upper extremities. In this case, it was used to disperse the excess in the Large Intestine meridian.

    B-12 is used for problems in the shoulder area, as well as the Lung meridian; needling tender points here serves to relax the neck and shoulder area. L-11 is the wood phase point of the Lung meridian; dispersing this point serves to control the reactive excess in the Liver meridian, which is common in cases of Lung deficiency. Pricking and squeezing a few drops of blood from L-11 is a technique I often use in cases of acute upper respiratory tract infections, as well as shoulder joint inflammation. Inserting regular acupuncture needles at localized areas of inflammation can aggravate the inflammation. For this reason, intradermal needles, which safely reduce the inflammation over time, are preferred.

Second Treatment (November 19): The spontaneous pain stopped, and the patient was able to sleep well through the night. Movement of the left arm was still painful and impaired. The area was somewhat less red, but the swelling was a little worse than the day before. Palpation showed that the tenderness at the points where the intradermal needles were retained had disappeared, and that the tender points themselves had moved about 1cm distal. The pulse with the patient in a supine position indicated Kidney deficiency.

Needles were retained superficially at five tender points on the left shoulder, and direct moxibustion with three very small cones was applied at two of these points. Acupuncture and moxibustion were used at local points because the inflammation had diminished somewhat. When the insertion of a needle is ineffective in relieving the tenderness or induration, I often follow it with moxibustion. Needles were retained superficially at K-7, and simple insertion was performed at L-5. K-7 and L-5 are the principal tonification points for the Kidney meridian. The same treatment as before was repeated on the intrascapular region. There was slight pain in the occipital region, especially on the affected side; simple insertion was therefore performed on the left side at B-60, and at a tender point just above B-10. The patient was instructed to avoid bathing.

Third Treatment (November 21): The patient slept very well the night before, and was able to fix breakfast that morning. The redness in the left shoulder was gone, and there was only slight swelling. The active range of motion of the shoulder in flexion was 10 degrees, and the passive range was about 30 degrees. Two tender points were found on the anterior side of the shoulder joint, but there were no other tender points, even with strong pressure. The pulse indicated Liver deficiency. Needles were retained superficially at Liv-8 and K-10 to tonify the Liver meridian. The remainder of the treatment was the same as the previous one, except that B-60 was not needled.

Fourth Treatment (November 22): The patient was able to raise her left arm 90 degrees in flexion, but there was a pulling sensation in the axilla. The pulse indicated deficiency in the Liver and Kidney positions. Palpating Liv-3 and Liv-8, there was more tenderness at Liv-8. A needle was retained superficially at Liv-8 on the left side only. The remainder of the treatment was similar to previous ones, except that an intradermal needle was placed in a tender point lateral to Sp-18 on the left side.

Fifth Treatment (November 25): The patient was able to actively raise her arm 150 degrees. When her arm was passively raised beyond this point, there was pain around LI-15. Some tenderness remained on the anterior aspect of the shoulder joint. The swelling was completely gone. There also seemed to be slight discomfort in the right shoulder joint. The pulse indicated Liver deficiency. The principal tonification points for Liver deficiency were needled, and then symptomatic treatment similar to previous ones was provided. The patient was informed that it was now permissible to bathe.

Sixth Treatment (November 28): There was no swelling at all in the left shoulder, and it seemed as if there were more wrinkles in the skin than in other areas. The patient also had no more problems using her left arm. The pulse indicated Liver deficiency. Roughly the same treatment as before was provided. The patient was instructed to do only about 70% of her normal work, and if this did not hurt her shoulder, to resume normal activity. However, if there was any discomfort at all, she was told to reduce the work load on the left arm until all discomfort was gone.

Observations: The patient asked me if the inflammation in the shoulder was caused by the injection that she had received a few hours before the onset of acute symptoms. I told her that the injection probably came right when the problem was ready to flare up, but was not the direct cause. Nevertheless, I suspect that the injection did have a negative impact. Based on my own experience with overstimulation of affected areas, it is hard to imagine that a thick hypodermic needle did not aggravate the problem. The palpatory findings of tenderness and induration on the back, however, suggested that the shoulder problem was chronic in nature. For some reason which was not clear to me, the chronic shoulder problem had become acute.

As for the treatment, I think that the intradermal needles in the tender points over the affected area were very effective in relieving the pain. In acute cases, I sometimes perform symptomatic treatment before root treatment. During the initial treatment, a good effect was obtained by first performing moxibustion to relax the patient, and then tonifying the Lung meridian and lightly sedating the Large Intestine meridian. It was interesting how the pattern changed from Lung deficiency to Kidney deficiency and then to Liver deficiency, where it stayed. This indicates that Liver deficiency was the fundamental pattern for this patient, and that Lung deficiency was the overlying pattern related to the shoulder problem. The evolution of the pattern through the generating cycle indicates that the progress of the disease was benign. As noted in chapter 53 of the *Classic of Difficulties:*

> "The classics say [diseases progressing through] seven transmissions [means] death, and [diseases progressing through] the organs in between [means] life, but what does this mean?
>
> It is as follows: [diseases progressing through] seven transmissions are those transmitted through the [organs that are] controlled, and [diseases progressing through] the organs in between are those transmitted through [the organs that are] the child. Why is this said? Take for example a disease [originating] in the Heart. [It is] transmitted to the Lung, the Lung transmits [it] to the Liver, the Liver transmits [it] to the Spleen, the Spleen transmits [it] to the Kidney, and the Kidney transmits [it back] to the Heart. One organ cannot be injured all over again, and thus [diseases progressing through] seven transmissions [means] death.
>
> [Diseases progressing through] the organs in between are those transmitted through the [organs that are] generated. Take for example a disease [originating] in the Heart. [It is] transmitted to the Spleen, the Spleen transmits [it] to the Lung, the Lung transmits [it] to the Kidney, the Kidney transmits [it] to the Liver, and the Liver transmits [it back] to the Heart. Thus, the disease is transmitted from mother to child, and when the end of the cycle is reached, it begins anew like a circuit without an end. It is therefore said that [diseases progressing through the organs in between means that] life [will be preserved]."

There are accordingly two basic ways in which disease is transmitted or progresses through the five yin organs of the five-phase cycle. In "seven transmissions," the disease is transmitted through the controlling cycle, with the controlling phase overrating on the controlled phase. This is a destructive cycle which successively exhausts the yin essence in each organ, and leads to death. In "organs in between," the disease is transmitted through the generating cycle, with the mother phase passing on the disease to the child phase. This is a benign cycle which enables the organs to retain their basic integrity, and allows the patient to live. In the normal destructive course of pathology, the disease is transferred from the affected organ to the controlled organ (two ahead in the generating cycle), but if the disease can be made to transfer to the organ in between (one ahead in the generating cycle), then there is a chance for recovery. The *Classic of Difficulties* stresses the importance of forestalling the destructive course of pathology by treating and strengthening that organ which is controlled by the diseased organ.

Case 2

FEMALE, 52 YEARS OLD

Chief Complaint: Pain and motor impairment in the left shoulder joint. The patient can slowly abduct her left arm about 90 degrees, but all other movement is impossible. The patient received treatment for "frozen shoulder" at another acupuncture clinic, and had just received her second treatment earlier on the same day that she came to my clinic. The pain, however, had worsened. She had in the past received acupuncture treatment for this condition, but it only became worse. She finally went to the hospital where she was given injections of cortisone and analgesics, after which she had apparently recovered. Her friend had strongly recommended my treatment, and despite some misgivings, she decided to give acupuncture another try.

Looking: No redness in the shoulder, but it seemed slightly swollen.

Pulse: The Lung and Spleen positions were deficient, and the Large Intestine position was excessive. The quality of the pulse was slightly floating.

Abdomen: Unremarkable.

Palpation: Tenderness at LI-15, SI-10, SI-12, B-13, B-14 and G-20 on the left side, and at a point below the spinous process of the fifth cervical vertebra.

Pattern: Lung deficiency and Large Intestine excess.

First Treatment: Only the affected side was treated. Needles were retained superficially at L-9 and Sp-3. Needles were also placed superficially at LI-4, a tender point anterior to LI-15, G-20, and G-21. Five small cones of direct moxa were applied at SI-11, and ten small cones at B-14 and B-15. Intradermal needles were placed at SI-10 and a point anterior to LI-15.

L-9 and Sp-3 are the principal tonification points for Lung deficiency. LI-4 is commonly used for problems of the upper extremities. As the source point of the Large Intestine meridian, it was also used here to correct the imbalance between the deficient Lung meridian and the excessive Large Intestine meridian. The tender point anterior to LI-15 was needled as the most sensitive local point. G-20 and G-21 are used to relax and facilitate the circulation of Qi in the neck and shoulder area. I often needle SI-11 to treat shoulder problems; in this case, moxa was applied to keep acupuncture stimulation to a minimum, since acupuncture had previously aggravated the problem.

Direct moxibustion was also used in the indurations at B-14 and B-15 on the affected side. Moxibustion at these points is known to be effective in reducing inflammation of the shoulder joint. Intradermal needles were placed at SI-10 and the tender point anterior to LI-15 to enhance and extend the effect of the treatment, especially because only minimal acupuncture stimulation was provided here.

Second Treatment: The pain was considerably relieved. The patient could extend her left arm, but abduction remained difficult. Some pain still occurred in the medial aspect of the upper arm during movement. Besides Lung deficiency, the pulse also indicated excess in both the Liver and Gallbladder meridians. Therefore, after first tonifying L-9 and Sp-3 bilaterally by retaining the needles superficially, G-38 was dispersed by simple insertion bilaterally. Direct moxibustion was applied at a tender point below the spinous process of the fifth cervical vertebra. Tenderness remained on the left side, so this was followed with simple needle insertion at the left lateral margin of the spinous process of the fifth cervical vertebra. Intradermal needles were placed at new tender points around the left shoulder.

Third Treatment: The patient could abduct her arm more than 100 degrees. The pain disappeared quickly after the last treatment, and the patient was amazed. The pulse indicated deficiency at both the Lung and Large Intestine positions. Therefore, L-9 and LI-11 on the left side were tonified. There was some itchiness at the points after needling, and some redness around the points. Abdominal diagnosis revealed tenderness at S-19 on the right side. This point overlies the liver and often becomes sensitive with Liver excess. Simple needle insertion was used here to treat this manifestation of excess directly. A few cones of direct moxa were also applied at tender points on the right shoulder.

Observations: I included this case because it was very similar to the previous one. The important difference was that both the Lung and Spleen positions were deficient, indicating a more long-standing case of Lung deficiency. In this case the deficiency pattern did not change as it had in the previous case, so it might have been easier to cure because the basic pattern remained consistent.

Nevertheless, this patient's problem had previously been aggravated by acupuncture, and her pulse was slightly floating. Care is required to reduce the depth of insertion and the amount of needling when the pulse is floating. I myself have aggravated problems in the shoulder joint by confusing arthritis with bursitis, and by overdoing the needle stimulation.

Bursitis in the shoulder, or "frozen shoulder" as it is called, is marked by the absence of inflammation, in contrast to acute arthritic shoulder conditions. In this case there were indurations at the upper back associated points, which indicated that it was a case of recurrent arthritis, even though the inflammation was not very apparent. Needle stimulation must be kept to a minimum in cases with inflammation, especially when using local points. Moxibustion should also be avoided directly over inflamed areas.

There are some questions that remain about this case, such as the lack of abdominal findings, the presence of Spleen symptoms, and the excess of the Large Intestine turning into deficiency. A more thorough examination and better record keeping would have been in order, but in any case, this is a typical example of shoulder problem related to the basic pattern of Lung deficiency.

Case 3

FEMALE, 44 YEARS OLD

Chief Complaint: Pain in the left ankle where amputated, and pain in the left leg. Pain occurs when extending the leg and while walking.

History: The patient's left foot was amputated through the ankle after an accident. She had six operations since then. A skin graft was placed on the amputated surface of the leg with skin taken from the medial aspect of the right calf around K-9. Her whole body was immobilized for a period to allow the graft to take. The pain in the left leg reached its present level after the last operation, and she came to the clinic for her first acupuncture treatment about six weeks later.

Looking: The area of the amputation and skin graft was reddish purple in color, and was warmer than other areas. The amputation was just below the lateral malleolus, and thus the end of the leg was around S-41. The calf muscle on the amputated side was slightly atrophied.

Pulse: The Liver and Kidney positions were deficient, and the Stomach, Bladder, and Gallbladder positions were excessive. Upon careful palpation at the superficial level the Gallbladder position was clearly more tense than the other positions. The Stomach position, though excessive, was soft compared to the Gallbladder position. The overall quality of the pulse was floating and slow. (The patient's respiration rate was a little faster than normal, but there were only 3-3.5 beats per breath.) The pulse also seemed slightly slippery.

Abdomen: The abdomen had good resiliency overall, but there was a little more resistance to pressure to the left of the navel. There was also some deficiency from the left flank region to the hypogastric region.

Palpation: Examining the legs, Liv-8 was tender bilaterally, and S-36, Sp-6, B-59, G-34, and G-39 were tender on the amputated limb. On the amputated part of the leg, one point just below S-41 and another on the lateral malleolus, as well as three points on the inferior surface contacting the artificial foot, showed tenderness. On the hips, B-32 bilaterally and M-BW-25 *(shi qi zhui xia)*, which is between the spinous process of the fifth lumbar and the sacrum, were tender. On the abdomen, S-19 on the right and CV-6 were also tender.

Pattern: Liver deficiency and Gallbladder excess.

Treatment: Needles were retained at Liv-8 and K-10. Needles were inserted at G-34 and G-39 on the left side. Needles were also retained at B-32, CV-6, and S-19 on the right side. Direct moxibustion with a few small cones was applied at Sp-6 and G-34, and the patient was instructed to do this once a day at home. One intradermal needle was imbedded at the tender point over the lateral malleolus.

    Liv-8 and K-10 are the principal tonification points for Liver deficiency. Because G-34 and G-39 were tender on the left side, dispersing these points served to correct the excess that was palpated in the pulse at the Gallbladder position. These points were therefore not needled on the right side. Tenderness or indurations often appear near B-32 when there is an arthritic condition affecting the lower limbs. Treating these tender points reduces the pain and inflammation. CV-6 and S-19, the tender points on the abdomen, were treated directly to improve the condition of the abdomen. Acupuncture at the principal tonification points is usually sufficient to correct the abdomen. When more treatment is necessary, tender or indurated points on the abdomen may be treated directly. G-34 and Sp-6 are key points for treating problems of the lower extremities. If they are tender or indurated, the use of moxibustion at these points is an effective way to increase circulation in the legs.

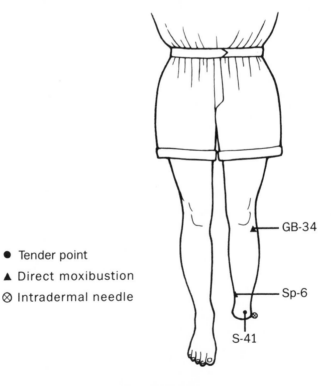

● Tender point
▲ Direct moxibustion
⊗ Intradermal needle

GB-34

Sp-6

S-41

Illustration 6-1
Palpatory Findings for Case 3

Treatment was performed at 3 p.m. At 6:30 the patient called to report that the pain was gone, and that she could stretch the leg and walk on it without any pain. She was so elated that she said she just had to call.

Observations: When I heard that the amputated surface of the leg was in pain, I first thought of the well-known case of Yanagiya treating pain in an amputated leg by using points on the opposite side. But after feeling the heat in the affected area, I decided that this was a case much like arthritis, where the lower extremity of the amputated limb had been irritated by walking and repeated surgery. Also, from the tenderness in the right hypochondriac region, I suspected that the liver had been adversely affected by the blood transfusions during surgery. Given these findings, I decided that rather than focusing on the area of pain, it was better to work on balancing the whole body.

I avoided treating the amputated surface of the leg because it was used in walking. The closest point to the site of the pain that I used was the intradermal needle inserted at the lateral malleolus. It appears that the root treatment of tonifying the Liver and Kidney meridians and dispersing the Gallbladder meridian had a beneficial effect overall. Acupuncture can be amazingly effective in cases of acute inflammation. The first two cases also illustrate this fact. The effect is comparable to steroids, but there are no side-effects.

The following things are important in deriving the most benefit from the anti-inflammatory effects of acupuncture:

► Make an accurate diagnosis based on the four examinations.
► Locate the acupuncture points carefully by searching for reactive points.
► Do not use too many points, and limit the amount of stimulation.

It may be possible to treat arthritis and inflammation simply by needling tender points, but the more comprehensive and systematic approach of meridian therapy seems far more practical and superior in its results.

Case 4

MALE, 48 YEARS OLD

Chief Complaint: Lower back pain and blood in urine.

History: **1.** Surgery for bladder stones; **2.** chronic hepatitis; **3.** chronic pancreatitis; **4.** whiplash injury; and **5.** the patient had a kidney stone removed, but the surgical scar became infected, and the left kidney had to be removed. There are still stones in the remaining kidney, but they are too large to pass down the ureter.

Examination: Blood pressure 140/90.

Questioning: The patient was not feeling well due to back pain. He often has cold feet.

Pulse: The pulse was deficient at the Liver, Kidney, and Heart positions. The yang meridians all seemed excessive, but the Bladder, Gallbladder, and Stomach meridians were the most excessive. The quality of the pulse was large, choppy, and slightly slow.

Abdomen: Soft under the navel and in the left flank region, and tender at CV-12 and K-16 on the left side.

Palpation: Pain when striking GV-5 and B-52 on the right side, tenderness on the right side of the back just lateral to GV-5, medial to B-24, and at B-24.

Pattern: Since the pulse was inconclusive, the back was examined and simple needle insertion was performed at B-20, B-23, and B-52 on the right. The Lung and Kidney positions were the most deficient when the pulse was checked again. Kidney deficiency was thus indicated by the pulse and abdominal signs, as well as by the symptoms of cold feet, lower back pain, and blood in the urine.

Treatment: The Kidney meridian was tonified by needling K-7 and L-5. When K-7 was needled on the left, the arrival of Qi was felt at a depth of 2mm, and there were intestinal sounds; the needle was therefore retained at this point. When K-7 on the right was needled, resistance was felt at just 1mm, and there were more intestinal sounds; the needle was therefore retained at this point as well. L-5 on the left was tonified, and the patient began to fall asleep. Needles were retained superficially at S-25 and S-24 on the right where there was sensitivity to pinching. Contact needling was performed at S-21 on the left where there was also sensitivity to pinching. A needle was inserted obliquely downward at CV-6, which was at the center of the depressed area below the navel, and the needle was twisted at a depth of 5mm. This caused more intestinal sounds, so the needle was briefly retained. The pulse at the deficient positions was somewhat stronger after treatment, but the general quality of the pulse did not improve much.

Observations: The pulse indicated deficiency in the Liver, Kidney, and Heart, but after needling a few points on the back, the Lung and Kidney positions were most deficient. Judging from the symptoms and abdominal signs, this was probably a case of Kidney deficiency from the beginning. One must be careful not to make too quick of a decision about the pattern when the pulse and other findings are inconsistent.

Retaining needles superficially at K-7 and L-5 seems to have had a very good effect in this case. The intestinal sounds occurred each time as I began to feel the arrival of Qi (a sensation of increased tension around the tip of the needle). This is a sign that Qi is moving and gathering at the point. The lower back pain was largely alleviated through effective tonification. The reason that the quality of the pulse did not change so much was perhaps because I did not use the right points on the yang meridians. I should have examined the pulse again after performing tonification to see which yang meridian was most excessive, and then dispersed that meridian. Some of the distal points on the Bladder or Stomach meridian probably should have been needled.

Case 5

MALE, 72 YEARS OLD

Chief Complaint: Pain and swelling of the right wrist, and pain in the index finger, brought on after pulling weeds three days previously. There was a grating sound

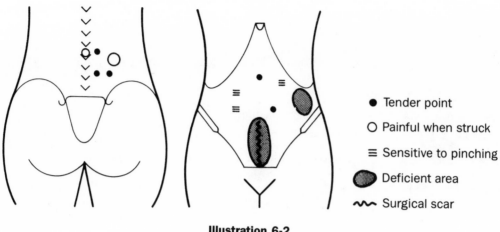

Illustration 6-2
Palpatory Findings for Case 4

• Tender point

○ Painful when struck

≡ Sensitive to pinching

Deficient area

∿ Surgical scar

together with pain when the index finger was flexed. This was probably a case of tenovaginitis.

Pulse: Clearly deficient at the Kidney position with no other notable feature.

Abdomen: Unremarkable.

Palpation: Induration at B-13 on the right, and tenderness at B-23 bilaterally.

Pattern: Kidney deficiency.

Treatment: Needles were retained superficially at K-7 and B-23 bilaterally. Needles were also retained at LI-11 and SI-11 on the right. Direct moxibustion with a few small cones was applied in the induration at B-13 on the right. An intradermal needle was placed at a tender point just distal to LI-6.

K-7 is the principal tonification point for Kidney deficiency. B-23 is the associated point on the back for the Kidney, and because this point was tender bilaterally, it was needled as an auxiliary point for tonifying the Kidney. LI-11 is commonly used for joint problems of the upper extremity. The pain and swelling in this case occurred along the course of the Large Intestine meridian, so LI-11 was also needled to disperse the excess on the affected side. SI-11 was needled because it was tender, and because it is an effective point for relaxing the shoulder and arm. The most tender and sore point over the affected area was just distal to LI-6. An intradermal needle was placed here to reduce the pain and inflammation by providing slight but prolonged stimulation.

Observations: This patient recovered after just one treatment. That is all I wrote down about the case. There is nothing about the pulse quality or abdominal findings, which means that they were unremarkable. In simple cases of deficiency like this, needling the principal tonification point alone can be very effective. Reviewing the points used in this treatment, tonifying K-7 served to raise the Qi in the Kidney and Lung meridians, and moxibustion at B-13 augmented the Qi in the Lung meridian and had a beneficial effect on the Qi along the Large Intestine meridian, the disruption of which was the cause of the complaint.

Case 6

FEMALE, 34 YEARS OLD

Chief Complaint: Stiffness in the shoulders, upper arms, and intrascapular region.

Looking: A thin physique.

Questioning: The patient had a baby six months previously, but before delivery had toxemia of pregnancy and had to be hospitalized.

Pulse: Deficiency at the Kidney position but otherwise unremarkable.

Abdomen: Tenderness at CV-6.

Palpation: Tenderness at B-13, B-23, G-20, and G-21.

Pattern: Kidney deficiency.

Treatment: Needles were retained superficially at K-7 and L-5. Needles were also retained in the tender points at CV-6, B-13, B-23, and G-21. Simple needle insertion was performed at G-20 and at two points slightly above B-10. Direct moxibustion with a few small cones was applied at G-21 and SI-11. Intradermal needles were placed in the auricular vertigo point (on the antitragus, just posterior to the asthma point).

Observations: This is another case where the symptoms were relieved after just one treatment. This treatment is typical of my approach in that a simple tonifying root treatment is coupled with a standard symptomatic treatment. Most of the points, except those on the Kidney and Lung meridians, were used for the symptomatic phase of treatment. This case also shows how incorporating the simple tonifying root treatment of meridian therapy enhances the overall effect of the treatment.

Case 7

MALE, 30 YEARS OLD

Chief Complaint: Pain on the right side of the lower back that began spontaneously one month previously. The pain occurred during movement. The patient had been visiting a local hospital for treatment that included traction and oral analgesics, but the pain remained unchanged.

Examination: Laségue's sign was positive at 45 degrees flexion of the right hip.

Pulse: The pulse indicated Liver meridian deficiency. The quality of the pulse was floating and wiry.

Abdomen: Tension in the area to the right of CV-12.

Palpation: There was tenderness with pressure and pain when striking M-BW-25 *(shi qi zhui xia)*, which is located between the spinous process of the fifth lumbar and the sacrum. There was also tenderness at B-52, B-37, B-58, and B-59 on the right side. These points are situated along the course of the sciatic nerve.

Pattern: Liver deficiency.

Treatment: With the patient in the prone position, direct moxibustion with ten small cones was applied at M-BW-25 *(shi qi zhui xia),* and five small cones were placed at B-59 on the right side. Simple needle insertion was performed at B-52 and B-58, and at a tender point on the gluteus maximus muscle on the right side. The patient was asked to bend forward at the waist to check the effect, but there was no improvement. He was then asked to assume a supine position with the knees flexed slightly. Needles were inserted superficially at Liv-8 and K-10 on the right side to tonify the Liver meridian. Special care was taken to insert the needles painlessly, as the skin around these points was very fine and sensitive. Also, since tenderness and induration was detected at G-38 on the right side, a needle was inserted here, and the needle was lifted and thrusted to disperse the excess in the yang meridian.

When the patient was again asked to bend forward, the pain was greatly relieved. However, there was still some discomfort at the medial aspect of the iliac crest. The treatment was concluded by simple needle insertion at a tender point along the iliac crest on the right side.

Observations: In this case symptomatic treatment was performed first. If it is just a matter of simple meridian pathology, most of the pain can be relieved by symptomatic treatment alone. In this case, however, there was no change at all in the subjective symptom of lower back pain with movement. Improvement came immediately after root treatment was performed on the affected side. It is possible that root treatment was more effective because I had already performed symptomatic treatment. Or it could have been that root treatment alone was sufficient.

Case 8

FEMALE, 58 YEARS OLD

Chief Complaint: Palpitations, chronic tension in the neck and shoulders, and chest pain extending from the back to the front on the left side.

Questioning: The patient has been diagnosed with a dysfunction in the autonomic nervous system since medical tests showed no abnormalities.

Looking: A thin physique.

Pulse: The Spleen position was deficient. The quality of the pulse was floating and almost flooding.

Abdomen: The abdomen was generally deficient with tension in the rectus abdominis muscle. The area around the navel was particularly soft, and there was slight hardness around CV-14.

Palpation: Tenderness at CV-17, K-24, and B-14. A tender point was located lateral to Sp-17 in the fifth intercostal space on the left side. There was also pain when striking GV-11.

Pattern: Spleen deficiency.

Treatment: Needles were retained superficially at Sp-3. Needles were also placed in the tender points at K-24 and B-14 on the left side. Needles were inserted shallowly and briefly retained at indurated points in the vicinity of G-20 and G-21. Direct moxibustion with three very small cones was applied at CV-17, and at SI-11 and B-14 on the left side. An intradermal needle was placed in the tender point lateral to Sp-17 on the left.

Sp-3 is the principal tonification point for Spleen deficiency. K-24 and B-14 on the left side were localized tender points that were needled to alleviate the chest pain. G-20 and G-21 are the principal points for reducing tension in the neck and shoulders. CV-17 is the accumulation point of the Pericardium meridian. It is used for disorders of the thoracic region, and for psychosomatic problems. In this case, because the pulse was floating, needle stimulation had to be kept to a minimum. Moxibustion was therefore used. SI-11 often becomes tender when there are problems in the upper extremities or thoracic region. Tenderness at SI-11 on the left side, and at CV-17 and B-14, indicates tension in the shoulders related to imbalances in the Pericardium meridian. Moxibustion was applied at B-14 to increase the tonifying effect of the treatment.

When there is pain or discomfort in the thorax, a tender point can often be found in the axillary region. This point is found anterior to the axillary line, and slightly above or below the level of the nipple. It is usually located along the course of the Spleen meridian, and its main indications are pain in the chest and flanks, coughing, and heart problems. Due to the sensitivity of this area, the point is only treated by the placement of an intradermal needle.

Observations: Tonification of P-7 was added at the beginning of subsequent treatments, but the rest of the treatment remained much the same. Retaining needles superficially at Sp-3 and P-7, the Spleen tonification points, was very beneficial for the symptoms of poor appetite, weight loss, palpitations, chest pain, and tension in the neck and shoulders. All of these symptoms were alleviated after just three treatments. The needle inserted just 1-2mm deep at B-14 on the left caused a sensation to radiate to the chest, and this seems to have helped greatly in relieving the symptom of chest pain. Though B-14 is a local point, since it is the associated point of the Pericardium, treating this point was significant both for root and symptomatic treatment. This patient has returned periodically for preventive treatments, but the symptoms have remained under control.

Case 9

MALE, 55 YEARS OLD

Chief Complaint: Polyuria of six months duration.

Questioning: The patient had to urinate about ten times an hour after getting up in the morning. During the day, the frequency of urination was about once an hour. There was a sensation of urine retention after urinating, but there was no pain during or after urination. Tests done at a hospital were all normal, and the physician was perplexed. The patient experienced a sensation of heat in the head and cold in the lower extremities, and also had occasional lower back pain. He had no palpitations, and his appetite was normal.

Looking: A red complexion with a tinge of dark blue. His eyelids were a little swollen.

Listening: Speech was slightly unclear.

Pulse: The difference between the positions was unclear, but the Lung and Kidney positions seemed slightly deficient. The quality of the pulse was large and flooding.

Abdomen: There was good resiliency overall, but the area around CV-4 was slightly soft, and there was tenderness and induration just above CV-6. Also, compared with other areas, the skin over the Kidney area appeared to be lacking in luster.

Palpation: There was tenderness at B-23 and B-32 on the left side, and pain when striking M-BW-25 *(shi qi zhui xia).*

Pattern: Kidney deficiency.

First Treatment: Needles were retained superficially at K-7 and L-5, and in the tender points at B-23 and B-32 on the left side. Simple needle insertion was performed at K-12. A needle was also inserted to a depth of four units at B-53. Direct moxibustion with five small cones was applied at M-BW-25 *(shi qi zhui xia).*

   K-7 and L-5 are the principal tonification points for Kidney deficiency. B-23 is the associated point for the Kidney meridian, and B-32 is just medial to B-28, which is the associated point of the Bladder meridian. Tenderness and indurations often appear in the vicinity of these points when the Kidney meridian is deficient. In this case, because only the points on the left side were tender, only those points were needled. K-12 is known to be effective in reducing urinary frequency. To use this point properly, one must locate a thin band of tension or induration about one finger-width lateral to CV-3, and insert the needle slowly to a depth of about 0.5 unit. When K-12 is needled properly, the needle sensation reaches the ureter and the upper part of the bladder. B-53 is commonly used for urogenital disorders. I use deep needle insertion at B-53 mostly for male urogenital problems such as impotence and prostatitis. A special long needle is inserted to a depth of 3-4 units so that the needle sensation reaches the genital area, the perineum, or the inguinal region. M-BW-25 is a point that I often use in cases of lower back pain, but on occasion this point becomes sensitive when there are disorders of the pelvic organs. Moxibustion at this point serves to improve circulation in the pelvic region, and to increase the effect of the acupuncture treatment.

Second Treatment: The patient returned for another treatment two days later. His symptoms had completely disappeared. He was confounded that only one acupuncture treatment could alleviate six months of suffering. The pulse indicated deficiency at the Lung and Spleen positions, and was slightly thinner than before. The hardness palpated at CV-6 had softened somewhat. Although the pulse indicated Lung deficiency, considering the abdominal findings and the remarkable effect of the last treatment, the patient was treated again for Kidney deficiency in much the same manner as before.

Observations: The expressions, "dropping the pulse and choosing the abdomen" and "dropping the abdomen and choosing the pulse," are used in describing the identification of the pattern. These expressions are mainly used in herbal medicine when the pulse and abdominal findings are in conflict, and one must choose between the two. However, they also apply in acupuncture. It would be ideal if the pattern could be determined based on six-position pulse diagnosis in all cases. If pulse diagnosis were so reliable, there would be no need for any other type of examination. Although pulse diagnosis is usually the primary focus of the examination, other findings must be used to confirm the diagnosis. For various reasons, sometimes the pattern cannot be based on pulse diagnosis. There are times, as in this case, when the abdomen is the key factor in determining the pattern. In other cases, the pulse is too weak to palpate clearly, and other signs and symptoms must be used to determine the pattern.

Case 10

FEMALE, 49 YEARS OLD

Chief Complaint: Lower back pain for three years.

Questioning: The pain was at its worst when getting up in the morning. It eased later as she moved around, but was aggravated by doing work. On bad days, there was spontaneous pain during the night. The patient also experienced stiffness in her neck and shoulders. According to physicians at a local hospital, there was no deformity in the lumbar vertebrae, and the rheumatoid factor was negative. It was therefore diagnosed as idiopathic neuritis.

Examination: Laségue's sign, Patrick's test, femoral nerve stretch test, and Babinski's sign were all negative. There was also no palpable deformity in the lumbar vertebrae.

Pulse: The diagnosis was unclear from the pulse, but it was taken to be either Kidney or Liver deficiency because the Lung, Kidney, and Liver positions were all weak. The quality of the pulse was submerged, slow, and deficient.

Abdomen: The abdomen was soft overall, but some induration and pulsation was felt around S-25 on the left side. The lower abdomen was also tense, and the patient complained of distention in the lower abdomen that increased with the lower back pain.

Palpation: The muscles in the lumbar area were tense and rigid. Some tenderness and induration was found at B-52, on the superior margin of the iliac crest, and inferior to the iliac crest on the left side. No tenderness or induration was found along the course of the sciatic nerve. Indurations were at B-15 on the left side, as well as at G-20 and G-21 bilaterally.

Pattern: The pattern could not be determined immediately, and symptomatic treatment was therefore performed first.

Treatment: Needles were retained at B-52, at the tender points superior to the iliac crest, and at the point inferior to the iliac crest on the left side. Needles were also retained at G-20 and G-21 bilaterally. Direct moxibustion with five small cones was applied at B-15 on the left side, and at B-52 and two tender points superior to the iliac crest bilaterally. B-52 is commonly used for lower back pain, especially when the point is tender or indurated. The tender point inferior to the iliac crest on the right side was needled as a local or *"ahshi"* point. G-20 and G-21 are commonly used for tension in the neck and shoulders. Needling indurated points here serves to reduce stiffness in the neck and shoulders. Moxibustion at B-15 is effective in relaxing the intrascapular region. In this case, direct moxibustion was applied at the induration on the left side.

Moxibustion was also applied at B-52 bilaterally since the lumbar area was very tight, and the tension was most pronounced around B-52. When there is lower back pain, I always look for tender or indurated points on the superior margin of the iliac crest (at the origin of the quadratus lumborum muscle). In acute cases, inserting a needle into the locus of sensitivity brings immediate relief. In chronic cases, when there are indurations and bands of tension, direct moxibustion works better than acupuncture in relaxing the lumbar area.

The pulse and abdomen were reexamined after the symptomatic treatment, and the pulse was clearly deficient at the Kidney and Liver positions. The tension in the lower abdomen had disappeared, but the pulsation at S-25 on the left could still be felt with deep pressure. The basic pattern was thus determined to be Liver deficiency, and needles were retained superficially at Liv-8 and K-10. Simple needle insertion was also performed at S-25 on the left side, and at tender points on the knee and elbow joints.

Liv-8 and K-10 are the principal tonification points for Liver deficiency. Because S-25 on the left side was indurated, this point was treated directly to further improve the condition of the abdomen. Tender points around the knee and elbow were also sought and treated since this patient seemed to suffer from a nonspecific arthritic condition. The tender points in this case were found on the medial inferior aspect of the patella, and on the margin of the medial epicondyle of the humerus.

Observations: It was previously noted that physical ailments can be relieved without the aid of meridian therapy. Treating symptoms by needling localized areas can sometimes bring improvement in the overall picture. It may seem contradictory that treatment of localized areas can bring overall improvement, but this is just as it should be. This case shows that one must not overlook appropriate symptomatic treatment. The only problem with symptomatic treatment is that, when a practitioner becomes preoccupied with only the local areas or symptoms, the total picture is likely to be forgotten. We must always keep in mind that the root is more important than the branches, and that patterns of deficiency and excess identified by the pulse and abdomen should be addressed first whenever possible.

Case 11

FEMALE, 49 YEARS OLD

Chief Complaint: Dizziness.

Looking: The patient was slightly plump, but her skin was soft and fine.

Questioning: The patient was a school teacher who had negotiated with her principal late into the night, and had accordingly built up a great deal of stress. The next day at school she suddenly became nauseous and dizzy, and therefore immediately came in for treatment. This patient liked acupuncture and had received many treatments in the past. With the dizziness she had tinnitus, and her hearing was reduced to the point of almost being unable to hear the sound of my fingers rubbing together next to her ear. She had also experienced occasional cramping in her calf muscles at night.

Pulse: The Liver and Kidney positions were deficient, and the Gallbladder position was excessive. The Bladder position was also slightly excessive.

Abdomen: Unremarkable.

Palpation: A point near Liv-8 on the right side was slightly tender. This point was about 5mm anterior to the standard Liv-8 location on the sartorius muscle when the knee was flexed. Tenderness was also found at G-38, and induration and tenderness was found at G-20, G-21, and B-10.

Pattern: Liver deficiency.

Treatment: After confirming the arrival of Qi, needles were retained superficially at Liv-8 (the alternative location 5mm anterior to the normal location) and at K-10 on the right side to tonify the Liver meridian. For symptomatic treatment, needles were retained at GV-22 and the auricular vertigo point. Reexamining the pulse, the Liver and Kidney positions seemed a little stronger. The patient said she was beginning to feel better. To treat the excess in the Gallbladder meridian, the tender points at G-38 were dispersed. The needles at Liv-8 and K-10 were removed after using slight rotation. Intestinal sounds were heard at this time. As additional symptomatic treatment to relax the neck and shoulders, needles were retained superficially in tender points at G-20, G-21, and B-10. The dizziness was cured in just one treatment, although the patient came in for two more follow-up treatments.

Observations: In this case the needling of Liv-8 on the right side seemed most effective in alleviating the dizziness and nausea. The point location for tonification was not standard, in that a point on the muscle rather than in the depression was needled, but it is often more effective to use the reactive point. Some practitioners say that reactions such as indurations or tenderness do not appear at the five-phase points on the yin meridians, but careful palpation often proves otherwise. It is very difficult to say which point — the standard or reactive — is more effective in providing root treatment. In my experience, however, the reactive point is usually more effective. This is why it is important to take time in locating points to detect any changes in the vicinity of standard acupuncture point locations.

Case 12

MALE, 54 YEARS OLD

Chief Complaint: Painful apthous stomatitis (canker sores) in the mouth and on the tongue, stiffness in the neck and shoulders, and some pain down the back.

Questioning: The patient had apthous stomatitis ever since undergoing an operation for gastric ulcer two years previously. Although his appetite was normal, he had lost weight since it was painful to eat. He had received some injections and medication at a hospital, but this had provided little relief.

Looking: There was a large sore on the inside of the right cheek, and five smaller ones on the tongue. There was also some swelling in the cervical lymph nodes.

Pulse: The Lung position was clearly deficient. The quality of the pulse was tight.

Abdomen: The entire abdomen above and below the navel was depressed and lacking in resiliency.

Palpation: There was tenderness at S-21, and tenderness and induration at G-20 and G-21. There was also strong tension at B-43, and tenderness at B-20.

Pattern: Lung deficiency.

First Treatment (April 10): Needles were retained superficially at L-9 and Sp-3. Needles were also retained at LI-11, S-21, G-20, G-21, B-43, and B-20. After removing the needles, direct moxibustion with five small cones was applied at B-20 bilaterally. The swollen lymph nodes were also needled very superficially in a few places.

L-9 and Sp-3 are the principal tonification points for Lung deficiency. LI-11 is the earth phase point of the Large Intestine meridian, and needling this point superficially tonifies that meridian. The tenderness at S-21 bilaterally was treated directly to affect the abdomen. G-20 and G-21 are commonly used for tension in the neck and shoulders. B-43 is commonly used for tension in the intrascapular region. B-43 is also known to improve the function of the Lung and Spleen, and to increase vitality. B-20 is the associated point of the Spleen meridian. Needling this point strengthens the Spleen and relaxes the back. Moxibustion was applied after needling B-20 to increase the tonifying effect. Superficially needling swollen lymph nodes disperses excessive Qi and often reduces the swelling. There is generally a correlation between the swelling of submaxillary nodes and the presence of apthous stomatitis.

Second Treatment (April 14): There was no appreciable change in any of the symptoms since the last treatment. The pulse and abdomen were the same as before. Basically, the same treatment was provided again. The area of the apthous stomatitis was also pricked lightly with a Chinese needle.

Third Treatment (April 17): The original area of the sores was reduced in size, but a large new sore had formed on the back of the tongue. The pulse indicated Liver deficiency, so Liv-8 and K-10 were tonified. There was some tenderness at CV-12 and an intradermal needle was placed at this point. The sores were pricked with a Chinese needle and bled slightly. Repeatedly pricking the ulcerated areas of the oral mucus membrane is effective for treating apthous stomatitis. This may cause some bleeding, but bleeding is actually beneficial in these cases.

Fourth Treatment (April 25): The original sores had healed to a large extent, and the new sore was substantially reduced in size. The pain from the sores was minimal during the previous week, and the patient was eating better. The pattern was still Liver deficiency so the same treatment as before was provided.

Fifth Treatment (May 2): The sores were reduced to the point where they were barely visible. The swelling in the cervical lymph nodes was also significantly reduced. The patient complained of dizziness when standing up. The pattern was still Liver deficiency so a similar treatment was provided.

Sixth Treatment (May 8): The patient had some denture work done and this led to the formation of another area of aphthous stomatitis in the mouth. He appeared to be gaining a little weight, and complained of some heartburn. The pulse indicated Lung deficiency. The abdomen felt firmer overall, but there was tenderness at S-20 on the right side. L-9 and Sp-3 were tonified, and tender points on the Stomach meridian were dispersed. An intradermal needle was imbedded at S-20 on the right side. Otherwise the treatment was similar to previous ones, including the pricking of the sore with a Chinese needle.

Observations: In this chronic case of apthous stomatitis, in which the patient lost weight because of the pain, the sores were alleviated in about a month. The improvement did not appear until after the second treatment, but then the sores began to heal rapidly. Although they did reappear, they did not become worse than before the treatment. I feel that the root treatment was very useful in making the symptomatic treatment of needling the cervical lymph nodes and pricking the sores more effective. In general, when the abdomen becomes firmer it is a very good sign that treatment has been effective on a core level.

This patient continued to receive treatments on a weekly basis for over a year, during which time he steadily gained weight. Although the sores did go away after the tenth treatment, they periodically reappeared. These sores, however, disappeared quickly with acupuncture. After the forty-fifth treatment, the sores disappeared and did not return. The patient nevertheless continues to receive periodic treatment to strengthen his digestive system.

Case 13

MALE, 39 YEARS OLD

Chief Complaint: Diarrhea and pain in the lower abdomen.

Questioning: The patient had recurrent diarrhea for several weeks, but this had been accompanied by pain in the lower abdomen since only the day before.

Looking: A thin physique, pale complexion, and rough skin.

Listening: Weak voice.

Pulse: The pulse was deficient at the Lung and Spleen positions, and excessive at the Liver position. The quality of the pulse was deep, slow, and slightly tight.

Abdomen: There was slight tension across the rectus abdominis muscle as well as tenderness around the navel, especially at CV-9 and S-25 on the right side.

Palpation: There was tenderness and induration at B-52, and tenderness at B-32.

Pattern: Lung deficiency.

Treatment: Needles were retained superficially at L-7 and Sp-3 to tonify the Lung meridian. Needles were also retained superficially at tender points in the vicinity of Sp-9. Tonifying Sp-9 (the water phase point) in this way prevented the earth phase from over-controlling the water phase. Needles were also retained at CV-9 and CV-12. CV-9 is within the diagnostic area of the Spleen on the abdomen, and this point is commonly used for urinary dysfunction and intestinal disorders. CV-12 is a controlling point of the yang organs and serves to reduce abdominal pain. Needles were also retained in the induration at B-52, and in the tender area at B-32. Finally, ten small cones of direct moxa were applied at CV-9 and B-52. Moxibustion at these two points warms the Spleen and Kidneys, facilitates water metabolism, and controls diarrhea.

Observations: The pain in the lower abdomen was relieved after just one treatment, and the diarrhea stopped after a few days. In this case, even though deficiency was apparent in three meridians in a row (Spleen, Lung, and Kidney), providing basic root treatment for the meridian in the middle (Lung deficiency) improved the balance in the pulse and reduced the Liver excess. Moxibustion at tender points on the Conception vessel and along the Bladder meridian in the lumbar region is a very effective symptomatic treatment for diarrhea in general; together with appropriate root treatment, it makes a winning combination.

Case 14

MALE, 40 YEARS OLD

Chief Complaint: The patient caught a cold and has had copious nasal discharge and a severe headache.

Questioning: The patient also had stiffness and pain in the neck and shoulders, and his left elbow (around LI-11) became tight whenever he played golf. After golfing, he felt very tired the following day. He suffered a whiplash injury two years previously.

Examination: The compression test for cervical spine impingement was positive. Some motor impairment was noted in the left shoulder joint. His temperature was 36.6 degrees centigrade.

Pulse: The Lung and Spleen positions were weak. The quality of the pulse was floating, rapid, and wiry.

Abdomen: L-1 was slightly tender, and there was some tension at CV-12.

Palpation: There was tension and tenderness at B-10, G-20, and G-21. There was also tenderness at GV-22, K-27, and at a point lateral to Sp-17 in the left axilla, as well as induration at SI-11.

Pattern: Lung deficiency.

First Treatment (January 8): The Lung meridian was tonified by superficial insertion at L-9 and Sp-3. Needles were then retained superficially at the auricular vertigo point, GV-22, K-27, and CV-12. The auricular vertigo point is effective for headaches as well as dizziness. Needling the tender point at GV-22 also relieves headaches. The patient reported that his headache was gone. Next an intradermal needle was placed at the left axillary tender point. This is effective in treating chest pain, colds, and coughing. Direct moxibustion with five small cones was applied at GV-23. This is known to be effective in stopping excessive nasal discharge. Needles were retained just after penetrating the skin at B-10, G-20, and G-21. These are all important points for relaxing the neck and shoulder region. Simple needle insertion was performed at SI-11 and L-1 as local treatment for the shoulder and arm. Needling L-1 also serves to tonify the Lung meridian. The treatment was concluded by applying fifteen medium sized cones of moxa at GV-14, which is known to be effective in the early stages of a cold.

Second Treatment (February 22): The headache never returned and the pain in his left arm was much better than before. There was still some tension in his neck and shoulders. The left elbow was tender around the lateral epicondyle of the humerus. The pulse still indicated Lung deficiency, but the quality was no longer floating or rapid, and the abdominal findings were unremarkable. Tonification was used at L-9 only. This was sufficient to balance the pulse. Tender points on the neck and shoulder were treated by retaining the needles superficially as before. Simple needle insertion was performed at the tender point on the lateral epicondyle of the left arm, and an intradermal needle was placed at LI-11 on the left.

Observations: The cause of this headache seems to have been more than just a cold. The tension in the neck and shoulders was one of the causes that was aggravated by the cold. The patient had a rapid pulse, but I retained the needles for symptomatic treatment. The quick effect in relieving his most annoying symptom made the patient believe in the efficacy of acupuncture. The other chronic problems of cervicobrachialgia, slight motor impairment in the shoulder joint, and tennis elbow can be taken care of later. The patient told me that he had been treated with acupuncture several years before, but had a bad experience. He said it was not so much the pain of the needle penetrating the skin that was intolerable, but the heavy needle sensation. Strong stimulation should generally be avoided because it can have an adverse effect on sensitive patients; moreover, in most cases good results can be obtained without it.

Case 15

FEMALE, 47 YEARS OLD

Chief Complaint: Hypertensive headaches.

Questioning: The patient suffered from high blood pressure and throbbing headaches. She also had multiple complaints including stiffness and pain in the neck and shoulders on the left side, cold extremities, shortness of breath, tonsillitis, lower back pain, nausea, stomach upset, and a tendency to become easily fatigued. She had been receiving treatment for chronic nephritis and had marked proteinuria. She also had an operation for a uterine leiomyoma five months previously.

Examination: Blood pressure was measured at 180/90.

Pulse: The Heart and Spleen positions were deficient, and the Liver position was excessive. The quality of the pulse was tight and slightly rapid.

Abdomen: The abdomen was generally tense, particularly around CV-12.

Palpation: There was tenderness at CV-22, LI-10, B-59, and G-38. Tenderness and induration was also found at B-10, B-23, G-20, and G-21.

Pattern: Spleen deficiency and Liver excess.

First Treatment (February 16): Needles were retained superficially at Sp-3 and Liv-3 to tonify the Spleen meridian. For symptomatic relief of the headache, needles were retained at GV-22 and the auricular vertigo points. Simple needle insertion was performed at CV-12, LI-10, and G-38. CV-12, the accumulation point of the Stomach meridian, was needled to reduce tension in the abdomen and harmonize the Stomach and Spleen. LI-10 is used for headaches in the Sawada school of acupuncture. G-38 was needled to disperse the excess Liver meridian indirectly through its paired yang meridian. An intradermal needle was placed at the auricular vertigo point on the left side. Needles were then retained at B-10, G-20, and G-21, which are important points for reducing stiffness in the neck and shoulders. Tenderness and induration on the back were treated to alleviate stagnation in the Kidney and Bladder meridians. Needles were retained at B-23 and B-59. B-23 is the associated point of the Kidney meridian. B-59 was used as a distal point coupled with B-10 to relieve the headache and tension in the back of the neck. Direct moxibustion with five small cones was applied at GV-10 and G-21. Direct moxibustion on tender points in the vicinity of GV-10 is known to have a calming effect on patients with a nervous disposition, and to bring relief to patients prone to multiple complaints. Moxibustion was also applied at G-21 to reduce the strong tension in the neck and shoulders.

Second Treatment (February 20): The patient experienced slight fatigue the day after treatment. The throbbing headache was reduced to a dull headache. The patient's blood pressure was 160/88. Although the pulse still indicated Spleen deficiency and Liver excess, the tense quality was gone from her pulse. The urine analysis done at the hospital the day before showed only trace amounts of protein in the urine. Almost the same treatment was provided as before.

Third Treatment (February 24): A dull headache still persisted and pain was felt in the back of her eyes. The patient also complained of pain in her lower back extending down to the left thigh. Her blood pressure was 160/85. The pulse indicated Liver deficiency instead of Spleen deficiency as before. The Liver meridian was therefore tonified by retaining needles at Liv-8 and K-10. The remainder of the treatment was similar to the one before, consisting of acupuncture and moxibustion at tender points on the cranium, shoulder, lower back, and legs.

Fourth Treatment (March 2): The headache was greatly improved after the third treatment, but the lower back pain was only slightly better. The patient's blood pressure was down to 150/82. The pulse again indicated Liver deficiency, so almost the same treatment as before was given.

Observations: This patient continued to receive weekly treatments for about three months. The headache diminished as her blood pressure lowered, so it was without a doubt a hypertensive headache. The nephritis and nausea were also closely related to the high blood pressure. The diminished protein in the urine and the steady reduction in blood pressure were good signs that the treatments were having an effect on a deep level, rather than simply relieving the symptoms. Nevertheless, despite the initial success, the patient's blood pressure began to rise again about a month after the first treatment, and the nephritis did not significantly improve. This is an example of a very difficult case in which chronic illness had depleted the Qi in the Kidney and Liver meridians.

Although the initial pattern was one of Spleen deficiency and Liver excess, it changed to Liver deficiency after one week of treatment, and subsequently alternated between Liver and Kidney deficiency. Thus, the fundamental pattern was Liver deficiency rather than Liver excess. The Spleen meridian was deficient for awhile, and this decline in the earth phase caused a temporary reactive excess in the Liver meridian, and made the water phase appear normal. While the pattern can change with repeated treatment, generally the most fundamental pattern related to the patient's predisposition will reestablish itself.

Case 16

MALE, 33 YEARS OLD

Chief Complaint: Headache of one week's duration.

Questioning: One week previously, along with a cold, the patient started vomiting and suffered a throbbing headache in the occipital and temporal regions, as well as on the temple above the eyebrows. A thorough examination at a neurological clinic turned up no abnormality, and he was diagnosed with a migraine. He received an acupuncture treatment at another clinic, but without effect. The headache got worse when he was in large crowds and when he ate; it eased when he lay down.

Pulse: The Liver and Kidney positions were deficient, and the Gallbladder position was excessive. The quality of the pulse was moderate.

Abdomen: Unremarkable.

Palpation: There were no notable findings except some tenderness in the temporal region and at G-20.

Pattern: Liver deficiency and Gallbladder excess.

First Treatment (May 28): Needles were retained superficially at Liv-8 and K-10 to tonify the Liver meridian. The Gallbladder meridian was dispersed by simple needle insertion at G-38 on the right side. Needles were retained at B-18 and B-23 to further strengthen the Liver and Kidney meridians because these points were slightly depressed. For symptomatic relief from the headache, needles were also retained at the local points GV-22, G-5, and GV-14, as well as the auricular vertigo point. LI-10 was needled as a distal point to aid in treating the symptoms. To relieve the tension in the neck and shoulders, needles were retained at B-10, G-20, and G-21, with B-59 serving as a distal point. Direct moxibustion with five small cones was applied at GV-10. The use of moxibustion at the tender points around GV-10 calms and relaxes individuals who are sensitive and prone to tension. An intradermal needle was placed in the auricular vertigo point on the right side to increase and extend the symptomatic relief.

Second Treatment (May 31): The headache was considerably better since the first treatment, and the nausea had disappeared. The pulse indicated the same Liver deficient pattern as before, so an almost identical treatment was provided, except that B-2 was needled instead of G-14, and moxibustion was applied at G-20 and G-5 instead of GV-10.

Third Treatment (June 5): The headache and nausea were completely relieved after the second treatment. The pulse indicated the same pattern, except that the Gallbladder excess was not as noticeable. The treatment was basically the same as before, except for dispersion of the Gallbladder.

Observations: This patient was diagnosed by a physician as having a migraine, but it could just as well have been a case of trigeminal neuralgia. In cases like this, where the headache is primarily related to excesses in yang meridians and there are no serious internal problems, the headache and other symptoms are easily resolved.

Afterword

This book has been a long time in the making, from its beginnings in 1980 as a serial feature in the *Journal of Japanese Acupuncture and Moxibustion,* to the present English edition. I am greatly relieved that it is at last completed. I am a little worried, however, about whether I have conveyed the essence of meridian therapy without error. I have written about the accomplishments of great acupuncturists of the past within the scope of my understanding. I only hope that I do not perpetuate any errors or inaccuracies because of limitations in that understanding. The responsibility of publishing this information abroad is a very heavy one, but the time is ripe to make this work available to acupuncturists outside of Japan.

I have written about meridian therapy in great detail, but there is still a considerable amount of material I have chosen not to include. This is as it should be, as this book is an introduction to meridian therapy, and not a comprehensive text. Sometimes it is better to keep things simple. There are also some things that just cannot be expressed in words. The main purpose of this book is to familiarize the reader with the general approach and methods used in meridian therapy, and to enable the practitioner to refine his or her own approach by applying the wisdom contained in the classics of acupuncture.

Many approaches to treatment have been developed in the long history of acupuncture and moxibustion, and through the centuries Japan has made important contributions to this ancient art. Every approach has its strengths and weaknesses, but any approach is most effective when applied in the specific situations for which it was intended. This being the case, it makes no sense to argue the merits of one approach over another, or to criticize another approach as being inferior or ineffective. It is far wiser to become familiar with a variety of approaches, and to learn to apply different approaches in a flexible manner. Through this book I trust that readers will gain an understanding of meridian therapy as a relatively new approach based on the earliest classics of acupuncture, and which also draws from the rich tradition of Japanese acupuncture. This book will have served its purpose if it broadens the reader's perspective and increases his or her options in treatment.

It is no easy matter to master pulse diagnosis without a teacher. But many individuals have no other choice. I would be most pleased if practitioners faced with this situation could use this book to further develop this skill. This book should be of interest even if read only as a record of one practitioner who mastered pulse diagnosis on his own through trial and error. It is most appropriately viewed as the result of one practitioner's attempt to understand meridian therapy, and to incorporate it into his own acupuncture practice.

Acupuncture is incredibly difficult to master. To this day, I can recall only a few cases in which I have been completely happy with the treatment, and wonder if I will ever become truly satisfied. Even if this never happens, I must still put my heart and soul into each and every needle I insert. Acupuncture is actually very much a spiritual practice, and no teacher can teach a person acupuncture in the real sense. It cannot even be transmitted from father to son. Each person must learn it for himself. The mastery of acupuncture is truly a solitary journey.

Acupuncture which is based on study alone will be ineffective. Acupuncture without any study will also be ineffective. Acupuncture becomes truly effective only through daily practice, and the secret to its mastery lies in nothing other than this. Daily practice is the essential element for understanding Oriental medicine, and is the key to all Oriental arts. The spirit of meridian therapy can be fully experienced only when this truth about the Oriental way is made your own.

Bibliography

Chinese Classics:

Anonymous, *Basic Questions (Su Wen)*, circa first century B.C.

Anonymous, *Vital Axis (Ling Shu)*, circa first century B.C.

Bian Que (attribution), *Classic of Difficulties (Nan Jing)*, circa second century A.D.

Gao Wu, *Gatherings from Eminent Acupuncturists (Zhen Jiu Ju Ying)*, 1529.

Hua Shou, *Elaboration of the Fourteen Meridians (Shi Si Jing Fa Hui)*, 1341.

Wang Shu-He, *Pulse Classic (Mai Jing)*, 280 A.D.

Japanese Classics:

Hara Nanyo, *Clarification of Acupuncture Points (Keiketsu Ikai)*, 1807.

Hongo Masatoyo, *A Precious Record of Acupuncture and Moxibustion (Shinkyu Chohoki)*, 1718. Reprinted by Ido-no-Nippon Company, 1959.

Manase Dosan, *Newly Compiled Addition to the Secrets of Pulse Diagnosis (Shinsen Zoho Maykuron Kuketsu)*, 1578. Reprinted by Japan Meridian Therapy Association, 1982.

Mubunsai, *Compilation of the Secrets of Acupuncture (Shindo Hiketsushu)*, 1685. Reprinted by Seibundo Oriental Medical Publications, 1980.

Sugiyama Waichi, *Sugiyama Style of Treatment in Three Parts (Sugiyamaryu Sanbusho)*, 1682. Reprinted by Ido-no-Nippon Company, 1976.

Wada Yoan, *Guide to the Secrets of Acupuncture (Shinkyu Kuketsu Shinan)*, 1728.

Yama Nobutoshi, *Handbook of Pulse Diagnosis (Myakuho Tebikigusa)*, 1770. Reprinted by Ido-no-Nippon Company, 1966.

Yoshimasu Shigenari, *Definitive Medicine (Idan)*, 1752.

Modern Texts and References:

Akabori Akira, *Study of Moxiustion Classic of Eleven Yin and Yang Meridians. Journal of Meridian Therapy (Keiraku Chiryo)*. No. 67, Oct. 1981.

Araki Shoin, *Chinese Herbal Therapy (Kampo Chiryo)*. Tokyo: Iwasaki Books, 1982.

Byodo Yoshiaki, Serizawa Katsusuke, et al. *Concise Dictionary of Acupuncture Medicine (Kanmei Shinkyu Igaku Jiten)*. Tokyo: Ishiyaku Publishing Company, 1981.

Committee for the study of silk manuscripts from the Han Dynasty tombs of Ma Wang Tui, *Treatment for Fifty Two Diseases (Wu shi er bing fang)*. Beijing: Wenwu Publishing Company, 1977.

Fujiki Toshiro, *The World of Basic Questions' Medicine (Somon Igaku no Sekai)*. Tokyo: Sekibundo, 1976.

Fukushima Kodo, *Compendium of Meridian Therapy (Keiraku Chiryo Yoko)*. Tokyo: Toyo Hari Igakukai, 1971.

___ . *Meridian Therapy Made Simple (Wakariyasui Keiraku Chiryo)*. Tokyo: Toyo Hari Igakukai, 1979.

Honma Shohaku, *Five Element Acupoint Chart (Shinkyu Hosha Yoketsu Nozu)*. Yokosuka: Ido-no-Nippon Company, 1941.

___ . *Point Selection Guide for Five Element Acupoint Chart (Shinkyu Hosha Yoketsu Nozu Setsumeisho fu Shuketsuron)*. Yokosuka: Ido-no-Nippon Company, 1941.

___ . *Discourse on Meridian Therapy (Keiraku Chiryo Kowa)*. Yokosuka: Ido-no-Nippon Company, 1949.

___ . *Study of the Classic of Difficulties (Nangyo no Kenkyu)*. Yokosuka: Ido-no-Nippon Company, 1965.

Ikeda Masakazu, Gomazaki Yo, *Illustrated Text of Acupuncture for Beginners (Zukai Shinkyu Igaku Nyumon)*. Yokosuka: Ido-no-Nippon Company, 1977.

Inoue Keiri, *On Needling Techniques Used for Meridian Therapy (Keiraku Teki Chiryo ni Okeru Shuho ni Tsuite)*. Oriental Medical Journal (Toho Igaku). Vol. 8, No.10, 1941.

___ . *Private Edition of Tapes on Inoue's Lecture about the Classic of Difficulties (Nangyo Kogi)*. Tokyo: Toyo Hari Igakukai, 1962.

___ . *Lecture on Meridian Therapy given by Inoue in Ohita (Ohita Koen)*. Meridian Therapy Association (Ohita branch), 1962.

Inoue K., Okabe S., Maruyama M. et. al. *Roundtable Discussion on Meridian Therapy (Keiraku Chiryo Zadankai). Journal of Japanese Acupuncture and Moxibustion (Ido-no-Nippon).* Vol. 20, No.2, Feb. 1961.

Inoue Masafumi, *Study of Pulse Quality Diagnosis (Myakujoshin no Kenkyu).* Tokyo: Shizensha, 1980.

___ . *Discussion on Pulse Diagnosis (Myakushin ni Tsuite). Oriental Medicine Journal (Toyo Igaku).* Vol. 13, No. 4, Aug. 1980.

Kamichi Sakae, *Doctor Takeyama and The Journal of Oriental Medicine (Takeyama-sensei to Tohoigaku). Journal of Acupuncture Medicine (Shinkyu Igaku).* No. 31, Apr. 1978.

Kuwahara Yoji, *Commentary on Medical Texts Excavated from the Han Dynasty Ma Wang Tui Tombs. Journal of Meridian Therapy (Keiraku Chiryo).* No. 44, Jan. 1976.

Maruyama Mamoru, *On Abdominal Diagnosis (Fukushin ni Tsuite). Journal of Japan Meridian Therapy Association (Keiraku Chiryo Gakkai).* Vol. 3, No. 5, Dec. 1976.

Nagahama Yoshio, *Outline of Oriental Medicine (Toyoigaku Gaisetsu).* Tokyo: Sogensha, 1978.

Okabe Sodo, *Study of Indurations in Relation to the Meridians (Koketsu no Keiraku Teki Kenkyu). Oriental Medical Journal (Toho Igaku).* Vol. 7, No. 5, 1940.

___ . *Acupuncture by Meridian Therapy (Shinkyu Keiraku Chiryo).* Tokyo: Sekibundo, 1974.

___ . *The Essence of Acupuncture Therapy (Shinkyu Chiryo no Shinzui).* Tokyo: Sekibundo, 1982.

Shanghai Institute of Traditional Chinese Medicine, *Acupuncture (Zhen Jiu Xue),* translated by Ikegaki Kiyoaki et al. Tokyo: Kenkodo Publishing, 1977.

Shimada Takashi, *Searching for the Essence of Classical Medicine (Koten Igaku no Honshitsu o Saguru). Journal of Acupuncture Medicine (Shinkyu Igaku).* No. 40, Nov. 1980.

Shiroda Bunshi, *The Clinical Study of Acupuncture Therapy (Shinkyu Chiryo Rin-shogaku).* Tokyo: Nippon Shobo, 1948.

Takeyama Shinichi, *What is Meant by Meridian Therapy? (Keirakuteki Chiryo towa Nanzoya?) Oriental Medical Journal (Toho Igaku).* Vol. 8, No. 6, Aug. 1941

___ . *Introduction to Meridian Therapy (Keiraku Chiryo Nyumon). Oriental Medical Journal (Toho Igaku).* Vol. 11, No. 1, Jan. 1944.

___ . *Overview of Meridian Thearpy (Keiraku Chiryo Soron). Journal of Meridian Therapy (Keiraku-Chiryo).* No. 1, Apr. 1965.

Toyota Hakushi, *Meridian Therapy Symposium (6) Symptomology (Byosho ni Tsuite). Journal of Meridian Therapy (Keiraku-Chiryo).* No. 29, Apr. 1972.

Yamashita Makoto, *Introductory Text of Acupuncture for Meridian Therapy (Keiraku Chiryo no Tameno Shinkyugaku Soron)*. Tokyo: Toyo Koten Igaku Kenkyusho, 1971.

____ . *Introduction to Pulse Diagnosis (Myakushin Nyumon)*. Tokyo: Ishiyaku Publishing Company, 1982.

Yanagiya Sorei, *Gateway to the Art of Acupuncture (Shinkyu Ijyutsu no Mon)*. Yokosuka: Ido-no-Nippon Company, 1948.

____ . *Illustrated Guide to Acupuncture Techniques (Zusetsu Shinkyu Jitsugi)*. Yokosuka: Ido-no-Nippon Company, 1948.

____ . *Simple Diagnosis Without Questioning (Kanmei Fumon Shinsatsugaku)*. Tokyo: Ishiyama Acupuncture Company, 1976.

____ . *Dissertations on Tonification and Sedation (Hosha Ronshu)*. Tokyo: Ishiyama Acupuncture Company, 1977.

____ . *Collected Works of Yanagiya Sorei (Yanagiya Sorei Senshu)*. Tokyo: Sekibundo, 1979.

Point Index

General Index